Cheryl Robertson
96
371-4746

The Relationship of Theory and Research

Second Edition

The Relationship of Theory and Research

Second Edition

Jacqueline Fawcett, Ph.D., F.A.A.N.
Florence S. Downs, Ed.D., F.A.A.N.
University of Pennsylvania
School of Nursing
Philadelphia, Pennsylvania

 F. A. DAVIS COMPANY • Philadelphia

Printed in the United States of America

Last digit indicates print number: 10 9 8 7 6 5 4 3 2 1

acquisitions editors: Robert G. Martone/Alan Sorkowitz
production editor: Gail Shapiro
cover design by: Donald B. Freggens

As new scientific information becomes available through basic and clinical research, recommended treatments and drug therapies undergo changes. The author(s) and publisher have done everything possible to make this book accurate, up to date, and in accord with accepted standards at the time of publication. The authors, editors, and publisher are not responsible for errors or omissions or for consequences from application of the book, and make no warranty, expressed or implied, in regard to the contents of the book. Any practice described in this book should be applied by the reader in accordance with professional standards of care used in regard to the unique circumstances that may apply in each situation. The reader is advised always to check product information (package inserts) for changes and new information regarding dose and contraindications before administering any drug. Caution is especially urged when using new or infrequently ordered drugs.

PREFACE

This book is meant to fill a major gap in the literature of most disciplines by presenting a detailed discussion of the relationship between theory and research. Emphasis in the second edition of the book continues to be placed on information needed by both novice and accomplished scholars for the analysis and evaluation of research reports and proposals for new studies.

The book is based on three related premises. First, in keeping with a postpositivist perspective, we believe that all observation is theory-laden. Second, we believe that theory without research and research without theory do little to advance knowledge in any meaningful way. And third, we believe that although it is true that the theoretical aspects of research have been neglected by many investigators in favor of an emphasis on methodology, it is not true that there is no basis for theory in existing research reports. Rather, we believe that the paucity of recognizable theory in some disciplines is due to investigators' failure to be explicit about the theoretical components of their studies.

The contents of this book extend what has been published in other texts that are concerned with either theory or research methods by focusing on the relationship between theory and research. Chapter 1 presents an overview of the relationship of theory and research. Included are the definitions, functions, and types of theory and research. Chapter 2 presents a comprehensive format for analysis of the theoretical elements of research reports. Chapter 3 includes an extensive discussion of criteria for evaluation of the relationship between the theoretical and methodological aspects of research reports. Chapter 4 describes formal procedures that can be used to integrate the findings of related studies and estimate the magnitude of research results. Chapter 5 presents a discussion of conceptual models and their influence on theory and research. Each of these chapters has been revised extensively for this edition of the book, and many new examples have been included.

Chapter 6 has been added to this edition. This chapter presents guidelines for preparation of research proposals and research reports. Examples are drawn from a funded research project and journal articles.

The Appendix, which illustrates the use of the format for analysis of theory and the criteria for evaluation of the relation between theory and research, has been expanded to include two descriptive studies, two correlational studies, and two experiments. Reprints of the studies are also included.

The book is best read in sequence, although each chapter can stand alone. Diagrams are used to illustrate narrative points in Chapters 1, 2, 3, 5, and 6. A table listing different kinds of theories and modes of inquiry is presented in Chapter 1. A table summarizing the criteria for evaluation of the relation between theory and research is included in Chapter 3. A table listing the criteria for evaluation of the linkage of conceptual models with theories and empirical indicators is presented in Chapter 5. A table also is included in Chapter 6 to summarize the guidelines for writing research proposals and reports. The reference list for each chapter is augmented by additional readings that we think readers will find helpful in forming their own ideas about the relationship between theory and research.

The book is intended for neophyte and mature scholars in all academic and professional disciplines. Theorists and researchers should find the chapters on analysis of theory and integration of research findings enlightening. Researchers seeking funding for their proposals and journal publication of their findings will find the chapter on writing proposals and reports particularly helpful. Consumers of research should find that the chapter on evaluation of the relation of theory and research facilitates their understanding of the content of research reports and provides a systematic approach to judgments about the applicability of research findings in practical situations. Educators should find that the book as a whole assists students to comprehend the essential connection between theory and research and improves their abilities to analyze and evaluate existing research reports and prepare coherent research proposals.

The questions about theory and research raised by our former colleagues and students at New York University and the University of Connecticut provided the impetus for this book. The responses to the first edition of the book from our colleagues and students at the University of Pennsylvania have challenged us to continue to refine and clarify our ideas. We also have been stimulated by the questions raised by students and faculty at the schools where we have held visiting professorships, including the University of San Diego, Vanderbilt University, the University of Alabama at Birmingham, Loyola University of Chicago, and Case Western Reserve University.

We acknowledge the contribution of Steven Kahn to our understanding of inductive and deductive reasoning. We also acknowledge the stimulation and assistance of Diane Cooper, which led to the preparation of Chapter 6.

We are grateful to our husbands, John S. Fawcett and William Downs, for the love and support they have steadfastly provided, no matter how distracted we have been by our writing and teaching. We continue to acknowledge the encouragement given us by the editor of the first edition of the book, Charles Bollinger. And, we gratefully acknowledge our current editor Robert G. Martone and F. A. Davis Company, Publishers, for their willingness to take on an out-of-print book and their support of our work. We also acknowledge the essential contributions of all the people who facilitated the production of this edition, noting the special contributions of Ruth De George, Alan Sorkowitz, Herbert J. Powell, Jr., and Gail Shapiro.

Jacqueline Fawcett
Florence S. Downs

CREDITS

Portions of Figures 2–4, 2–5, 2–7, 2–8, and 2–12 were adapted with permission of The Free Press, a Division of Macmillan, Inc. from *Contemporary theories about the family. Vols. 1 and 2*, Wesley R. Burr, Ruben Hill, F. Ivan Nye, & Ira L. Reiss, Editors, Copyright 1979 by The Free Press.

Figure 2–13 was reprinted with permission from B. Weiner, the role of affect in rational (attributional) approaches to human motivation. *Educational Researcher, 9*(7), 9. Copyright 1980 by the American Educational Research Association.

Portions or all of Figures 2–1, 2–2, 2–5, 2–6, 2–9, 3–1, 6–1, 6–2, and 6–3, Tables 6–2, 6–4, 6–5, 6–6, 6–7 and numerous quotations in Chapters 2 and 6 were reprinted or adapted from research reports in *Nursing Research* with permission of the American Journal of Nursing Company.

A portion of Figure 2–9 was adapted with the permission of Margaret E. Hardy.

Portions of Figures 2–10, 2–11, and 2–12 were adapted with permission of Prentice-Hall, Inc.

Figure 5–3 was adapted with permission of Blackwell Scientific Publications.

Duffy, M. E. (1984). Transcending options: Creating a milieu for practicing high-level wellness. *Health Care for Women International, 5*, 145–161 was reprinted with permission of Hemisphere Publishing Corporation.

Carter, S. L. (1989). Themes of grief. *Nursing Research, 38*, 354–358 was reprinted with permission of the American Journal of Nursing Company.

Christman, N. L. (1990). Uncertainty and adjustment during radiotherapy. *Nursing Research, 39*, 17–20, 47 was reprinted with permission of the American Journal of Nursing Company.

Hubbard, P., Muhlenkamp, A. F., & Brown, N. (1984). The relationship between social support and self-care practices. *Nursing Research,*

33, 266–270 was reprinted with permission of the American Journal of Nursing Company.

MacVicar, M. G., Winningham, M. L., & Nickel, J. L. (1989). Effects of aerobic interval training on cancer patients' functional capacity. *Nursing Research, 38*, 348–351 was reprinted with permission of the American Journal of Nursing Company.

Riesch, S. K., & Munns, S. K. (1984). Promoting awareness: The mother and her baby. *Nursing Research, 33*, 271–276 was reprinted with permission of the American Journal of Nursing Company.

CONTENTS

1

An Overview of Theory and Research

This chapter presents an overview of the relationship of theory and research. The discussion is focused on the definitions, functions, and kinds of theory and research. Emphasis is placed on the selection of appropriate research designs for development of different types of empirical theories.

DEFINITIONS OF THEORY

Theorists and researchers frequently attach different meanings to the same term or use different terms to mean the same thing. This lack of congruence precludes assuming that one author's use of a term is the same as either another author's or the reader's. One of the best ways to be sure about the meaning of any term is to determine how the author used it in the context of the work. The definitions of "theory" presented here are typical of the variability in the scope of the word's meaning.

> A theory is a statement that purports to account for or characterize some phenomenon. (Barnum, 1990, p. 1)

A theory is a provisional explanatory proposition, or set of propositions, concerning some natural phenomena and consisting of symbolic representations of (1) the observed relationships among (measured) events, (2) the mechanisms or structures presumed to underlie such relationships, or (3) [any] inferred relationships and underlying mechanisms intended to account for observed data in the absence of any direct empirical manifestation of the relationships. (Marx, 1976, p. 237)

A theory is a set of interrelated constructs (concepts), definitions, and propositions that present a systematic view of phenomena by specifying relations among variables, with the purpose of explaining and predicting the phenomena. (Kerlinger, 1986, p. 9)

Not until one has [concepts], and propositions stating the relations between them, and the propositions form a deductive system—not until one has all three does one have theory. (Homans, 1964, p. 812)

These definitions place various restrictions on what is considered to be theory. Barnum's definition is the least restrictive, because it does not require that a theory state a relationship, nor does it preclude statements of relationships. Also, her definition is the only one that does not require a theory to take more than one concept into account, nor does it limit the theory to just one concept. This lack of restriction permits descriptions of one concept to be considered theory.

Marx's and Kerlinger's definitions are more restrictive in that they require a theory to state a relationship between two or more concepts. Descriptions of just one concept would not be considered theory according to their definitions.

Homans's definition is the most restrictive, because it requires not only that relationships be stated but also that a deductive system of propositions be evident. Thus, theories that are developed by means of induction would not be considered legitimate theories. The restrictions imposed by Homans would, therefore, preclude all but the most elaborate deductively developed formulations from being considered theory.

Barnum's definition of theory is used in this book. The lack of restrictions imposed by her definition is advantageous in that descriptions, explanations, and predictions all may be considered theory.

THE FUNCTION OF THEORY

Theories represent intelligible and systematic patterns for observations. The value of these patterns lies in the ability to "unite phenomena which, without the theor[ies], are either surprising, anomalous, or wholly unnoticed" (Hanson, 1958, p. 121). Theories, then, provide structures for the interpretation of initially puzzling behavior, situations, and events.

Many theories are required to account for the vast array of experiences encountered by human beings. Each theory addresses a relatively specific and concrete phenomenon by stating what the phenomenon is, how it occurs, or why it occurs. The function of a theory, therefore, is to describe, explain, or predict phenomena.

It is important to point out that theories are not real entities. They are not tangible or concrete; rather, they are tentative constructions of the mind, plausible statements about what might in fact be the case (Achinstein, 1974). Their tentative nature means that theories represent "knowledge under conditions of uncertainty" (Selltiz, Wrightsman, & Cook, 1976, pp. 47–48).

DEFINITIONS OF RESEARCH

Research, like theory, has several meanings. Here are some typical definitions.

> Research is a systematic, formal, rigorous, and precise process employed to gain solutions to problems and/or to discover and interpret new facts and relationships. (Waltz & Bausell, 1981, p. 1)

> Research is the process of looking for a specific answer to a specific question in an organized, objective, reliable way. (Payton, 1979, p. 4)

> Research is systematic, controlled, empirical, and critical investigation of natural phenomena guided by theory and hypotheses about the presumed relations among such phenomena. (Kerlinger, 1986, p. 10)

These definitions, like those of theory, vary in their restrictiveness. Waltz and Bausell's is the least restrictive because it does not require, and does not preclude, that the study be empirical. Thus, it does not call for a single mode of inquiry for the development of knowledge. Yet it is a strong definition that, like the others, requires research to be rigorous and systematic.

Payton's definition is more restrictive in that it requires research to be objective. That could be interpreted to mean that subjective methods of inquiry, such as phenomenology, are not considered research.

Kerlinger's definition is distinctive in that it emphasizes the connection between theory and research. It is, however, also the most restrictive definition, for it requires study of relationships and thereby excludes investigation of single concepts. Furthermore, it requires direct experience or observation of data, that is, the empirical method. This requirement implies that nonempirical works, such as some philosophical inquiries, are not considered research. Finally, it requires the testing of existing theories and hypotheses. This requirement implies that inquiry directed toward the generation of theories would not be considered research.

The lack of restrictions, combined with rigor, makes Waltz and Bausell's definition the most useful; furthermore, their definition permits the use of the term "inquiry" as a synonym for research. For those reasons, their definition is used in this book.

THE FUNCTION OF RESEARCH

Research is frequently viewed as a systematic process employed to answer questions. The process is often regarded as sterile — a linear series of steps to be surmounted in the search for solutions to problems. Research is, however, much more than a method of problem solving. In fact, the function of research is to generate or test theory. Research designed to generate theory seeks to identify a phenomenon, discover its dimensions or characteristics, or specify the relationships between the dimensions. Research designed to test theory seeks to develop evidence about hypotheses derived from the theory.

THE RELATIONSHIP BETWEEN THEORY AND RESEARCH

The close connection between theory and research was noted in Kerlinger's (1986) definition of research and was implied in the discussion of the function of research. Stated explicitly, although the initial impetus for research is usually the desire to understand some phenomenon, theory comes with understanding. Thus, theory development relies on research, and research relies on theory. The relationship between theory and research is a dialectic: a transaction whereby the theory specifies the boundaries of the phenomenon being studied, the definition of the phenomenon and its dimensions, as well as what data are to be collected. Research findings provide challenges to accepted theories (Brown, 1977).

Research, then, is neither more nor less than the vehicle for theory development. Indeed, research is just one part of a cycle, the part that supplies the data. The other part of the cycle, theory, gives meaning to the data (Lavee & Dollahite, 1991). In other words, research is the method used to gather the data needed for a theory. That is true whether the purpose of the research is to generate a theory or to test one. When the purpose is theory generation, the phenomenon of interest suggests things to look for. For example, if a theory of women's reactions to different modes of childbirth were to be generated, one source of data would be the women's statements about their labor and delivery experiences. Conversely, if the purpose is theory testing, the theory dictates the data to be collected. For example, if a theory proposes that support provided by family members and friends is one explanation for a woman's functional status after childbirth, then the data to be collected include the amount and type of support provided by relatives and friends as well as the level of functional status.

Kinds of Theory and Research

The definitions of theory and research used in this book permit discussion of various kinds of theory and various kinds of research or, more generally, modes of inquiry. A comprehensive typology of theory and inquiry has been developed by Carper (1978) and refined by Chinn and Kramer (1991). Although this typology was derived from the nursing literature, it is likely that the same or a similar typology could be extracted from the literature of other disciplines with a practice component such as social work, education, or medicine.

Carper proposed that practice requires four patterns of knowing: empirics, ethics, personal knowledge, and esthetics. Each pattern of knowing can be viewed as a different kind of theory. Chinn and Kramer elaborated on the four kinds of theory and identified the mode of inquiry used to generate and test each kind. The characteristics of each kind of theory and its associated mode of inquiry are summarized in Table 1–1.

Each kind of theory is an essential component of the knowledge base for professional practice, and no one kind of theory should be used in isolation from the others (Jacobs-Kramer & Chinn, 1988). The emphasis in this book, however, is on empirics and scientific, or empirical, research. Readers are referred to the seminal works by Carper (1978) and Chinn & Kramer (1991) for detailed discussions about ethics, personal knowledge, and esthetics.

TABLE 1–1. Four Kinds of Theory and Modes of Inquiry

Kind of Theory	Characteristics	Mode of Inquiry
Empirics	Factual descriptions, explanations, or predictions based on subjective or objective group data. Publicly verifiable. Discursively written as scientific theory.	Scientific research
Ethics	Emphasizes the values of nurses and nursing. Focuses on the value of changes and outcomes in terms of desired ends. Addresses questions of moral obligation, moral value, and nonmoral value. Discursively written as standards, codes, and normative ethical theories.	Dialogue about justness
Personal knowledge	Concerned with the knowing, encountering, and actualizing of the self. Also concerned with wholeness and integrity in the personal encounter between nurse and patient. Addresses the quality and authenticity of the interpersonal process between each nurse and each patient. Expressed as the authentic and disclosed self.	Reflection on the congruity between the authentic and disclosed selves
Esthetics	Focuses on particulars rather than universals. Emphasizes the nurse's perception of what is significant in the individual patient's behavior. Also addresses manual and technical skills. Expressed as the art-act of nursing.	Critique of the act of nursing

Empirical Theories and Scientific Research

Empirical theories generally are classified as descriptive, explanatory, or predictive. The scientific research designs that generate and test these types of theories are descriptive, correlational, and experimental.

Descriptive Theory and Descriptive Research. Descriptive theories are the most basic type of theory. They describe or classify specific dimensions or characteristics of individuals, groups, situations, or events by summarizing the commonalities found in discrete observations. They state "what *is*." Descriptive theories are needed when nothing or very little is known about the phenomenon in question.

There are two categories of descriptive theory: naming and classification (Barnum, 1990). A *naming theory* is a description of the dimensions or characteristics of some phenomenon. A *classification theory* is more elaborate in that it states that the dimensions or characteristics of a given phenomenon are structurally interrelated. The dimensions may be mutually exclusive, overlapping, hierarchical, or sequential. Classification theories frequently are referred to as *typologies* or *taxonomies*.

Descriptive theories are generated and tested by descriptive research. This type of research is also called *exploratory research*. It is directed toward answering such questions as:

> What *is* this? (Diers, 1979, p. 103)

> What are the existing characteristics of the real world relative to the specific question? (Payton, 1979, p. 44)

Descriptive studies involve observation of a phenomenon in its natural setting. Data are gathered by participant or nonparticipant observation, as well as by open-ended or structured interview schedules or questionnaires. The raw data gathered in a descriptive study may be qualitative and/or quantitative. Qualitative data may be analyzed by means of content analysis. This technique is used to sort data into a priori categories or into categories that emerge during the analysis. Quantitative data are analyzed by various measures of central tendency and variability, such as the mean, median, mode, standard deviation, and range.

Descriptive research encompasses case studies, grounded theory, ethnographies, phenomenologic studies, and surveys. Case studies are intensive and systematic investigations of many factors for a small number of individuals, a group, or a community. The case study is an excellent research method for the initial exploration of clinical problems. Fruehwirth (1989), for example, used the case study approach to describe the behavior patterns of participants in a support group for caregivers of Alzheimer's disease patients. The descriptive theory in this example is a taxonomy of caregivers' behaviors.

The method of grounded theory yields a description of processes occurring in social situations. Every piece of data is constantly compared with every other piece in order to discover the dominant social process that characterizes the phenomenon under study. An example of this method is Van Dongen's (1990) study, which generated a descriptive theory of the questioning behavior of relatives of suicide victims.

Ethnography yields a theory of cultural behavior for a particular society or societal group. Emphasis is placed on describing the group's way of life from the perspectives of the group members. For example, Germain (1982) conducted an ethnography of an adult oncology unit in a community hospital. It yielded a descriptive theory that identified the various roles nurses played, the problems and stresses they faced, their ways of trying to cope with these problems, and the consequences of their behaviors.

The method of phenomenology yields a description of human experiences. The investigator gathers data without preconceived expectations or a priori definitions of terms. Emphasis is placed on understanding individuals' cognitive, subjective perceptions and the effect of those perceptions on behavior. Banonis (1989), for example, used a phenomenologic approach to develop a descriptive theory of recovery from chemical addiction. The theory described recovering from addiction as "a lived experience of choosing the struggle to pull self out of a well of darkness into the comfort of light" (Banonis, 1989, p. 42).

Surveys yield factual and accurate descriptions of an intact phenomenon, such as attributes, attitudes, knowledge, and opinions. Surveys use both open-ended and structured interview schedules or questionnaires for data collection. One example of survey research using an open-ended approach is Strumpf and Evans's (1988) study, which yielded a descriptive theory that identified the frequency and types of physical restraints used with elderly patients and classified patients' and nurses' reasons for and responses to use of restraints. Another example is the study conducted by Lauver, Barsevick, and Rubin (1990). Their study results revealed a descriptive theory dealing with the frequency of spontaneous causal searching about abnormal Papanicolaou test results. The survey conducted by Hayden, Davies, and Clore (1982) yielded data from a structured questionnaire. These data were the basis for a descriptive theory that identified factors that facilitated and those that inhibited implementation of the nurse practitioner role in hospital emergency departments.

Explanatory Theory and Correlational Research. *Explanatory theories* specify relations between dimensions or characteristics of individuals, groups, situations, or events. They explain how the parts of a phenomenon are related to one another. These theories can be developed only after the parts of the phenomenon have been identified, that is, only after descriptive theories have been developed and validated.

Explanatory theories are developed by correlational research. This type of research seeks to answer the following question:

> To what extent do two (or more) characteristics tend to occur together? (Payton, 1979, p. 44)

Correlational studies require measurement of the dimensions or characteristics of phenomena in their natural states. Interviews and surveys are two frequently used approaches. Data usually are gathered by nonparticipant observation or self-report measures. Instruments may include fixed-choice observation checklists, rating scales, or standardized questionnaires, as well as open-ended questionnaires or interview schedules. The use of fixed-choice instruments is possible because the dimensions or characteristics of the phenomenon are believed to be known. These instruments yield qualitative or quantitative data. When quantitatively based explanations are desired and qualitative data have been collected, numbers must be attached to the raw data so that statistical procedures can be used. Statistical analyses employ various nonparametric or parametric measures of association, such as the contingency coefficient and the Pearson product moment coefficient of correlation. More sophisticated statistical analyses include multiple regression, canonical correlation, path analysis, and causal modeling.

Christman's (1990) study is an example of correlational research. She developed a theory to address the relationship of uncertainty, hope, preference for control, and symptom severity to psychosocial adjustment in women receiving radiation therapy for breast cancer. Another example is McClowry's (1990) study, in which a theory of temperament was tested by correlating school-age children's temperament with their pre- and posthospitalization behaviors. More specifically, the study tested the theory that the child's temperament would explain behavioral responses to hospitalization.

Predictive Theory and Experimental Research. *Predictive theories* move beyond explanation to the prediction of precise relationships between dimensions or characteristics of a phenomenon or differences between groups. This type of theory addresses cause and effect, the "why" of changes in a phenomenon. Predictive theories may be developed after explanatory theories have been formulated.

Predictive theories are generated and tested by experimental research. The question answered by this type of research is:

What will happen if . . . ? (Diers, 1979, p. 145)

Experimental research involves the manipulation of some phenomenon to determine its effect on some dimension or characteristic of another phenomenon. Experimentation encompasses many different designs. These include preexperiments such as the pretest-posttest – no control group design, quasiexperiments such as the nonequivalent pretest-posttest – control group design and time series analysis, and true experiments such as the Solomon Four Group and the posttest-only designs.

As correlational research, experimental research requires quantifiable data. That is because numbers are needed to determine if an experimental treatment makes a difference and, if so, how much difference. Typically, these data are collected by standardized research instruments with calibrated scores. Statistical analyses involve various nonparametric and parametric measures of differences, such as the McNemar test, Mann-Whitney U test, t-test, and F-ratio.

Experimental research is exemplified by the study conducted by Miller and her associates (1990). Their experiment was designed to determine the effectiveness of a nursing intervention based on the theory of reasoned action for promotion of medical regimen compliance by myocardial infarction patients. Another example of experimental research is Kolanowski's (1990) study of the effects of broad-spectrum versus warm-white fluorescent lighting on activation and motor activity in healthy elderly men and women. This study was designed to test a theory predicting the influence of lighting on restlessness.

Choice of a Research Design

The choice of a research design depends on the question asked. This means that "the method chosen should not become an end in itself, but rather must be appropriate for answering the question'' (Moody & Hutchinson, 1989, p. 292). In turn, the question asked depends on the current state of knowledge as expressed in theory. Thus, if little is known about the phenomenon to be investigated, descriptive theory-generating research is needed. If the phenomenon has been adequately described but its relationships to other phenomena are not known, correlational studies are required. If the phenomenon has been adequately described and its relationships to other phenomena are well known, experiments would be appropriate.

As can be seen in Figure 1–1, theory development is primarily a sequential process (Lewis, cited in Bobbitt, 1990) that begins with descriptive studies employing qualitative methods such as grounded theory, ethnography, and phenomenology. The results of qualitative descriptive research are descriptive theories that can be tested by means of another qualitative study or by quantitative descriptive studies. Theory development then proceeds to generation of explanatory theories by means of qualitative explanatory research and/or quantitative correlational studies. Correlational procedures are then used to test explanatory theories, but they may also be employed to generate predictive theories. Finally, experimental research is employed to generate and test predictive theories.

The progression of theory development from descriptive through correlational to experimental research may seem self-evident. However, because the pressure to solve practical problems is so great, especially in the professional practice disciplines, it is tempting to begin with experiments that will determine the efficacy of actions taken by practitioners, despite the absence of theoretical explanations for the effects of the

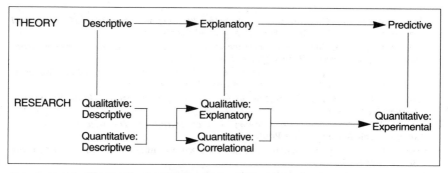

Figure 1–1. Progression of theory and research.

actions. Although the heuristic value of such studies cannot be denied, the temptation to rush to experiments should be resisted if the goal of the discipline is development of a logical and meaningful body of knowledge.

That is not to say, however, that the sequential process of progressing from qualitative description to quantitative experimentation must always be linear. Rather, either qualitative or quantitative methodology may be used to enrich and enhance the theory obtained from the primary study approach. A combination of qualitative and quantitative methods can be a very effective theory development strategy. That is because qualitative and quantitative methods "are mutually supportive. Qualitative knowing can benefit from quantitative knowing, and together they can provide a depth of perception or a binocular vision that neither can provide alone" (Bobbitt, 1990, p. 4). Murphy (1989), for example, used both methods in her program of research designed to generate a theory of recovery from disaster-caused loss.

CONCLUSION

This chapter lays the groundwork for the remainder of the book. The close connection between theory and research will continue to be emphasized in subsequent chapters by focusing on analysis and evaluation of theories and evaluation of the methods used to generate and test them.

REFERENCES

Achinstein, P. (1974). Theories. In A. C. Michalos, *Philosophical problems of science and technology* (pp. 280–297). Boston: Allyn and Bacon.

Banonis, B. C. (1989). The lived experience of recovering from addiction: A phenomenological study. *Nursing Science Quarterly, 2,* 37–43.

Barnum, B. J. S. (1990). *Nursing theory: Analysis, application, evaluation* (3rd ed.). Glenview, IL: Scott, Foresman/Little, Brown Higher Education.

Bobbitt, N. (1990). A holistic profession requires holistic research. *Home Economics Forum, 4*(2), 3–5.

Brown, H. I. (1977). *Perception, theory and commitment: The new philosophy of science.* Chicago: Precedent Publishing.

Carper, B. A. (1978). Fundamental patterns of knowing in nursing. *Advances in Nursing Science, 1*(1), 13–23.

Chinn, P. L., & Kramer, M. K. (1991). *Theory and nursing: A systematic approach* (3rd ed.). St. Louis: Mosby Year Book.

Christman, N. J. (1990). Uncertainty and adjustment during radiotherapy. *Nursing Research, 39*, 17–20, 47.

Diers, D. (1979). *Research in nursing practice.* Philadelphia: Lippincott.

Fruehwirth, S. E. S. (1989). An application of Johnson's behavioral model: A case study. *Journal of Community Health Nursing, 6*, 61–71.

Germain, C. (1982). *The cancer unit.* Rockville, MD: Aspen.

Homans, G. C. (1964). Bringing men back in. *American Sociological Review, 29*, 809–818.

Hanson, N. R. (1958). *Patterns of discovery.* New York: Cambridge University Press.

Hayden, M. L., Davies, L. R., & Clore, E. R. (1982). Facilitators and inhibitors of the emergency nurse practitioner role. *Nursing Research, 31*, 294–299.

Jacobs-Kramer, M. K., & Chinn, P. L. (1988). Perspectives on knowing: A model of nursing knowledge. *Scholarly Inquiry for Nursing Practice, 2*, 129–139.

Kerlinger, F. N. (1986). *Foundations of behavioral research* (3rd ed.). New York: Holt, Rinehart & Winston.

Kolanowski, A. M. (1990). Restlessness in the elderly: The effect of artificial lighting. *Nursing Research, 39*, 181–183.

Lauver, D., Barsevick, A., & Rubin, M. (1990). Spontaneous causal searching and adjustment to abnormal Papanicolaou test results. *Nursing Research, 39*, 305–308.

Lavee, Y., & Dollahite, D. C. (1991). The linkage between theory and research in family science. *Journal of Marriage and the Family, 53*, 361–373.

Marx, M. H. (1976). Formal theory. In M. H. Marx & F. E. Goodson (Eds.), *Theories in contemporary psychology* (2nd ed., pp. 234–260). New York: Macmillan.

McClowry, S. G. (1990). The relationship of temperament to pre- and posthospitalization behavioral responses of school-age children. *Nursing Research, 39*, 30–35.

Miller, Sr. P., Wikoff, R., Garrett, M. J., McMahon, M., & Smith, T. (1990). Regimen compliance two years after myocardial infarction. *Nursing Research, 39*, 333–336.

Moody, L. E., & Hutchinson, S. A. (1989). Relating your study to a theoretical context. In H. S. Wilson, *Research in nursing* (2nd ed., pp. 275–332). Redwood City, CA: Addison-Wesley Health Sciences.

Murphy, S. A. (1989). Multiple triangulation: Applications in a program of nursing research. *Nursing Research, 38*, 294–297.

Payton, O. D. (1979). *Research: The validation of clinical practice.* Philadelphia: F. A. Davis.

Selltiz, C., Wrightsman, L. S., & Cook, S. W. (1976). *Research methods in social relations* (3rd ed.). New York: Holt, Rinehart & Winston.

Strumpf, N. E., & Evans, L. K. (1988). Physical restraint of the hospitalized elderly: Perceptions of patients and nurses. *Nursing Research, 37*, 132–136.

Van Dongen, C. J. (1990). Agonizing questioning: Experiences of survivors of suicide victims. *Nursing Research, 39*, 224–229.

Waltz, C., & Bausell, R. B. (1981). *Nursing research: Design, statistics and computer analysis.* Philadelphia: F. A. Davis.

ADDITIONAL READINGS

Aamodt, A. M. (1982). Examining ethnography for nurse researchers. *Western Journal of Nursing Research, 4*, 209–221.

Babbie, E. R. (1990). *Survey research methods* (2nd ed.). Belmont, CA: Wadsworth.

Burr, W. R., Hill, R., Nye, F. I., & Reiss, I. R. (1979). Metatheory and diagramming conventions. In W. R. Burr, R. Hill, F. I. Nye, & I. R. Reiss, (Eds.), *Contemporary theories about the family. Vol. 1. Research-based theories* (pp. 17–24). New York: The Free Press.

Crosby, F. E., Ventura, M. R., & Feldman, M. J. (1989). Determination of survey methodology: Dillman's total design method. *Nursing Research, 38,* 56–58.

Denzin, N. (1970). Strategies of multiple triangulation. In N. Denzin (Ed.), *The research act* (pp. 229–313). New York: McGraw-Hill.

Dickoff, J., & James, P. (1968). A theory of theories: A position paper. *Nursing Research, 17,* 197–203.

Diesing, P. (1971). *Patterns of discovery in the social sciences.* New York: Aldine, Atherton.

Glaser, B., & Strauss, A. (1967). *The discovery of grounded theory.* Chicago: Aldine.

Hutchinson, S. A. (1990). The case study approach. In L. E. Moody (Ed.), *Advancing nursing science through research* (Vol. 2, pp. 177–213). Newbury Park, CA: Sage.

Krippendorff, K. (1980). *Content analysis. An introduction to its methodology.* Newbury Park, CA: Sage.

Lincoln, Y. S., & Guba, E. G. (1985). *Naturalistic inquiry.* Beverly Hills: Sage.

Meier, P., & Pugh, E. J. (1986). The case study: A viable approach to clinical research. *Research in Nursing and Health, 9,* 195–202.

Mitchell, E. S. (1986). Multiple triangulation: A methodology for nursing science. *Advances in Nursing Science, 8*(3), 18–26.

Munhall, P. L. , & Oiler, C. J. (Eds.). (1986). *Nursing research: A qualitative perspective.* Norwalk, CT: Appleton-Century-Crofts.

Myers, S. T., & Haase, J. E. (1989). Guidelines for integration of quantitative and qualitative approaches. *Nursing Research, 38,* 299–301.

Omery, A. (1983). Phenomenology: A method for nursing research. *Advances in Nursing Science, 5*(2), 49–63.

Stern, P. N. (1980). Grounded theory methodology: Its uses and processes. *Image, 12,* 20–23.

Strauss, A., & Corbin, J. (1990). *Basics of qualitative research. Grounded theory procedures and techniques.* Newbury Park, CA: Sage.

2
Analysis of Theory

Research that generates or tests theory is reported in books, journals, and monographs. Regardless of the form of publication, however, all research reports have similar content. This chapter presents a description of the content of each section of the research report and a comprehensive format for analysis of the report's theoretical elements.

CONTENT OF RESEARCH REPORTS

Research reports are generally divided into these sections: introduction, method, results, and discussion of the results. The introduction, which may be labeled the conceptual framework or model, the theoretical framework or rationale, the review of the literature, the background, and/or the significance of the study, presents the theoretical structure for the study. In this section, the reasons why the research was undertaken and how the study fills gaps in current knowledge or extends previously developed theory are explained. Theory-generating studies emphasize the lack of theory in a particular substantive area and explain the theoretical significance of the study in the introductory section. Theory-testing studies include a critical discussion of previous research that both supports and refutes the theoretical assertions, as well as the theoretical basis for hypotheses.

The method section presents a detailed discussion of how the study was conducted. The subsections under method include descriptions of the sample of subjects, the research instruments and equipment used, and the procedures for data collection.

The results section includes an explanation of how the data were analyzed, a summary of the data that were collected, and a presentation of the outcomes of any statistical tests. The discussion section presents an interpretation of the results and their implications. In theory-generating studies, the major concepts and propositions are usually summarized in this section. In theory-testing studies, conclusions regarding the support or refutation of hypotheses and the empirical adequacy of the theory are drawn.

THEORY FORMALIZATION

Theories are made up of one or more concepts and the propositions that state something about the concepts. A *concept* is a word or phrase that describes an abstract idea or mental image of some phenomenon. A *proposition* is a statement about a concept or the relationship between concepts.

Several forms of theories are evident in research reports. In theory-generating studies, the theory frequently is presented in the form of one or more newly discovered concepts, the dimensions of the concept(s), and relevant propositions. For example, data from Mishel and Murdaugh's (1987) qualitative study of family adjustment to heart transplantation led to formulation of the theory called "redesigning the dream." The theory is made up of the concepts "immersion," "passage," and "negotiation," along with the dimensions of the three concepts and the propositions that define and describe the concepts and their dimensions. The concepts and dimensions of the theory of redesigning the dream are illustrated in Figure 2–1.

Other forms of theory are evident in theory-testing studies. One form is the established theory, such as role theory, body image theory, the theory of reasoned action, or social learning theory, that is tested in a new setting or with a new population. Research designed to test an established theory is exemplified by Lowery, Jacobsen, and McCauley's (1987) study. The investigations tested attribution theory in the real-world clinical situations of arthritis, diabetes, hypertension, and myocardial infarction to determine its generalizability from controlled laboratory situations.

Another form of theory, usually referred to as a theoretical rationale or theoretical framework, uses the findings from previous empirical re-

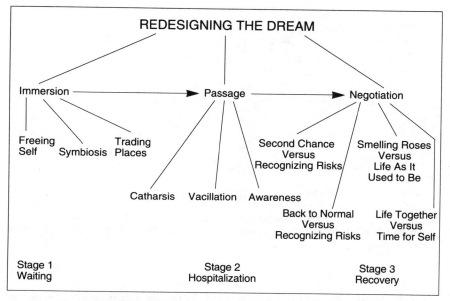

Figure 2–1. The theory of redesigning the dream: Concepts and their dimensions. (From Mishel & Murdaugh, 1987, p. 334, with permission.)

search to develop testable propositions. For example, Tobey and Schraeder (1990) used the findings from several related studies to develop a theory of the association between daily stress and life strain experienced by caretakers and the behavior of very low birth weight children during their preschool years.

In some instances, the theoretical framework or model combines some elements of an established theory with findings from previous research. An example is the theory of the relationship between antepartum stress and family functioning developed by Mercer and her associates (1986). The theory, which is depicted in Figure 2–2, is made up of concepts and propositions from family development theory and other concepts and propositions identified through a review of studies dealing with stress and pregnancy.

Regardless of the form, theories are not always presented as explicit sets of concepts and propositions in research reports. In fact, sometimes the theory that is contained in a research report is presented as an "untidy and inelegant" narrative (Marx, 1976, p. 235). The narrative must, there-

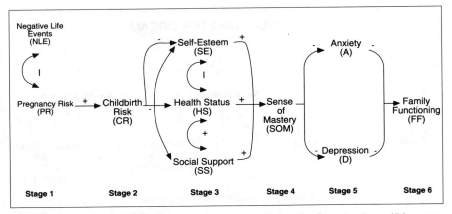

Figure 2–2. Theory of antepartum stress and family functioning. (Diagram adapted from Mercer, May, Ferketich, & DeJoseph, 1986, p. 341, with permission.)

fore, be analyzed systematically to identify the concepts and propositions that make up the theory.

Identification of the theory components is accomplished by the technique of theory formalization, which is also called theoretical substruction. *Theory formalization* is used to determine exactly what a theory says. It is a way of extracting an explicit statement and diagram of a theory from the narrative research report.

Theory formalization is similar to grammatical parsing of a sentence. Just as parsing identifies the nouns, verbs, adjectives, adverbs, and other parts of a sentence, so theory formalization permits identification of the concepts and propositions that make up a theory. Theory formalization may even involve the translation of a narrative theory into mathematic or computer language, which means that symbols are substituted for concepts and equations for propositions. The result of theory formalization is a concise and polished version of the theory that sets forth its components clearly, concisely, pictorially, and if desired, symbolically.

Several of the examples used in this chapter are taken from published research reports that present at least some theory components in a formal manner. In some instances, minor modifications were made to enhance the clarity of the example. Complete formalizations of the theoretical elements of descriptive studies, correlational studies, and experiments are presented in the Appendix.

Concepts

The first step in formalization of a theory is the identification and classification of the theory's major concepts. The concepts summarize actual observations and experiences that seem to be related. Babbie (1989) explains:

> Although the observations and experiences are real, our concepts are only mental creations. The terms associated with concepts are merely devices created for purposes of filing and communication. . . . Ultimately, [the concept] is only a collection of letters and has no intrinsic meaning. (p. 111)

A concept, then, is a tool and not a real entity. It facilitates observation and understanding of a real phenomenon (Bates, 1987). Furthermore, a concept refers to the properties of a phenomenon, not to the phenomenon itself. It gives meaning to what can be seen, heard, tasted, smelled, and touched. Thus, a concept enables us to categorize, interpret, and structure the phenomenon. The concepts of a theory represent its special vocabulary.

Pragmatics of Concept Identification

If the concepts are not immediately evident, then the research report must be read carefully to identify and categorize the key ideas. At times, it may be difficult to distinguish between the ideas that are integral to the theory and those that are part of the supporting narrative.

Accurate identification of concepts may require repeated readings of the research report. The final selection of major concepts is aided by identifying the concepts contained in the title of the report, the stated purpose of the study, the research questions, and the hypotheses (if any). In theory-generating studies that use such qualitative methods as grounded theory, ethnography, and phenomenology, the concepts are frequently not evident until the results of the data analysis are presented.

Classification of Concepts

Once the concepts have been identified, they must be classified on the basis of their variability, the extent of their observability, and their measurement characteristics.

Classification by Variability. Concepts represent nonvariable or variable phenomena. When the concept has only one dimension, when it simply labels a phenomenon, it is referred to as a *nonvariable*. The mental image evoked by a nonvariable concept is of one and only one form of the phenomenon. When the concept has more than one dimension, it is referred to as a *variable*. A variable concept evokes a mental image of more than one form of the phenomenon. Numerical scores are usually assigned to the dimensions of a variable. That is, of course, mandatory when statistical analyses are desired. An example of a nonvariable concept is "female." The nonvariable female is simply present; nothing is implied about the kind or amount of "femaleness." In contrast, the concept "femininity" is a variable because it can encompass several dimensions. One measure of femininity might yield the categorical scores 1, 2, and 3 representing the dimensions of feminine, androgenous, and masculine. Another measure might yield continuous scores ranging from 1 to 10, wherein a score of 1 represents the lowest and a score of 10 the highest degree of femininity.

Classification by Observability. Kaplan (1964) classified concepts on a continuum of observability. He identified four points on the continuum.

Observational Terms. At one end of the continuum is the observational term, which refers to a property that is a directly observable empirical referent. The property is observed by means of the senses, especially the visual and auditory senses. A patient's statement that he is anxious about impending open-heart surgery is an observational term because the statement can be directly observed through the sense of hearing. Nurses cannot see the patient's anxiety, but they have no difficulty in recognizing it when the patient reports it: The patient says he is anxious. The precise concept in this example, then, is report of anxiety.

Indirect Observable Terms. Next in line is the indirect observable term, which refers to a property that must be inferred. In contrast to the concept report of anxiety, the concept "anxiety" cannot be directly observed, but it can be inferred by a combination of signs and symptoms exhibited by a person, such as restlessness and perspiration. The indirect observable term is more subject than the observational term to misinterpretation. For example, restlessness and perspiration are symptoms of shock due to blood loss as well as signs of anxiety about impending surgery. Misinterpretation of the indirect observable term can be reduced or eliminated by designating a proxy observational term. For example, the observational term "report of anxiety" can be designated as the proxy for the indirect observable term "anxiety." Thus, when a concept is classified as indirectly observable, the proxy observational term also must be identified.

Constructs. Next in line is the construct, which refers to a property that is neither directly nor indirectly observed. Constructs are invented for special scientific purposes. Although they have intrinsic theoretical meaning, they have empirical meaning only when proxy observational terms are designated. An example of a construct is social support, which was invented to describe a property of a person, namely, the amount of support the person received from others. The construct "social support" cannot be observed; it is inferred through designation of a proxy observational term, such as an individual's reports of the amounts of emotional and financial support received from relatives, friends, and colleagues.

Theoretical terms. At the far end of the continuum is the theoretical term, which refers to a complex, global property that is even more abstract than a construct. A theoretical term is impossible to observe, but it can be interpreted through its relationship to a construct. Thus, a theoretical term ultimately is observed through its connection to the proxy observational term designated for the construct. Self-concept, for example, cannot be observed, but it can be interpreted in a theory through its relationship to such constructs as self-esteem and body attitude, which are thought to be components of self-concept. Self-esteem and body attitude, in turn, can be observed through reports of feelings about one's self and one's body.

A theoretical term also can be interpreted through the role it plays in a theory. For example, self-concept is viewed differently in different theories. Coombs and Snygg (1959) postulated that how individuals behave is determined by their perceptions of themselves, which are dependent on the ideas they have of themselves and their abilities, that is, their self-concepts. In contrast, Mead (1934) postulated that self-concept is determined through interactions with others. That is, individuals' self-concepts are based on what people think others think about them. Thus, individuals behave in accord with what they think others expect of them.

Kaplan's classification schema, although widely cited, is not particularly easy to use. Distinctions among the four types of concepts are somewhat unclear and can be confusing. Acknowledging this lack of clarity, Kaplan (1964) stated:

These four types of terms are usually treated as two, the first two being combined as "observational" and the last two as "symbolic"; or else, the first three are lumped together as "empirical" or "descriptive" and contrasted with the "theoretical." However the lines are drawn, it is important to recognize that drawing them is to a significant degree arbitrary. The distinctions are vague, and in any case a matter of degree. (p. 57)

Observables and Constructs. Willer and Webster (1970) argued that there is no justification for the assumption that concepts exist in any sort of continuum. They classified concepts as either observables or constructs. *Observables*, which are also called descriptive terms, are the result of sensation. They are, then, immediately accessible to or very close to being immediately accessible to direct sensory observations. Gender and race are examples.

Constructs, which refer to abstract properties of phenomena, are the result of thought. They are not immediately accessible to direct sensory observation and so, like Kaplan's constructs, must be connected to an observable concept to test a theory empirically. According to Willer and Webster, constructs have greater generality. They pointed out that most mature sciences use constructs to build theory. They note the examples of mass and specific gravity from physics, bonds and valences of molecules from chemistry, and heredity, natural selection, and genes from biology. Another example is social support.

Classification by Measurement Characteristics. Dubin (1978) classified concepts according to their measurement characteristics. He identified five types of units, the term he used for concept.

Enumerative Units. The enumerative unit is a property of a phenomenon in all its conditions. It is always present, regardless of its condition; it can never take a zero or absent value. If the enumerative unit is nonvariable, it is always present. Gender is an example of a nonvariable enumerative unit. In contrast, if the enumerative unit is a variable, it is always present to some extent. Height and weight are examples of variable enumerative units.

Associative Units. The associative unit is a property of a phenomenon in only some of its conditions. It can have a real zero or absent value, as well as positive and negative numerical values. Associative units that are nonvariable, such as employed and unemployed, are either present or absent. Associative units that are variables are either present to some degree or not present at all. Job satisfaction is an example.

Relational Units. The relational unit is a property of a phenomenon that can be determined only by the relations among properties. In effect, it is a property of two or more properties. One type of relational unit reflects an interaction among properties, such as marital adjustment. In this example, a wife and a husband, when they interact, reflect one property called marital adjustment. Another type of relational unit reflects a combination of properties. For example, adolescent pregnancy is a combination of the properties age and reproductive status. Relational units also may encompass plural properties and entities. Sibling rivalry is an example; the plural properties are the child-child relationship and the parent-child relationship, and the plural entities are children and parents.

Statistical Units. The statistical unit is a property of a phenomenon that summarizes the distribution of the property. The label for this unit comes from the statistical terms for measures of central tendency and dispersion. There are three classes of statistical units. One class of statistical units summarizes the central tendency in the distribution of a property. An example is mean functional status, which is calculated from the score the individual receives for each item; that is, a mean score is determined for each individual. The second class of statistical units summarizes the dispersion of a property in a group as a whole. For example, the ethnicity of people in a town may be designated as homogeneous or diverse. The third class of statistical units designates the relative position in the distribution of a property. An example is the percentage of time an individual was able to remain at home, rather than in a hospital, from onset of terminal illness until death.

It is important to understand what statistical unit is the unit of analysis in a study. For example, when the mean is used to summarize central tendency in the distribution of a property, the individual's mean score is the unit of analysis. A mean of the individual means is then determined for descriptive and inferential purposes.

Summative Units. The summative unit is a global unit that refers to an entire complex phenomenon. Like Kaplan's theoretical term, this unit draws together several properties of the phenomenon and gives them a label that emphasizes one of the more important properties. Self-concept is an example; it reflects one's overall perception of oneself, including feelings about body, intellectual ability, morality, and goodness and worth as a human being.

Pragmatics of Concept Classification

The classification of concepts requires three steps. First, variability of the concept must be determined by identifying the number of dimensions of the concept. Care must be taken to distinguish between a concept that is a variable and the dimensions of the concept. Consider the example of quality of life. The concept, which is a variable, is "quality of life." One set of dimensions that this variable can take is low, moderate, and high quality of life, but they are the dimensions of the concept of interest, not the concept itself. It is important to note that a term may be a nonvariable concept in one study and a dimension of a variable concept in another study. For example, in a study limited to full-term infant subjects, a concept is the nonvariable, "full-term infant." In a study including full-term and preterm infants, however, a concept is the variable "length of gestation." "Full-term infant" is then one of the two dimensions of the variable, and "preterm infant" is the other.

Second, the empirical observability of the concept is determined. This requires the application of Kaplan's or Willer and Webster's schema. If a major concept is not directly observable, then the way it is made directly observable has to be determined. For example, if the concept of interest is the indirect observable term "depression," the research report must be reviewed to determine how depression was actually observed.

Third, the measurement characteristic of each concept is determined by applying Dubin's schema, which requires classification of each concept *as it is used in the research report being analyzed*. This point cannot be overemphasized; for many concepts do not have fixed measurement characteristics. Rather, classification is determined by how the concept is used in the study. For example, the concept "depression" is classified as an enumerative unit in a study limited to patients who exhibit signs of depression. In contrast, "depression" is classified as an associative unit in a study that compares depressed and nondepressed patients.

Furthermore, care must be taken in the classification of relational units because the units often appear to be associative or enumerative. Care must also be taken to classify statistical units correctly. In this case, the measure of central tendency or dispersion must be the raw score for the individual study subject; group means, for example, are not the basis for classification.

Successful classification of concepts according to their measurement characteristics is dependent on the information given in the research report. If scoring procedures and the range of possible scores on a measurement device are not described, it may not be possible to apply Dubin's schema.

Propositions

The second step in theory formalization is specification of the propositions as they are given in the research report. A proposition is a declarative statement about one or more concepts, a statement that purports or asserts what is the case (Achinstein, 1974).

Types of Propositions

The statements that describe or link concepts encompass nonrelational and relational propositions. Although definitions are sometimes treated as separate components of a theory, here they are more accurately identified as one category of nonrelational propositions.

Nonrelational Propositions. Propositions that say something about one concept are called *nonrelational propositions*. There are two categories of these propositions: those that state the existence of a concept and those that define a concept.

Existence Propositions. Existence propositions assert the existence or level of existence of a phenomenon. An example of a proposition that asserts the existence of a phenomenon is:

> There is a phenomenon known as bereavement.

An example of a proposition that asserts the level of existence of a phenomenon is:

> The majority of the sample experienced intense grief reactions.

Definitional Propositions. Definitional propositions go beyond statements of existence by describing the characteristics of a phenomenon. Concepts are the basic building blocks of theories and, therefore, must be precisely defined so that the meaning of one concept can be distinguished from the meaning of another. A definition is a statement of intention to use a concept in a particular way. Although definitions are arbitrary labels that are not verifiable, they are usually determined by convention. At any given stage of theory development, some definitions of concepts are taken as understood and others are newly introduced. Usually, a new theory adds only a few newly defined concepts; instead, it uses definitions taken from existing theories.

Two kinds of definitional propositions are needed to make the concepts of a theory empirically testable. The *constitutive definition* provides concepts with theoretical meaning. This type of definition is also called a theoretical definition, a nominal definition, or a rational definition. A constitutive definition states what a concept means by defining it with one or more other concepts. Perceived uncertainty, for example, can be constitutively defined as "the individual's perception of a situation as ambiguous" (Wineman, 1990, p. 294). In this example, the concept "perceived uncertainty" is defined by the concept "ambiguous."

The *operational definition* provides the concept with empirical meaning by defining it in terms of observable data, such as the activities necessary to measure the concept or to manipulate it. This type of definition is also called an epistemic definition, a real definition, or rules of correspondence or interpretation. Operational definitions identify the proxies for nonobservable concepts. Operational definitions are measurement-oriented interpretations of constitutive definitions. Kerlinger (1986) identified two classes of these definitions, which he called measured and experimental. The *measured* operational definition states how a concept will be measured. An example is: "Daily stress was measured by the Hassles Scale" (De Maio-Esteves, 1990, p. 361).

The *experimental* operational definition spells out the details or operations required to manipulate or vary the dimensions of the concept. An example of an experimental operational definition is taken from Holtzclaw's (1990) study of the effects of extremity wraps on amphotericin B (AmB)-induced shivering. [Amphotericin B is a drug used to treat life-threatening systemic fungal infections. One side effect is violent febrile shivering.]

Experimental Condition: The wraps consisted of three terry cloth towels, applied lengthwise to each extremity, from toes to groin and from fingertips to axillae. Towels were joined at the top of the extremity and edges rolled and clamped with plastic clips to form a seam and folded down at the ends to resemble mittens or boots. Blood pressure cuff tubing and intravenous lines were accommodated through the clipped seams of the wraps. Wraps were applied prior to the start of the AmB infusion. Patients wore pajamas and light covering and remained in bed except for short walks to the commode. Care was taken not to expose the patient's skin during measurement procedures.

Control Condition: Subjects in the control group were monitored by exactly the same protocol as the treatment group. They also wore pajamas and were allowed to use additional covering as they chose. Actions taken to

bundle up or add covers were noted on the record, and care was taken not
to expose the patient's skin during measurement. (p. 282)

Operational definitions are necessary regardless of the type of research. This is true whether the operational definition identifies the
paper-and-pencil questionnaire used in a survey or the domain of the
researcher-informant experience of an ethnography. Although operational definitions are needed for all types of research, they are a legacy of
the experimental method. Development of theory by experimentation
depends on actual operations with the variables involved. In fact, Bridgman (1927), the originator of operationism, viewed a concept as nothing
more than a set of unique operations or procedures necessary to produce
an observation. His view of the one-to-one correspondence of concepts
and operational definitions has been superseded by the view that no one
operational definition can "capture the rich and complex ideas contained in a [concept]" (Kidder, Judd, & Smith, 1986, p. 41). Indeed,
many concepts have multiple operational definitions. For example, functional status is measured by many different instruments (Moinpour,
McCorkle, & Saunders, 1988).

Empirical Indicators. Operational definitions state how concepts are
to be measured. Empirical indicators are the actual instruments, experimental conditions, and/or procedures that are used in a study. Strictly
speaking, operational definitions and empirical indicators are not part of
a theory, although they are mandatory elements of the research enter-
prise. Their crucial function is to link constitutively defined concepts to
the real world by indicating how the concepts are measured or observed.
Figure 2–3, which is adapted from the works of Gibbs (1972) and
Margenau (1972), illustrates the linkage of constitutively defined concepts to empirical indicators by means of operational definitions. The
diagram may depict any number of concepts ($C_1 \ldots _n$), operational
definitions (— — —), and empirical indicators ($EI_1 \ldots _n$). The example shown in Figure 2–3 is a formalization of components of Ragsdale
and Morrow's (1990) study of the association between HIV classification
and quality of life. Ragsdale and Morrow's use of two instruments to
measure quality of life illustrates the fact that a concept can have more
than one operational definition and, hence, more than one empirical
indicator.

Relational Propositions. Propositions that link two or more concepts
are said to be relational: they are declarative statements that express an

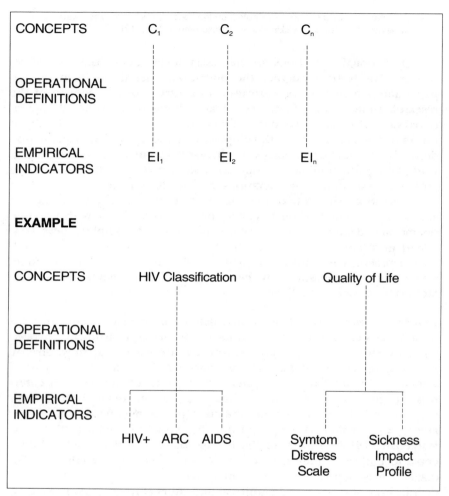

Figure 2–3. Linkage of concepts to empirical indicators by operational definitions. (Diagram for example constructed from Ragsdale & Morrow, 1990.)

association between concepts. More specifically, relational propositions state patterns of covariation between concepts that are variables; that is, they state that variation in one variable is systematically accompanied by variation in another. In correlational studies, the relationship between variables is expressed as a correlation between variables. In experimental studies, the relationship is frequently expressed as the effect of the experimental treatment. Thus, the phrases used to indicate a relationship include "relationship with," "related to," "associated with," "correlated with," and "effect of."

Several types of assertions about a relational proposition can be made. In fact, the more assertions that can be made about a proposition, the more that is known about the nature of the relationship.

Existence of a Relationship. The most basic assertion that can be made about a relationship is that it exists. A relational proposition asserting the existence of a relationship indicates that the association between two or more concepts is a recurring phenomenon rather than a unique event. The general form of this assertion is:

> There is a relationship between X and Y.

An example of a proposition asserting the existence of a relationship is: There is a relationship between functional status and psychological state (Tulman & Fawcett, 1990). Here it is simply asserted that the relationship exists.

Direction of a Relationship. A proposition that asserts the direction of a relationship states that the association between two concepts is positive (direct) or negative (indirect, inverse). The two general forms of a directional proposition are:

> There is a positive (negative) relationship between X and Y.
>
> X is positively (negatively) related to Y.

An example of a directional proposition is: Functional disability is negatively related to adaptation (Wineman, 1990). Another example is: Providing information to new mothers about infant behavior is directly related to their sense of maternal competence (Flagler, 1988).

Shape of a Relationship. A proposition that asserts the shape of a relationship states that the association between concepts is linear or curvilinear and, if curvilinear, is quadratic, cubic, quartic, or another shape. The general form of a linear relationship is:

> There is a linear relationship between X and Y such that as the numerical values of X increase, the numerical values of Y also increase (decrease).

An example of a linear relationship is that between stress and blood pressure; it is such that an increase in stress is associated with an increase in blood pressure.

The general form of a quadratic relationship is:

> There is a quadratic relationship between X and Y such that, when the values of X are low and high, the values of Y are low (high) and, when the values of X are moderate, the values of Y are high (low).

An example of a quadratic relationship is that between marital satisfaction and husband's income. This relationship is such that high and low incomes are associated with low marital satisfaction and moderate income is associated with high marital satisfaction (Voydanoff, 1980).

Relationships taking other shapes are stated in the same general form as linear and quadratic relationships, and the particular shape is specified.

Strength of a Relationship. A proposition that asserts the strength of a relationship identifies the magnitude of the relationship between two concepts. Magnitude is quantified by the effect size of a relationship, which is a standardized measure of the association between concepts or difference between two groups. Formulas for the effect sizes for several statistics are given by Cohen (1977), among others. The general form of the proposition is:

> There is a small (moderate, large) relationship between X and Y.

An example of this type of proposition is: There is a relationship between relaxation techniques and clinical symptoms, with large effects for headache and hypertension, moderate effects for insomnia, low or moderate effects for chronic pain and anxiety, and low effects for acute pain (Hyman, Feldman, Harris, Levin, & Malloy, 1989).

Symmetry of a Relationship. A proposition asserting the symmetry of a relationship states that the association between two concepts is either asymmetrical or symmetrical. An *asymmetrical relationship* is irreversible; only one idea is conveyed (X is related to Y). The general form of an asymmetrical relationship is:

If X, then Y; but if no X, no conclusion can be drawn about Y.

An example of an asymmetrical relationship is: There is a positive relationship between employment status and physical health (Ross, Mirowsky, & Goldsteen, 1990). This proposition indicates that being employed is associated with better physical health. Ross and her colleagues explained that recent research has revealed that the relationship is not due to selection, whereby healthy people work outside the home and unhealthy people do not, but rather that participation in the work force improves health.

A *symmetrical relationship* is also called a reversible or reciprocal relationship; it contains two separate ideas (X is related to Y and Y is related to X) that require two separate empirical tests. The general form of a symmetrical relationship is:

If X, then Y; and if Y, then X.

The following are examples of symmetrical relationships: (1) There is a positive relationship between post–high school educational plans and occupational plans, and vice versa. (2) There is a negative relationship between post–high school educational plans and marital plans, and vice versa. Otto (1979) noted that plans for post–high school education influence occupational plans and marital plans and that, conversely, marital plans or occupational plans influence educational plans.

Still another example is the reciprocal relationship between functional status and psychological state; it illustrates the fact that more than one assertion may be made about a relationship. Earlier in this chapter, the relationship between functional status and psychological state was given as an example of existence of a relationship. Now it can be asserted that the relationship exists and is symmetrical.

Concurrent and Sequential Relationships. A proposition that asserts the concurrent or sequential nature of a relationship refers to the period of time that elapses between the appearance of one concept and the appearance of another. If both concepts appear at the same time, the relationship is said to be *concurrent* or *coextensive*. The general form of a concurrent relationship is:

If X, then also Y.

An example of a concurrent relationship is the association between functional status and psychological state; it illustrates the fact that several assertions about a relationship can be made. Previously, the relationship between functional status and psychological state was given as an example of existence of a relationship and then as an example of a symmetrical relationship. Now it can be asserted that the relationship exists, is symmetrical, and is concurrent.

If one concept appears prior to the other, the relationship is said to be *sequential*. The general form of a sequential relationship is:

If X, then later Y.

An example of a sequential relationship is the association between relaxation techniques and hypertension. This is another example of the fact that several assertions can be made about a proposition. The information given by Hyman and her associates (1989) indicates that the relationship exists and is negative (i.e., use of a relaxation technique reduces hypertension), asymmetrical, sequential, and large in strength (average effect size$_d$ = 1.15).

Deterministic and Probabilistic Relationships. A proposition that asserts the deterministic or probabilistic nature of a relationship refers to the degree of certainty of occurrence of the relationship. *Deterministic relationships* state what always happens in a given situation. One type of deterministic relationship is the *universal truth or law*, the general form of which is:

If X, then always Y.

An example of a law is the relationship between the number of family members M and the number of reciprocal interactions R in the family. This relationship states that whenever a member is added to a family (as through birth or adoption of a child), the number of reciprocal interactions increases according to the formula $R = [M(M-1)] \div 2$ (Broderick & Smith, 1979).

Another example of a law is the relationship between the physical magnitude of a stimulus and the magnitude of the sensory response. Nield and Kim (1991) explained:

In mathematical terms, sensory magnitude is related to physical magnitude by a power function $Y = kX^n$, where Y is the intensity of the response or sensory magnitude, k is a constant, X is the stimulus intensity or physical magnitude, and n is the power function. The exponent n serves as an expression of the individual's perceptual sensitivity. (p. 17)

Laws are common in the physical sciences but rare in the behavioral sciences. Moreover, any law can be made untrue by just one instance. For example, if you wished to upset the law that all swans are white, you would not have to show that no swans are white; it would be sufficient to prove that a single swan is black.

Another type of deterministic relationship is the *tendency statement*, which is concerned with what always happens in a given situation in the absence of interfering conditions (Gibson, 1960). This means that there are certain conditions or circumstances which when present negate the relationship. Tendency statements are more common in the behavioral sciences than are laws. The general form of a tendency statement is:

If X, then always Y if there are no interfering conditions.

An example of a tendency statement is the relationship between family size and educational attainment of male children. This relationship states that there is an inverse relationship between family size and male children's educational attainment. The conditions that interfere with the occurrence of this relationship are sibling position (in large families, younger male children have greater educational attainment; in small families, older males have greater educational attainment), family intellectual environment (the greater the favorable intellectual environment, the greater the male children's educational attainment), and stability of the parents' marriage (having both parents present is related to greater educational attainment of male children; having one or none present is related to lower educational attainment) (Aldous, Osmond, & Hicks, 1979).

Probabilistic, or *stochastic*, *relationships* are concerned with the chances or probability of something happening in a given situation. The general form of a probabilistic relationship is:

If X, then probably Y.

An example is: Uncertainty about one's illness may influence psychological outcomes (Wineman, 1990).

Necessary and substitutable relationships. A proposition asserting the necessary or substitutable nature of a relationship refers to the need for a particular concept in the relationship. Relationships that are classified as *necessary* state that if one concept occurs, and only if that concept occurs, the other concept will occur. The first concept must be present to bring about the relationship. The general form of this proposition is:

If X, and only if X, then Y.

An example of a relationship that can be classified as necessary is this: Information about sensations associated with surgery given preoperatively reduces postoperative distress (Johnson, 1984).

Relationships that are classified as *substitutable* state that if one concept occurs, the other concept will occur. In this kind of relationship, however, if some other similar concept occurs, the second concept will also occur. The general form is:

If X_1, but also if X_2, then Y.

An example of a relationship that can be classified as substitutable is: High state anxiety *or* lack of studying is related to a low score on an examination.

Sufficient and Contingent Relationships. A proposition that asserts the sufficient or contingent nature of a relationship refers to the conditional nature of a concept in the relationship. Relationships that are classified as *sufficient* state that when a given concept occurs, a certain other concept will occur, regardless of anything else. The general form of this proposition is:

If X, then Y, regardless of anything else.

An example of a relationship that can be considered sufficient is: Procedural, sensory, and coping behavior information given preoperatively will reduce postoperative distress. Previously, the need for sensory information was given as an example of a necessary relationship. Now it can be asserted that sensory information is necessary for reduction of postoperative distress, but it is not sufficient. Rather, three types of information (procedural, sensory, and coping behaviors) are required to reduce distress (Johnson, 1984).

Propositions that are classified as *contingent* state that the relationship between two concepts X and Y is influenced by the presence of some third concept. The third concept is referred to as an intervening variable C. The general form of a contingent relationship is:

If X, then Y, in the presence of C.

One form of contingent relationship occurs when the intervening variable C is directly in the path between two other concepts X and Y; thus the three concepts form a chain. Wineman (1990), for example, theorized that functional disability is positively related to perceived uncertainty, which in turn is negatively related to adaptation. This proposition is still another example of the fact that more than one assertion about a relationship can be made. Here the direction of the relationship is given, as well as its status as contingent.

Another form of contingent relationship occurs when the values taken by the intervening variable affect the strength of the relationship between X and Y. An example is the strength of the positive relationship between marital status and physical health. This relationship is contingent on gender, such that it is stronger in men than in women (Ross et al., 1990).

Another example was given by Yarcheski and Mahon (1986). This proposition asserts that the strength of the contingent relationship between perceived stress and symptom patterns is affected by the amount of social support. In this case, the strength of the positive relationship between perceived stress and level of symptom patterns increases when social support is low. Conversely, the strength of the relationship decreases when social support is high.

A third form of contingent relationship occurs when the direction or even the existence of the relationship between X and Y is affected by the numerical values taken by the intervening variable or by a characteristic of the study subjects, such as age, gender, or race. The relationship between household structure and labor force participation, which is contingent on marital status and race, is an example. The relationship between household structure (live alone or with extended family) and labor force participation (employed or looking for work versus nonemployed) is negative for never married black mothers of preschool age children but positive for formerly married black mothers. Furthermore, there is no relationship between household structure and labor force participation of white mothers of preschool age children regardless of marital status (Rexroat, 1990). Another example is the relationship between psychosocial attributes and perceived stress, which Leidy (1990) found to be contingent on gender: The relationship is positive for males and negative for females.

The Hypothesis. Hypotheses are special types of propositions that represent conjectures about concepts stated in empirically testable forms. They are expectations about the way things are in the world if theoretical assertions are correct. A hypothesis is derived from a proposition by linking one or more constitutively defined concepts with the empirical indicators identified in the operational definitions (Fig. 2–3). Technically, a hypothesis is a prediction about one or more empirical indicators; more specifically, it is a prediction about the scores obtained from the empirical indicator(s) (Dubin, 1978; Gibbs, 1972). The numerical scores from the empirical indicators are what are compared when statistical tests are conducted.

Although most research reports state the hypothesis by using only the names of the concepts, examination of the report should determine what empirical indicators are included in the actual hypotheses. Like operational definitions and empirical indicators, hypotheses are, strictly speaking, not part of a theory.

An example of a nonrelational proposition and its derived hypothesis is taken from Pollock and Duffy's (1990) work:

> **Proposition:** The phenomenon known as health-related hardiness encompasses the dimensions of control, commitment, and challenge.

> **Hypothesis:** The 51 items of the Health-Related Hardiness Scale can be categorized into three subscales: Control, 21 items; Commitment, 15 items; and Challenge, 15 items.

An example of a relational proposition and its derived hypothesis is taken from Wineman's (1990) study of adaptation to multiple sclerosis:

> **Proposition:** The greater the satisfaction with social support, the greater the adaptation.

> **Hypothesis:** The higher the satisfaction score on the Social Network List and Support System Scale, the higher the score on the Purpose-in-Life Test.

Pragmatics of Proposition Identification and Classification

Propositions are not always presented clearly in research reports. Therefore, the report may have to be reviewed several times before all propositions are identified. Propositions are identified by listing all statements —sentences or phrases— that include the concepts already identified as central to the theory. The propositions should be listed exactly as they are stated in the research report. After all propositions are listed, they can be restated in a more formal manner (e.g., X is defined as . . . ; or X is related to Y) if that enhances the analysis. However, only the propositions presented in the research report should be listed, even if some concepts included in the theory are not accounted for in the list. Although it may be tempting to add the needed propositions, that should not be done as part of the analysis of a theory.

Identification of the propositions is followed by their classification. The first step in classification is to determine if each proposition is nonrelational or relational. Nonrelational propositions are further classified as existence or definitional propositions. Existence propositions are rarely stated in the formal manner of "There is a phenomenon known as . . ."; instead, they are reflected in the substance of the research report. For example, formalization of the theory presented in Carter's (1989) research report revealed existence propositions dealing with the phenomenon of bereavement.

Definitions of concepts, like concepts themselves, may not be readily identifiable. That is because definitions are not always labeled as such in a research report. Constitutive definitions can be extracted from the narrative discussion of the concepts or from the discussion of the empirical indicators (i.e., the research instruments, experimental conditions, and procedures). Operational definitions can usually be determined from the discussion of the empirical indicators or from the description of the research procedure. The research report must be carefully reviewed to determine which concepts are defined and how they are defined. The type of definition—constitutive or operational—also must be determined.

Relational propositions are further classified according to the assertions that can be made about them (existence, direction, strength, and so on). The second step is to determine which propositions are hypotheses. If desired, the hypotheses can be restated by substituting the empirical indicators for the concept names.

Hierarchies of Propositions

The third step in theory formalization is the hierarchical ordering of the propositions into sets. A proposition set provides a concise justification for the existence of a phenomenon or an explanation of why a particular relationship exists. Proposition sets can be arranged hierarchically according to level of abstraction, inductive reasoning, or deductive reasoning.

Hierarchies by Level of Abstraction

Propositions can be arranged on a continuum from abstract to concrete. Abstract propositions are concerned with more general phenomena or a wider class of objects than are concrete propositions, which are concerned with more specific phenomena or a narrower class of objects. Gibson (1960) referred to abstract statements as unrestricted propositions and to concrete statements as restricted propositions. He noted that the distinction arises from the limits of space and time within which the proposition applies. The proposition set, therefore, consists of statements arranged from most abstract to most concrete.

Propositions that can be arranged according to level of abstraction are most often found in reports of tests of a general theory in a specific situation. The following example, drawn from a test of the theory of reasoned action (Miller, Wikoff, Garrett, McMahon, & Smith, 1990), illustrates how propositions become more specific and narrow in scope as they become more concrete. The most abstract proposition is part of the general theory of reasoned action. The first concrete proposition narrows the relationship to the situation of medical regimen compliance. The second concrete proposition specifies the behaviors prescribed for the myocardial infarction patient and designates for the patient's significant others.

Abstract proposition: Perceived beliefs of others are related to behavior.

Concrete proposition: Action that the individual believes others think he or she should perform is related to medical regimen compliance.

More concrete proposition: The myocardial infarction patient's perception of a significant other's beliefs about the patient's following prescribed behaviors (diet, medications, activity, smoking, and stress in home, work, sports, and social environments) is related to the patient's self-assessment of prescribed behaviors (following diet, taking medications, performing activity, stopping smoking, and modifying responses to stress in home, work, sports, and social environments).

Hierarchies by Inductive Reasoning

Inductive reasoning is evident when a conclusion summarizes a series of discrete observations about a phenomenon. Each observation represents evidence for the conclusion (Crossley & Wilson, 1979). The inductive proposition set consists of a series of observations followed by a conclusion.

Inductive reasoning is most often found in reports of qualitative research designed to generate descriptive theories. An example is taken from Swanson's (1991) report of the development of her theory of caring. The theory, which includes the caring processes of knowing, being with, doing for, enabling, and maintaining belief, was induced from the findings of phenomenological studies of the experiences of childbearing families. The example includes two observations from which the process of knowing was induced.

> Observation₁: When things weren't right, I could say that things were fine and it was only a matter of time. I mean the nurse would ask certain questions and there would be no way that I could be consistent without telling the truth. And then we would talk, and pretty soon instead of saying it was fine, I would start out with what was really wrong. [Quotation from a mother who described how the nurse worked with her to help her to express her true feelings.]

> Observation₂: They thought at first that we were being like resistive to learning . . . and it wasn't until they found out that this was the third time in three years we've been here . . . [that] they started to figure out that the most important thing we wanted to find out immediately was the major things. We weren't so concerned about movement and that kind of stuff, the major things we were concerned with was the oxygen, the respirators, and how they were doing feeding . . . I was going in there daily. We'd wash up, she'd reach in and touch them first and I'd go right to the charts and start reading. [Quotation from a father whose prematurely born twin sons were in a neonatal intensive care unit. The parents had previously experienced the deaths of two other premature infants.]

> Conclusion: Knowing is striving to understand an event as it has meaning in the life of the other. When one is operating from a basis of knowing, the care provider works to avoid a priori assumptions about the meaning of an event, centers on the one cared for, and conducts a thorough, ongoing cue-seeking assessment of the experience of the one cared for. (p. 163)

Hierarchies by Deductive Reasoning

Deductive reasoning is evident when a conclusion necessarily follows from one or more statements that are taken as true (Crossley & Wilson, 1979); it is most frequently found in reports of theory-testing research. Hierarchical ordering of the propositions of a deductively developed theory requires that some statements be identified as initial starting points and others as deductions from the starting points.

The propositions that represent the starting points for deduction are called axioms, premises, or postulates. They are taken as givens in a theory and therefore do not have to be proved or tested. A proposition that is deduced from two or more axioms is called a theorem or conclusion. A theorem is a supposition. Its logical and empirical adequacy must be determined. Thus, the deductive proposition set is made up of a series of axioms followed by a theorem.

The transitive rule of relationships is used to deduce a theorem from axioms. According to the transitive rule, if X is related to Y (axiom) and if Y is related to Z (axiom), then X is related to Z (theorem).

An example of deduction using the transitive rule is taken from a study of adjustment in persons having radiotherapy for cancer (Christman, 1990). In this example, X is represented by symptom severity (i.e., the severity of side effects of radiotherapy), Y by uncertainty about illness-related events, and Z by psychosocial adjustment problems.

> *Axiom₁:* If there is a positive relationship between symptom severity and uncertainty, and
>
> *Axiom₂:* if there is a positive relationship between uncertainty and psychosocial adjustment problems,
>
> *Theorem:* then there is a positive relationship between symptom severity and psychosocial adjustment problems.

Although axioms are usually statements of relationships, sometimes one or more axioms may be nonrelational, definitional propositions. Hypotheses stated in the vocabulary of empirical indicators are developed through this form of deduction. In this case, the nonrelational, definitional propositions are axioms that identify the empirical indicators (X′ and Y′) of concepts X and Y. The proposition set in this case consists of axioms and the hypothesis.

An example of hypothesis derivation is taken from Wineman's (1990) study of adaptation to multiple sclerosis. This example illustrates the derivation of the hypothesis testing the relationship between functional disability and depression. Here X is represented by functional disability, X′ by the Incapacity Scale, Y by depression, and Y′ by the Beck Depression Inventory.

> *Axiom₁:* If functional disability is positively related to depression, and
>
> *Axiom₂:* if functional disability is measured by the Incapacity Scale, and
>
> *Axiom₃:* if depression is measured by the Beck Depression Inventory,

Hypothesis: then the higher the scores on the Incapacity Scale, the higher the scores on the Beck Depression Inventory and, conversely, the lower the scores on the Incapacity Scale, the lower the scores on the Beck Depression Inventory.

Sign of a Relational Proposition. The direction, or sign, of an axiom, if known, was established in previous research. The sign of a deduced theorem, however, must be calculated by means of the so-called sign rule, which is based on mathematical logic. This rule states that the sign of the deduced relationship (the theorem) is the algebraic product of the signs of the postulated relationships (the axioms). That is, the sign of the deduced relationship between X and Z is found by multiplying the sign of the relationship between X and Y by the sign of the relationship between Y and Z.

Various possible combinations of signs are:

Axiom₁: If X is positively (+) related to Y, and

Axiom₂: if Y is positively (+) related to Z,

Theorem: then X is positively (+) related to Z.

Axiom₁: If X is negatively (−) related to Y, and

Axiom₂: if Y is negatively (−) related to Z,

Theorem: then X is positively (+) related to Z.

Axiom₁: If X is negatively (−) related to Y, and

Axiom₂: if Y is positively (+) related to Z,

Theorem: then X is negatively (−) related to Z.

Axiom₁: If X is positively (+) related to Y, and

Axiom₂: if Y is related to Z in an unknown (?) direction,

Theorem: then X is related to Z in an unknown (?) direction.

Use of the sign rule is exemplified by restating the proposition set drawn from Christman's (1990) study.

Axiom₁: If there is a positive relationship (+) between symptom severity and uncertainty, and

Axiom₂: if there is a positive relationship (+) between uncertainty and psychosocial adjustment problems,

Theorem: then there is a positive relationship (+) between symptom severity and psychosocial adjustment problems.

Pragmatics of Hierarchical Ordering of Propositions

The arrangement of propositions in hierarchical order is frequently the most difficult step in theory formalization. That is because research reports usually do not present a theory in the formal manner of proposition sets. Furthermore, a hierarchical arrangement of proposition sets according to inductive or deductive reasoning may not be possible because space limitations in journals often preclude the development of full inductive or deductive arguments.

Selection of the method of hierarchy development depends on the purpose of the study and the information given in the research report. If the purpose of the study was to generate a theory by using an inductive method, then an attempt should be made to arrange the propositions as inductive sets of observations and conclusions. On the other hand, if the study purpose was to test a theory, then the propositions can be arranged according to level of abstraction or as deductive sets of axioms, theorems, and hypotheses. Arrangement of propositions according to level of abstraction is possible when a general theory was tested in a particular situation or when more abstract concepts, such as theoretical terms or summative units, are part of a theory. Arrangement of propositions as deductive sets of axioms and theorems requires that some statements were regarded as givens and others were deduced from those statements. Arrangement of propositions as deductive sets of axioms and hypotheses requires that operational definitions were given for the concepts making up at least one relational proposition.

The task of hierarchical ordering is accomplished by first arranging the propositions found in the research report in groups according to the concept or concepts included in each proposition. For example, all propositions about concept X could be placed in one group, all propositions about concept Y could be placed in another group, and all propositions about concepts X and Y could be placed in still another group.

Once the propositions are grouped, they can be arranged according to the type of hierarchy that is evident. If level of abstraction is evident, then the more abstract propositions are separated from the more concrete ones. If induction has been used, then the propositions that are observations are separated from those that are conclusions. If deduction has been used, then the propositions that are used as axioms are separated from those that are theorems and those that are hypotheses. Finally, the proposition sets are created by listing the propositions in the appropriate hierarchical order.

The arrangement of deductive proposition sets in appropriate hierarchical order is facilitated by listing each hypothesis in its narrative form (i.e., the theorem) or in its operational form (i.e., using empirical indicators for concept names). The hypothesis is the final step in the deductive process, and so the other propositions are arranged in the order that leads to that end point. Additional examples of hierarchical ordering of proposition sets are presented in the Appendix.

Diagrams

The final step in theory formalization is the construction of a diagram of the theory. A diagram helps to determine how all the concepts and propositions of the theory were brought together. It is the final aid to understanding exactly what the theory says and what it does not say. It also facilitates the identification of gaps and overlapping ideas or redundancies in the theory.

Diagramming Conventions for Propositions

Conventions for diagramming the relationships between concepts have been suggested by several authors (Blalock, 1969; Burr, Hill, Nye, & Reiss, 1979; Hardy, 1974; Lin, 1976). The conventions for illustrating the existence and direction of a relationship and for asymmetrical and symmetrical relationships are shown in Figure 2–4, along with examples from works by Tulman and Fawcett (1990), Ross et al., (1990), and Otto (1979) that were discussed on pages 29 to 31. The existence of a relationship is illustrated by an unbroken line (—) connecting the two concepts X and Y. An arrowhead at one end of the line indicates an asymmetrical relationship (→). Arrowheads at both ends of the line indicate a symmetrical relationship (↔). The direction of the relationship is indicated by a plus sign (+) for a positive relationship or a minus sign (−) for a negative, or inverse, relationship. If the direction of the relationship is not known, no sign is required, although a question mark (?) may be used.

Conventions for diagramming contingent relationships and examples of these types of relationships are illustrated in Figures 2–5 to 2–8.

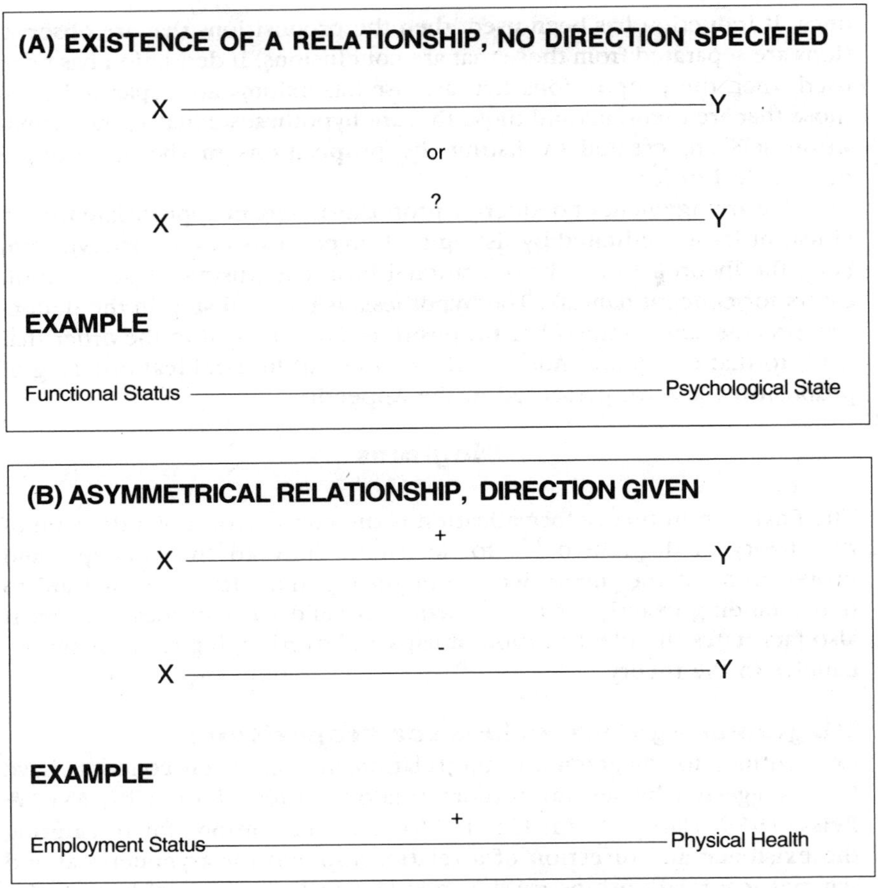

(A) EXISTENCE OF A RELATIONSHIP, NO DIRECTION SPECIFIED

X ——————————————————————————— Y

or

X ————————————————?—————————— Y

EXAMPLE

Functional Status ——————————————————————— Psychological State

---

(B) ASYMMETRICAL RELATIONSHIP, DIRECTION GIVEN

X ————————————————+—————————— Y

X ————————————————-—————————— Y

EXAMPLE

Employment Status———————————+——————————— Physical Health

Figure 2–4. Conventions for diagramming relationships between concepts (Diagramming conventions adapted from Burr, Hill, Nye, and Reiss, 1979, p. 23, with permission.) [(*A*), Diagram for example adapted from Tulman & Fawcett, 1990, p. 98, with permission. (*B*) Diagram for example constructed from Ross, Mirowsky, and Goldsteen, 1990. (*C*) Diagram for example adapted from Otto, 1979, p. 114, with permission.]

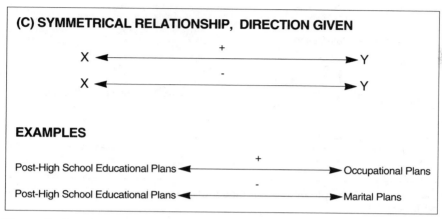

Figure 2–4. *Continued*

Figure 2–5 shows the three concepts in a chain. The intervening variable C comes between concepts X and Y. The direction of each relationship is indicated by a plus (+) or minus (−) sign. The example, taken from Wineman's (1990) study of adaptation to multiple sclerosis, was discussed on page 35. Chains can include more than three concepts. Diagrams that depict the theoretical frameworks or models tested by means of path analysis and causal modeling, for example, are chains that contain

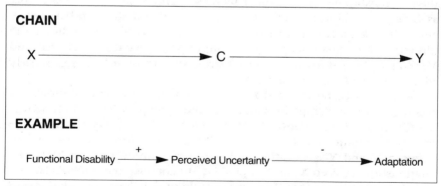

Figure 2–5. Diagramming conventions for contingent relationships: Chains (see above Fig. 2–4.) (Diagram for example adapted from Wineman, 1990, p. 297, with permission.)

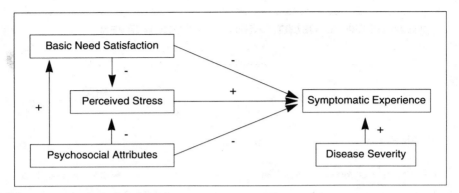

Figure 2-6. Example of a causal model diagram. (From Leidy, 1990, p. 232, with permission.)

many intervening variables (Pedhazur, 1982). An example of this kind of diagram is presented in Figure 2-6. This example illustrates the concepts and propositions of the theory tested by use of causal modeling techniques in Leidy's (1990) study of the relationships between stress, psychosocial resources, and symptomatic experience in chronic illness.

Figure 2-7 shows the diagramming conventions and examples for contingent relationships in which the intervening variable C influences the strength of the relationship between X and Y. The symbol ↑S indicates that as the intervening variable C increases in magnitude, the strength of the relationship between X and Y increases. The symbol ↓S indicates that as C decreases in magnitude, the strength of the relationship between X and Y increases. A plus (+) or minus (−) sign is used to indicate the direction of the relationship. The example was drawn from Yarcheski and Mahon's (1986) study of perceived stress and symptom patterns in early adolescents and was discussed on page 35.

Figure 2-8 shows the diagramming conventions and examples for contingent relationships in which the intervening variable C influences the direction of the relationship between X and Y. The symbols Lo = − and Hi = + indicate that if the magnitude of C is low, the relationship between X and Y is negative and if the magnitude of C is high, the relationship between X and Y is positive. In contrast, the symbols Lo = + and Hi = − indicate that if the magnitude of C is low, the relationship between X and Y is positive and if the magnitude of C is high, the relationship between X and Y is negative. If the intervening variable is a characteristic of the study subjects, the characteristic is substituted for Hi

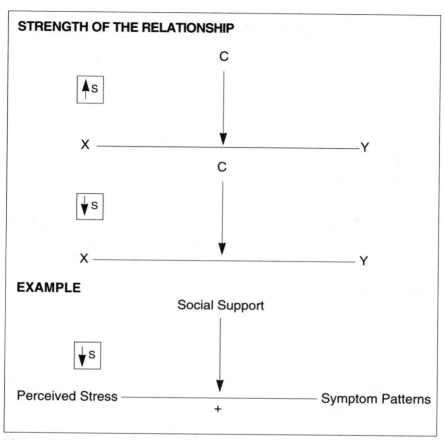

Figure 2–7. Diagramming conventions for contingent relationships: Strength of the relationship (see Fig. 2–4.) (Diagram for example constructed from Yarcheski & Mahon, 1986.)

and Lo. The symbol 0 is used when a certain value of the intervening variable eliminates the existence of the relationship between X and Y. The example was taken from Rexroat's (1990) study of labor force participation, which was discussed on pages 35 and 36.

Inventories of Concepts and Propositions
The diagramming conventions can be used to illustrate each proposition of a theory, as discussed above, or they can be used in inventories that

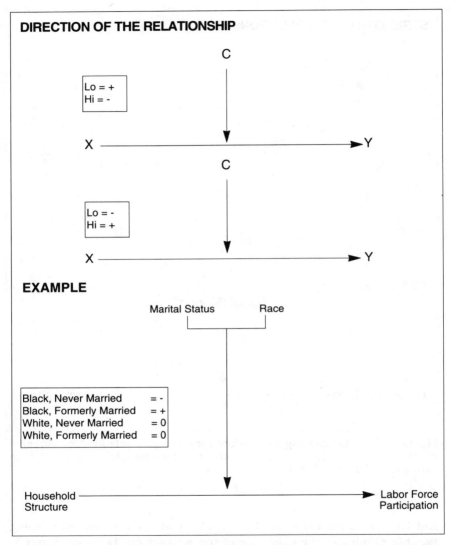

Figure 2–8. Diagramming conventions for contingent relationships: Direction (see Fig. 2–4) of the relationship. (Diagram for example constructed from Rexroat, 1990.)

depict all of the concepts and propositions that make up a theory. Inventories take six different forms.

Concepts and Empirical Indicators. One form of an inventory is a diagram of concepts and their empirical indicators. This form of an inventory was depicted in Figure 2-3. The vertical broken lines (- - -) indicate operational definitions. Horizontal unbroken lines (——), arrowheads (◀▶), and signs (+ - ?) can be added to the figure to illustrate the linkages between concepts of the theory and between empirical indicators.

Matrix of Concepts. The second form of an inventory is a matrix of concepts. The matrix, which is adapted from the matrix format used to display correlation coefficients, is used to illustrate the stated relationships between concepts in a theory and to uncover the unstated relationships. The number of cells in the matrix is determined by the number of concepts in the theory. The matrix may include checkmarks (✓) to indicate which concepts have been linked. It may also include the signs for the direction of the relationships (+ -) if they are known or a question mark (?) if the direction of a relationship is not known. Blank spaces indicate that the concepts are not linked in the theory. The matrix format is shown in Figure 2-9, along with an example given by Crawford (1985) to depict the relationships between concepts in the theory of support network conflict experienced by new mothers.

Inventory of Causes. The third form of an inventory, displayed in Figure 2-10, is a diagram of the relationships between a concept of interest (Y) and its antecedents ($X_1 \ldots {}_n$). The antecedent form of an inventory links the concept of interest to other concepts that precede it either theoretically or in time. The unbroken lines with arrowheads (→) indicate asymmetrical relationships. The sign for the direction of the relationship (+ -) may be included if known, or a question mark (?) may be used if the direction is unknown. The concept of interest is the dependent variable, and the antecedent concepts are the independent variables. This convergent structure is usually called an inventory of determinants or of causes. The example given in Figure 2-10 was developed from the narrative report of a study of psychosocial predictors of maternal depressive symptoms in single-parent families (Hall, Gurley, Sachs, & Kryscio, 1991).

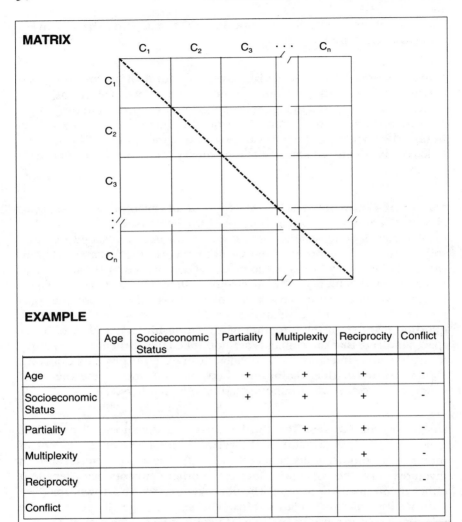

Figure 2–9. The matrix form of inventory. (Diagram adapted from Hardy, 1974, p. 103, with permission. Diagram for example adapted from Crawford, 1985, p. 102, with permission.)

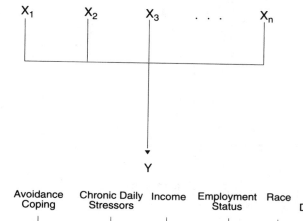

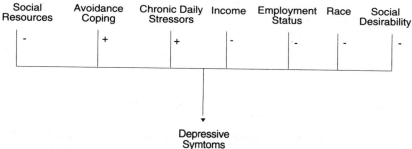

Figure 2-10. Inventory of causes. (Diagram adapted from Blalock, 1969, p. 35, with permission. Diagram for example constructed from Hall, Gurley, Sachs, & Kryscio, 1991.)

Inventory of Effects. The fourth form of an inventory, shown in Figure 2-11, is a diagram of the relationships between a concept of interest (Y) and its consequent concepts ($Z_1 \ldots n$). This inventory links the concept of interest with other concepts that follow it either theoretically or in time. The unbroken lines with arrowheads ($\rightarrow$) indicate asymmetrical relationships. The sign for the direction of the relationship ($+ -$) may be included if it is known, or a question mark (?) may be used if the direction is unknown. Here, the concept of interest is the independent variable and the consequent concepts are the dependent variables. This divergent structure is usually called an inventory of results or of effects. The example seen in Figure 2-11 was developed from the narrative report of a meta-analysis of the long-term consequences of parental divorce for adult well-being (Amato & Keith, 1991).

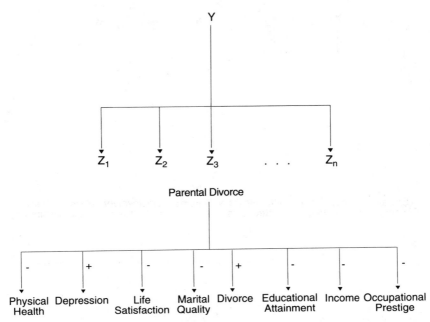

Figure 2-11. Inventory of effects. (Diagram adapted from Blalock, 1969, p. 41, with permission. Diagram for example constructed from Amato & Keith, 1991.)

Inventory of Causes and Effects. The fifth form of an inventory, which is depicted in Figure 2-12, is a diagram of the relationships between a concept of interest (Y) and both antecedent (X_1 . . . $_n$) and consequent (Z_1 . . . $_n$) concepts. The antecedent-consequent form of an inventory links the concept of interest with other concepts that precede it and still others that follow it theoretically or in time. As in the other inventories, the unbroken lines with arrowheads ($\rightarrow$) indicate asymmetrical relationships. Again, the sign for the direction of the relationship (+ −) may be included if it is known, or a question mark (?) may be used if the direction is unknown. This combined convergent-divergent structure is usually called an inventory of causes and effects. The example shown in Figure 2-12 illustrates antecedents and consequences of family size (Gecas, 1979).

Conceptual Maps. The sixth form of an inventory is the conceptual map. Although Moody (1989) used the term "conceptual map" to refer

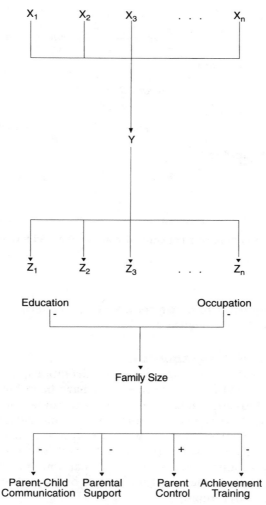

Figure 2–12. Inventory of causes and effects. (Diagram adapted from Blalock, 1969, p. 42, with permission. Diagram for example adapted from Gecas, 1979, p. 384, with permission.)

to any type of inventory, Artinian's (1982) discussion of conceptual maps emphasized illustration of the consequences of different values taken by independent variables. More specifically, the map depicts the effects of the various dimensions or numerical scores taken by each independent variable. Intervening variables also can be included in the map. An exam-

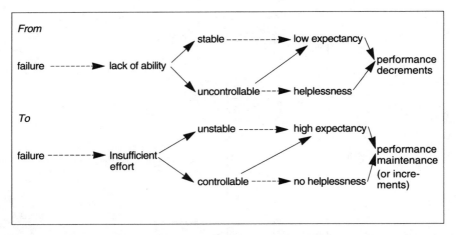

Figure 2–13. Example of a conceptual map. (From Weiner, 1980, p. 9, with permission.)

ple of a conceptual map drawn from Weiner's (1980) studies of causal attributions is given in Figure 2–13.

Pragmatics of Diagramming

Diagramming is done after the concepts, definitions, and propositions have been identified and the propositions have been hierarchically ordered. The various approaches to diagramming can be used separately or in combination. The choice of approach is an individual one. No one approach is better than another. Whatever approach makes clear what concepts are included in the theory and which of these concepts are linked in propositions should be selected. Caution must be taken, however, not to include in the diagram concepts or propositions that are not given in the research report.

CONCLUSION

In this chapter, theory formalization is described as a technique consisting of four steps. Step 1 involves the identification and classification of concepts. Step 2 involves the identification and classification of propositions. Step 3 is the hierarchical ordering of propositions. Step 4 is the construction of a diagram of the theory.

The use of the technique of theory formalization facilitates understanding the exact content of a theory and the way it was operationalized in research. In theory-generating research, the technique of theory formalization is applied to the results of the study to determine the concepts and propositions that were discovered. In theory-testing research, the technique is applied to the introductory section of the research report to determine what concepts and propositions constituted the theory that was tested, and also to the results of the study to determine what concepts and propositions were retained. Examples of theory formalization for both theory-generating and theory-testing studies are given in the Appendix.

The results of theory formalization are drawn upon when the theory is evaluated. Evaluation of the content of research reports is the focus of Chapter 3.

REFERENCES

Achinstein, P. (1974). Theories. In A. C. Michalos, *Philosophical problems of science and technology* (pp. 280–297). Boston: Allyn and Bacon.

Aldous, J., Osmond, M. W., & Hicks, M. W. (1979). Men's work and men's families. In W. R. Burr, R. Hill, F. I. Nye, & I. L. Reiss (Eds.), *Contemporary theories about the family. Vol. 1. Research-based theories* (pp. 227–256). New York: The Free Press.

Amato, P. R., & Keith, B. (1991). Parental divorce and adult well-being: A meta-analysis. *Journal of Marriage and the Family, 53,* 43–58.

Artinian, B. M. (1982). Conceptual mapping: Development of the strategy. *Western Journal of Nursing Research, 4,* 379–393.

Babbie, E. (1989). *The practice of social research* (5th ed.). Belmont, CA: Wadsworth.

Bates, J. E. (1987). Temperament in infancy. In J. D. Osofsky (Ed.), *Handbook of infant development* (2nd ed., pp. 1101–1149). New York: Wiley.

Blalock, H. M., Jr. (1969). *Theory construction: From verbal to mathematical formulations.* Englewood Cliffs, NJ: Prentice-Hall.

Bridgman, P. W. (1927). *The logic of modern physics.* New York: Macmillan.

Broderick, C. B., & Smith, J. (1979). The general systems approach to the family. In W. R. Burr, R. Hill, F. I. Nye, & I. L. Reiss (Eds.), *Contemporary theories about the family. Vol. II. General theories: Theoretical orientations* (pp. 112–129). New York: The Free Press.

Burr, W. R., Hill, R., Nye, F. I., & Reiss, I. L. (1979). Metatheory and diagramming conventions. In W. R. Burr, R. Hill, F. I. Nye, & I. L. Reiss (Eds.), *Contemporary theories about the family. Vol. 1. Research-based theories* (pp. 17–24). New York: The Free Press.

Carter, S. L. (1989). Themes of grief. *Nursing Research, 38,* 354–358.

Cohen, J. (1977). *Statistical power analysis for the behavioral sciences* (rev. ed.). New York: Academic Press.

Coombs, A., & Snygg, D. (1959). *Individual behavior: A perceptual approach to behavior.* New York: Harper and Row.

Crawford, G. (1985). A theoretical model of support network conflict experienced by new mothers. *Nursing Research, 34,* 100–102.

Christman, N. J. (1990). Uncertainty and adjustment during radiotherapy. *Nursing Research, 39,* 17–20, 47.

Crossley, D. J., & Wilson, P. A. (1979). *How to argue: An introduction to logical thinking.* New York: Random House.

De Maio-Esteves, M. (1990). Mediators of daily stress and perceived health status in adolescent girls. *Nursing Research, 39,* 360–364.

Dubin, R. (1978). *Theory building* (rev. ed.). New York: The Free Press.

Flagler, S. (1988). Maternal role competence. *Western Journal of Nursing Research, 10,* 274–290.

Gecas, V. (1979). The influence of social class on socialization. In W. R. Burr, R. Hill, F. I. Nye, & I. L. Reiss (Eds.), *Contemporary theories about the family. Vol. 1. Research-based theories* (pp. 365–404). New York: The Free Press.

Gibbs, J. (1972). *Sociological theory construction.* Hinsdale, IL: Dryden Press.

Gibson, Q. (1960). *The logic of social enquiry.* New York: Humanities Press.

Hall, L. A., Gurley, D. N., Sachs, B., & Kryscio, R. J. (1991). Psychosocial predictors of maternal depressive symptoms, parenting attitudes, and child behavior in single-parent families. *Nursing Research, 40,* 214–220.

Hardy, M. E. (1974). Theories: Components, development, evaluation. *Nursing Research, 23,* 100–107.

Holtzclaw, B. J. (1990). Effects of extremity wraps to control drug-induced shivering: A pilot study. *Nursing Research, 39,* 280–283.

Hyman, R. B., Feldman, H. R., Harris, R. B., Levin, R. F., & Malloy, G. B. (1989). The effects of relaxation training on clinical symptoms: A meta-analysis. *Nursing Research, 38,* 216–220.

Johnson, J. E. (1984). Coping with elective surgery. In H. H. Werley & J. J. Fitzpatrick (Eds.), *Annual review of nursing research* (Vol. 2, pp. 107–132). New York: Springer.

Kaplan, A. (1964). *The conduct of inquiry.* San Francisco: Chandler.

Kerlinger, F. N. (1986). *Foundations of behavioral research* (3rd ed.). New York: Holt, Rinehart & Winston.

Kidder, L. H., Judd, C. M., & Smith, E. R. (1986). *Research methods in social relations* (5th ed.). New York: Holt, Rinehart & Winston.

Leidy, N. K. (1990). A structural model of stress, psychosocial resources, and symptomatic experience in chronic physical illness. *Nursing Research, 39,* 230–236.

Lin, N. (1976). *Foundations of social research.* New York: McGraw-Hill.

Lowery, B. J., Jacobsen, B. S., & McCauley, K. (1987). On the prevalence of causal search in illness situations. *Nursing Research, 36,* 88–93.

Margenau, H. (1972). The method of science and the meaning of reality. In H. Margenau (Ed.), *Integrative principles of modern thought* (pp. 3–43). New York: Gordon and Breach.

Marx, M. H. (1976). Formal theory. In M. H. Marx & F. E. Goodson (Eds.), *Theories in contemporary psychology* (2nd ed., pp. 234–260). New York: Macmillan.

Mead, G. H. (1934). *Mind, self, and society.* Chicago: University of Chicago Press.

Mercer, R. T., May, K. A., Ferketich, S., & DeJoseph, J. (1986). Theoretical models for studying the effect of antepartum stress on the family. *Nursing Research, 35,* 339–346.

Miller, Sr., P., Wikoff, R., Garrett, M. J., McMahon, M., & Smith, T. (1990). Regimen compliance two years after myocardial infarction. *Nursing Research, 39,* 333–336.

Mishel, M. H., & Murdaugh, C. L. (1987). Family adjustment to heart transplantation: Redesigning the dream. *Nursing Research, 36,* 332–338.

Moinpour, C. M., McCorkle, R., & Saunders, J. (1988). Measuring functional status. In M. Frank-Stromborg (Ed.), *Instruments for clinical nursing research* (pp. 23–45). Norwalk, CT: Appleton and Lange.

Moody, L. E. (1989). Building a conceptual map to guide research. *Florida Nursing Review, 4*(1), 1–5.

Nield, M., & Kim, M. J. (1991). The reliability of magnitude estimation for dyspnea measurement. *Nursing Research, 40,* 17–19.

Otto, L. B. (1979). Antecedents and consequences of marital timing. In W. R. Burr, R. Hill, F. I. Nye, & I. L. Reiss (Eds.), *Contemporary theories about the family. Vol. 1. Research-based theories* (pp. 101–126). New York: The Free Press.

Pedhazur, E. J. (1982). *Multiple regression in behavioral research* (2nd ed.). New York: Holt, Rinehart & Winston.

Pollock, S. E., & Duffy, M. E. (1990). The Health-Related Hardiness Scale: Development and psychometric analysis. *Nursing Research, 39,* 218–222.

Ragsdale, D., & Morrow, J. R. (1990). Quality of life as a function of HIV classification. *Nursing Research, 39,* 355–359.

Rexroat, C. (1990). Race and marital status differences in the labor force behavior of female family heads: The effect of household structure. *Journal of Marriage and the Family, 52,* 591–601.

Ross, C. E., Mirowsky, J., & Goldsteen, K. (1990). The impact of the family on health: The decade in review. *Journal of Marriage and the Family, 52,* 1059–1078.

Swanson, K. M. (1991). Empirical development of a middle range theory of caring. *Nursing Research, 40,* 161–166.

Tobey, G. T., & Schraeder, B. D. (1990). Impact of caretaker stress on behavioral adjustment of very low birth weight preschool children. *Nursing Research, 39,* 84–89.

Tulman, L., & Fawcett, J. (1990). A framework for studying functional status after diagnosis of breast cancer. *Cancer Nursing, 13,* 95–99.

Voydanoff, P. (1980). *The implications of work-family relationships for productivity.* Scarsdale, NY: Work in American Institute.

Weiner, B. (1980). The role of affect in rational (attributional) approaches to human motivation. *Educational Researcher, 9*(7), 4–11.

Willer, D., & Webster, M., Jr. (1970). Theoretical concepts and observables. *American Sociological Review, 35,* 748–757.

Wineman, N. M. (1990). Adaptation to multiple sclerosis: The role of social support, functional disability, and perceived uncertainty. *Nursing Research, 39,* 294–299.

Yarcheski, A., & Mahon, N. E. (1986). Perceived stress and symptom patterns in early adolescents: The role of mediating variables. *Research in Nursing and Health, 9,* 289–297.

ADDITIONAL READINGS

Dulock, H. L., & Holzemer, W. L. (1991). Substruction: Improving the linkage from theory to method. *Nursing Science Quarterly*, *4*, 83–87.

Hinshaw, A. S. (1979). Theoretical substruction: An assessment process. *Western Journal of Nursing Research*, *1*, 319–324.

Jacox, A. (1974). Theory construction in nursing: An overview. *Nursing Research*, *23*, 4–13.

Reynolds, P. D. (1971). *A primer in theory construction*. Indianapolis: Bobbs-Merrill.

Rodgers, B. L. (1989). Concepts, analysis and the development of nursing knowledge: The evolutionary cycle. *Journal of Advanced Nursing*, *14*, 330–335.

Walker, L. O., & Avant, K. C. (1988). *Strategies for theory construction in nursing* (2nd ed.). Norwalk, CT: Appleton and Lange.

Zetterberg, H. (1965). *On theory and verification in sociology* (3rd ed.). Totowa, NJ: Bedminster Press.

3

Evaluation of the Relation between Theory and Research

The close connection between theory and research mandates evaluation of the theoretical elements of a research report as well as the methodology used to generate or test the theory. This chapter presents criteria for the evaluation of the theoretical and methodologic aspects of research reports that draw on the results of analysis of theory, which was the subject of Chapter 2.

CRITERIA FOR EVALUATION OF RESEARCH REPORTS

Criteria for the evaluation of theory and the critique of research are available in the literature of almost every discipline. Review of the criteria indicates considerable agreement about what should be expected of theory and research methods. Few criteria, however, emphasize the relationship between theory and research. The evaluation criteria presented in this chapter highlight the commonalities found in the literature and emphasize the essential connection between the theoretical and methodologic aspects of research. An attempt has been made to develop the criteria so that they are appropriate for evaluation of descriptive, correlational, and experimental studies.

Judgments regarding the extent to which the content of a research report satisfies certain criteria are most readily and accurately made after an analysis of the theoretical elements has been completed. A detailed discussion of the analytic technique of theory formalization was presented in Chapter 2. As explained there, theory formalization yields a clear and concise listing of the concepts and propositions that make up a theory. In theory-generating research, formalization involves identification and classification of the concepts and propositions that emerge from the study findings. In theory-testing research, formalization encompasses two phases. The first phase focuses on identification and classification of the concepts and propositions that entered into the empirical test; the second involves identification and classification of the concepts and propositions that were retained after testing.

Evaluation of Theory

The first component of the evaluation of a research report focuses on the theory that was generated or tested by the study. Criteria include the significance, internal consistency, parsimony, and testability of the theory.

Significance of a Theory

The criterion of significance requires theories to reflect theoretical and social significance. Theoretical significance is evident when the theory addresses a phenomenon of interest to a discipline by extending or filling in gaps in knowledge about that phenomenon. For example, the phenomena of interest to nursing are considered by many to be person, environment, health, and nursing (Fawcett, 1984). "Person" refers to the recipient of nursing care; "environment," to the significant others and the surroundings of the person, as well as to the setting in which nursing care occurs; "health," to the wellness or illness state of the person at the time that nursing care occurs; and "nursing," to the goals of nursing care and the actions taken by nurses on behalf of or in conjunction with the person. Broad categories of theories that are considered significant to the discipline of nursing focus on:

- The life process, well-being, and optimum function of human beings, sick or well
- The patterning of human behavior in interaction with the environment in normal life events and critical life situations
- The processes by which positive changes in health status are affected (Donaldson & Crowley, 1978; Gortner, 1980)

Social significance is evident when a theory addresses a problem of particular interest to society. Such a problem can be identified at any given time by reference to priorities for research set by expert panels sponsored by government agencies, professional organizations, or clinical specialty organizations.

Although it is generally agreed that a significant theory provides a new insight into a phenomenon or a new way to view a phenomenon, the judgment of significance can be relative: What seems significant to one person may not be significant to another. The ultimate jury usually is the relevant scientific community, which, however, is not always unbiased. Some theories may generate considerable attention from the scientific community for reasons that have little or nothing to do with their intrinsic merit. For example, the theory of the efficacy of topical insulin for treatment of pressure sores was adopted enthusiastically by clinicians and highly recommended by the authors of nursing textbooks despite conflicting research findings and negative clinical outcomes. Speculating on the reason for that, Gerber and Van Ort (1981) stated, "Perhaps as we desperately seek a cure for the problems associated with these chronic wounds we are blinded to the potential dangers of some drug-containing therapies" (p. 1159). Similarly, a theory may gain wide acceptance in the public sector yet be a misleading or even false explanation of a phenomenon. Gall's theory of phrenology and Reich's theory of orgone energy are historical examples.

Conversely, a theory may be scorned by scientists and/or the public because it goes against current thinking or because it represents such a major leap in knowledge that it cannot be comprehended. An example of the former is Darwin's theory of evolution; an example of the latter is McClintock's theory of gene transposition. Everyone knows about Darwin's theory; McClintock's may not be so familiar. McClintock, the winner of a 1983 Nobel Prize, found that genes are not fixed on the chromosome but rather can move around in an unpredictable manner and cause unexpected changes in heredity. Although her gene transposition ("jumping genes") theory was first published more than 35 years ago, its significance has been widely acknowledged only in the past decade.

Precision in Prediction and Explanatory Power. The significance criterion requires that a theory not only reflect theoretical and social significance but also provide both precision in prediction and explanatory power. "Precision" refers to the ability of a theory to accurately predict something about a phenomenon — its occurrence, its relationship to another phenomenon, the numerical scores that will be taken by one variable given the scores of another variable, and so on. Precision is objective, and it may be expressed in mathematical equations. "Explanatory power" refers to the degree to which a theory contributes to understanding. "A theory that provides a good explanation of some phenomenon can be said to rate highly on explanatory power because it produces a [subjective] feeling of understanding in those who study it" (Goodson & Morgan, 1976, p. 297).

Both precision and explanatory power are needed because, no matter how precise the statements about concepts might be, they are neither meaningful nor significant unless they are understood. However, the contrast between the objectively stated precision of a theory and the more subjective, experiential condition of understanding that represents explanation gives rise to two paradoxes (Dubin, 1978).

The precision paradox states that it is possible for a theory to achieve high precision in prediction without explaining how the predicted outcome was achieved. For example, there is a predictable strong relationship (effect size$_d$ = 1.12) between use of relaxation techniques and reduction of headache (Hyman, Feldman, Harris, Levin, & Malloy, 1989). The explanation for this relationship, however, is not well understood.

The power paradox states that it is possible for a theory to achieve high explanatory power without the concomitant ability to predict precise outcomes. For example, although a relatively complete understanding of the risk factors associated with cardiac disease exists, a precise prediction of when an individual will experience a myocardial infarction or develop congestive heart failure is not possible.

Theories with high precision tend to be narrow in scope, and those with high explanatory power tend to be broad in scope. That is problematic because a theory of extremely narrow scope is so tied to one or a few individuals at a given time or in a given place that it may be trivial, and a theory of extremely broad range, a so-called grand theory, may be so abstract that it tends to explain everything and at the same time explain nothing. Theories must, therefore, be somewhat general and complex yet encompass a small number of well-defined concepts. Such formulations frequently are referred to as *middle-range theories*.

A middle-range theory tends to resolve the precision and power paradoxes by limiting the scope of a theory, although not to the point that the theory becomes trivial. A middle-range theory may also resolve the paradoxes by simplifying relationships through such statistical controls as analysis of covariance or through such methodologic controls as sample limitations. Finally, a middle-range theory can resolve the paradoxes by increasing the number of assertions that can be made about the relationships between concepts such as direction, shape, and strength.

Application of the Criterion of Significance. In theory-generating research, the significance criterion is applied to the theory that is presented by the results of the study; in theory-testing research, it is applied to the theory that was tested as well as to the version that was retained after testing.

Internal Consistency of a Theory

The internal consistency criterion encompasses three major requirements: semantic clarity, semantic consistency, and structural consistency.

Semantic Clarity. The internal consistency criterion requires concepts to reflect semantic clarity, that is, to be clearly defined. Semantic clarity is more likely to occur when both constitutive and operational definitions are given for each concept making up the theory than when no definitions are given or when just one type of definition is stated. The inclusion of both constitutive and operational definitions enhances semantic clarity, especially when the same term can take several meanings. "Functional status," for example, can refer to and be measured by various behaviors ranging from walking to driving a car to working as a volunteer for a charitable organization.

Semantic clarity also is more likely to occur when concepts are not redundant. Dubin (1978) proposed the four rules listed below for the use of concepts (units) that, if followed, render the theory free of concept redundancy.

1. Enumerative units may be used alone in a theory in any logically consistent manner. Associative, relational, or statistical units also may be used alone in a theory.
2. Enumerative units and associative units may be used together in a theory without any restriction other than logical consistency.
3. Relational units may not be combined in the same theory with

enumerative or associative units that are themselves properties of the relational unit. Redundancies can easily occur when the relational unit is based on a combination such as a composite score. A redundancy would occur if, for example, the composite score of number of children who are properly secured in a car seat and who are in the correct type of seat was correlated with the number of children properly secured in car seats or with the number of children in the correct type of seat (Goebel, Copps, & Sulayman, 1984).

4. A statistical unit, which is by definition a property of a collective such as a group of study subjects, may not be combined with any enumerative, associative, or relational unit that describes a property of individual members of the same collective. For example, suppose it is known from a study of elderly people that, on the average, depression scores decrease 3 points with every increase of 1 point in self-transcendence scores (Reed, 1991). The knowledge based on the collective "elderly people" cannot be used to predict the depression score of any one elderly woman or man.

Semantic Consistency. The internal consistency criterion requires concepts to reflect semantic consistency, that is, consistent use of the same term and the same definition for a concept throughout the narrative presentation of the theory. This means that different words or phrases should not be used for the same concept and that different explicit or implicit definitions should not be used for a concept in any one theory. For example, the terms "functional ability" and "functional status" should not be used interchangeably in the same theory. That is because "functional ability" refers to the person's capability to perform activities, whereas "functional status" refers to the level at which the person is performing the activities. Thus, "functional ability" is an antecedent to "functional status."

Chinn and Kramer (1991) pointed out that semantic clarity and consistency are related. In particular, clarity is obscured if messages are inconsistent, and consistency is difficult to determine if messages are unclear.

Structural Consistency. The internal consistency criterion also requires propositions to reflect structural consistency. Flaws in the structural consistency of a theory can result in incomplete sets of propositions. Incompleteness, which is also called discontinuity, occurs in deductive proposition sets when some propositions are not explicit. For example, consider a theory stating only that (1) high role overload is associated with high role strain and (2) high role strain is associated with low cooperation. This theory is incomplete because the linkage between role overload and cooperation is not stated explicitly, even though the linkage can be deduced from the propositions that are given (Hardy, 1988).

Flaws in structural consistency can also result in redundant propositions. Redundancy occurs when one axiom can be deduced from another and, therefore, is not independent. Consider a theory stating that (1) burnout is a manifestation of stress, (2) stress results in high employee turnover rates, and (3) burnout results in high employee turnover rates. Propositions 2 and 3 are redundant because "stress" and "burnout" are equivalent concepts in this theory. The redundancy can be corrected by eliminating either proposition 2 or 3.

Furthermore, flaws in structural consistency can result in violations of inductive or deductive reasoning. Thus, inductive and deductive proposition sets must be related to each other in accordance with the appropriate rules of logic. Adherence to the rules of logic cannot, however, guarantee structural consistency. That is because a conclusion arrived at by means of induction can exceed the available observations, or a logically deduced theorem can be reached from a faulty premise. Thus, when an inductive structure is evident, the strength of the evidence offered for the conclusion should be evaluated. More specifically, the observations should be evaluated to determine if they represent sufficient, unbiased, and relevant evidence for the conclusion (Crossley & Wilson, 1979). Moreover, when a deductive structure of axioms and theorems is evident, the veracity of the axioms must be judged. In other words, the axioms, which are regarded as givens, must be evaluated to determine if each one has sufficient support to be regarded as knowledge that is believed to be true (Hardy, 1988).

Mixing of inductive and deductive reasoning almost always obscures the structural consistency of a theory and, therefore, should be avoided. An exception is retroduction, or abduction — a theory development strategy that combines inductive and deductive methods in a logical and sequential manner (Hanson, 1958).

Application of the Criterion of Internal Consistency. In theory-generating research, the internal consistency criterion is applied to the theory that was generated, as presented in the study findings. In theory-testing research, the criterion is applied to the theory that was tested as well as to the version that was retained after testing. In the case of theory-testing research, the two-phase application of the criterion permits a comparison of the completeness of proposition sets before and after evidence is obtained.

Parsimony of a Theory

The parsimony criterion, sometimes referred to as Occam's razor or Lloyd Morgan's canon, requires a theory to be stated in the most economical way possible. This means that the fewer the concepts and propositions needed to describe, explain, or predict a phenomenon the better. Marx (1976) claimed that parsimony has both historic and logical bases.

> Historically, scientists have learned that the more [theoretical statements] that are involved—or the more complex a theory is—the greater likelihood there is of error. And once a serious error creeps in, the whole theoretical superstructure may be fatally weakened. . . . Logically, the reason for the greater effectiveness of the simple solution is, in large part, that science mainly consists of a more or less feeble groping toward ''truth,'' or factualness, and that most of our original ideas are doomed to extinction. On a probability basis alone, therefore, the fewer the links in the chain, the less the likelihood of serious error. (p. 251)

Parsimonious *inductive* theories include a minimum number of concepts and propositions to describe a phenomenon; parsimonious *deductive* theories include a minimum number of independent axioms from which theorems can be derived. The minimum number of axioms is reached when each axiom makes a unique contribution to the theory and is essential to the deductive structure.

The parsimony criterion is not, however, to be confused with oversimplification of the phenomenon. Parsimony that does not capture the essential features of a phenomenon is false economy. Skinner's theory stating that reinforcement accounts for all changes in behavior is considered by many psychologists to be an example of parsimony achieved by oversimplification (Goodson & Morgan, 1976). Thus, a theory should be evaluated to determine whether the most parsimonious statement clarifies rather than obscures the phenomenon and whether it effectively deals with all of the data about the phenomenon.

Application of the Criterion of Parsimony. Like the preceding two criteria, the parsimony criterion is applied to the results of theory-generating studies. Similarly, in theory-testing research, the criterion is applied to the theory that was tested as well as to the version that was retained after testing. The two-phase application in the case of theory-testing research permits a judgment regarding enhanced or decreased parsimony, especially when some propositions have been rejected or when the addition of new concepts and propositions is recommended.

Testability of a Theory

The testability criterion requires the components of a theory to be empirically observable. A theory is testable if its concepts can be observed empirically, if its propositions can be measured, and if its derived hypotheses can be falsified. Concepts are empirically observable if they are connected to empirical indicators by operational definitions. Concepts that lack operational definitions must be connected to those that are operationally defined. Propositions are measurable when they are stated as hypotheses. More precisely, propositions are measurable when empirical indicators are substituted for concept names in the hypotheses. When a hypothesis states a relationship between empirical indicators, all assertions about that relationship must be testable. For example, if a hypothesis states that empirical indicator X' is asymmetrically and positively related to empirical indicator Y', such that when the score of X' increases 1 unit, the score of Y' increases 2 units, the symmetry, direction, and magnitude of change in scores must all be empirically testable.

Popper (1965) maintained that the goal of theory testing is to refute or falsify hypotheses. Scientific progress is hindered by a hypothesis that cannot be falsified because it cannot be modified or replaced by another hypothesis. Conversely, a falsifiable hypothesis can be improved or replaced by a better one. A falsifiable hypothesis is sufficiently precise that incompatible empirical results can be easily identified. For example, the hypothesis stating that all middle-aged men score high, medium, or low on a test of risk factors for cardiac disease cannot be refuted because it does not rule out any logically or practically possible findings. In contrast, the hypothesis stating that all middle-aged men score high on the risk factors test can be refuted because it asserts that middle-aged men will not have midrange or low scores on the test.

The requirements for testability can be summarized by reference to a masterpiece of satire written by Shearing (1973). He claimed that because theories frequently are presented in an untestable form in research reports, investigators might as well learn to make theories untestable. To that end, he then offered the following guidelines:

1. Make certain that no empirically refutable statements can be deduced from the theory. This may be done in the following ways:
   a. Provide no operational definitions for any of the concepts in the theory.

b. Provide no propositions in the theory.

c. If propositions are stated, ensure that the relationships between concepts remain as unclear as possible.

2. Ensure that the theory is internally inconsistent.

The converse of each of these guidelines is, of course, needed to meet the criterion of testability.

Alternative Requirements for Testability. Testability is frequently regarded as the primary characteristic of a scientifically useful theory. Marx (1976) maintained, "If there is no way of testing a theory it is scientifically worthless, no matter how plausible, imaginative, or innovative it may be" (p. 249). This view of testability is admittedly a strict one that is in keeping with the classic view of operationism (Bridgman, 1927). One alternative is a criterion stating that testability does not have to be direct. This criterion is appropriate in areas of inquiry in which active manipulation of variables usually is not feasible, such as astronomy and archeology. Another alternative is a criterion requiring theories to be potentially testable. It is particularly appropriate for theories that are generated by means of qualitative methods, such as grounded theory, ethnography, and phenomenology. That is because the empirical indicators needed to test the theory may not be available, yet it is believed that they can be developed.

Still another alternative is a criterion requiring theories to be testable through imaginary or thought experiments rather than by empirical means. This criterion is appropriate when a theory cannot be empirically tested because of the time or cost involved, the unavailability of empirical indicators, technical impossibility, or ethical prohibitions. For example, although technological limitations have prevented the empirical testing of components of Einstein's theory of relativity, the theory has been tested by means of thought experiments that involved mathematical equations and arguments based on logic (Cohen, Sarill, & Vishveshwara, 1982). Similarly, the existence of the Higgs boson, a hypothetical class of particles, cannot be empirically tested until a high-energy collider, such as the Superconducting Super Collider, is constructed (Mann, 1989).

Empirical testability is not, of course, an appropriate criterion for theories developed by such nonempirical methods as some philosophic inquiries, and it may not be an appropriate criterion for some types of historical research. Rather, these methods include their own rules for theory testing.

Application of the Criterion of Testability. Like the preceding three criteria, the testability criterion is applied to the results of theory-generating studies. Here the question is whether the concepts and propositions could be empirically tested in future studies. In contrast, in the case of theory-testing research, the application of this criterion is limited to the theory that was tested. In other words, judgments are confined to the empirical testability of the concepts and propositions that the investigator planned to study.

Evaluation of Research Design

Theory directs every aspect of a study. Thus, the second component of evaluation of a research report focuses on the congruence between theory and study design. The criterion is operational adequacy.

Operational Adequacy

The operational adequacy criterion requires the research design used to generate or test a theory to be congruent with the theory. Every aspect of design, including the sample, instruments, data collection procedures, and data analysis techniques, must be evaluated to determine whether the theory is accurately reflected and appropriately operationalized.

The sample should be appropriate for the theory that was generated or tested and for the study procedures. More specifically, the sample should represent the population for which the theory is being developed. That is true whether the sample is made up of human beings, animals, events, or the content of publications. In theory-generating studies using qualitative methods, nonprobability or convenience sampling, which is frequently called theoretical sampling, is appropriate. In theory-generating studies using quantitative methods and in theory-testing studies, probability sampling that includes random selection and/or assignment of subjects is more appropriate. Regardless of the sampling procedure, however, representativeness of the sample is the most important point to consider.

The research instruments, or empirical indicators, should be appropriate for eliciting the data needed to generate or test the theory of interest to the investigator. Each instrument should be a valid measure of the intended concept as constitutively defined in a given study. This point cannot be overemphasized, because many concepts have different constitutive as well as different operational definitions. For example, the Katz Index of Activities of Daily Living is a valid measure of functional status when constitutively defined as the extent of independence in bathing, dressing, toileting, transfering, continence, and feeding (Katz, 1983). The Katz Index, however, is not a valid measure of functional status when it is constitutively defined as the extent of assistance required for performance of usual daily activities and social role activities. The latter definition is operationalized by the Enforced Social Dependency Scale (Benoliel, McCorkle, & Young, 1980). Thus, the constitutive definition of each concept must be carefully considered when evaluating the validity of any empirical indicator.

Each instrument should also be a reliable measure for the population of interest and for the specific study subjects. A questionnaire that has demonstrated test-retest and internal consistency reliability for one sample may not be reliable with another sample, even when drawn from the same population. That is because measurement error, variability of scores, and other factors affecting the reliability of an instrument can vary from sample to sample.

The research procedure should be appropriate for the theory that the researcher wishes to generate or test and for the type of research that was conducted. For example, if a theory predicts differences between two distinct groups on a measure, the research procedure must include a comparison between the groups. Each type of theory (descriptive, explanatory, predictive) is developed by a particular type of research that has its own set of standards and safeguards for investigators and subjects. Detailed discussions of descriptive, correlational, and experimental methods are presented in several good research texts, including those by Babbie (1990), Cook and Campbell (1979), Kerlinger (1986), and Moody (1990).

The data analysis procedure should be appropriate for the theory being developed. Descriptive theory development frequently employs such summary statistics as frequency counts, percentages, medians, means, and ranges. Explanatory theory development requires such measures of association as correlation coefficients. Predictive theory development usually requires such measures of differences as analysis of variance procedures. The data analysis procedure should also be appropriate for the kind of data obtained. Narrative data usually are analyzed by means of a content analysis procedure, and numerical data usually are subjected to nonparametric or parametric statistical procedures. The selection of a particular nonparametric or parametric statistic depends on the measurement scale of the numerical data (nominal, ordinal, interval, or ratio). Narrative data can, of course, be transformed to numerical scores and then be analyzed statistically.

Application of the Criterion of Operational Adequacy. In theory-generating research, the operational adequacy criterion is applied to the results of the study. In theory-testing research, the application of this criterion is limited to the version of the theory that was tested. The judgment, therefore, focuses on the extent to which the empirical indicators are appropriate proxies for the concepts and the procedures are the appropriate methods to observe the propositions proposed by the investigator.

Evaluation of Research Findings

Research findings direct theory development. Therefore, the third component of evaluation of a research report emphasizes the influence of study results on theory generation or refinement. The criterion is empirical adequacy.

Empirical Adequacy

The empirical adequacy criterion requires theoretical claims to be congruent with empirical evidence derived from research. In theory-generating studies, the concepts and propositions that emerge from the data analysis should clearly reflect the raw data. In theory-testing studies, the interpretation of tests of hypotheses is especially important. The logic of scientific inference dictates that if the empirical data do not conform to the hypothesized expectation, it may be appropriate to conclude that the hypothesis is false. Conversely, if the empirical data conform to the expectation stated by the hypothesis, it may be appropriate to tentatively accept the hypothesis as empirically adequate.

The logical form that permits rejection of a hypothesis when empirical findings do not conform to expectations, called *modus tollens*, states that a single negative instance is sufficient to falsify a hypothesis: (1) If A then C; (2) Not C; (3) Therefore, not A (Crossley & Wilson, 1979, p. 271).

Acceptance of a hypothesis as the truth when findings conform to expectations, called the *fallacy of affirming the consequent*, takes this logical form: (1) If A then C; (2) C; (3) Therefore A (Crossley & Wilson, 1979, p. 272). The argument is fallacious because "the positive result does not give unequivocal support to the . . . hypothesis" (Phillips, 1987, pp. 14–15). In fact, it is always possible that exceptions can occur. Thus, the argument underscores the logical flaw that occurs when extraneous variables that could have influenced the findings are ignored.

For example, if study findings reveal a significant difference in cardiac output between a group that performed aerobic exercises and a group that did not, one must ask if both groups were equivalent in such other respects as age, ordinary activity, and pretest physical health. Of course, extraneous variables also could account for negative findings. Consequently, the empirical adequacy of hypotheses and their parent theories is based on probability rather than certainty.

It is unlikely that any one test of a hypothesis or theory will provide the definitive evidence needed to establish empirical adequacy. Thus, decisions about empirical adequacy should take the findings of all related studies into account. Formal procedures for integrating the results of related studies are discussed in detail in Chapter 4. Suffice it to say here that the more tests of a theory that yield supporting evidence, the more adequate the theory.

Alternative Methodologic and Substantive Explanations. Regardless of the empirical adequacy of a theory, competing or alternative explanations for empirical findings must be taken into account. Two alternative explanations that always must be considered are methodologic. One explanation is that the findings were produced by the research design, especially by the sample of observations or measurements actually made out of all those that could have been made. The other explanation is that the findings were produced by many small errors of measurement, such as perceptual and coding errors associated with subjects' and investigators' use of the research instruments.

Other explanations are substantive; they attempt to account for the study findings by recommending the elimination of some concepts, the addition of other concepts, and/or different linkages between concepts. A substantive explanation may also include the recommendation of an entirely different theory to account for the findings.

Alternative methodologic and substantive explanations are given in Schepp's (1991) research report. Schepp tested a theory of the effects of predictability of events, control, and anxiety on coping effort in a sample of mothers of acutely ill, hospitalized children. She found that the data did not provide support for two of the four hypotheses that were tested. More specifically, she found that, contrary to hypothesized expectations, 100 percent of control and 65 percent of anxiety were not explained by the other variables in the theoretical model.

Methodologic explanations for the lack of support for the two hypotheses focused on sample anomalies and instrument weakness. Schepp explained:

It is highly probable that previous research findings cannot be generalized to this population group. At the time of the interview, the mothers were experiencing extraordinarily high levels of stress. Their children's hospitalizations were unplanned. . . . The mothers were also quite young, had limited parenting experience, and [had] little or no previous experience with the hospitalization of their children.

The unexpected findings related to control may reflect comments made by many of the subjects that they had no control, or very little control, over the events that they were asked to rank proportionately. The instrument indexing control may, therefore, have lacked construct validity under the assumption that the potential for control existed when, in the minds of the subjects, it did not. (pp. 44–45)

One substantive explanation offered by Schepp emphasized the need to eliminate the concept of control from the theoretical model. As part of that explanation, Schepp stated:

The concept of control as defined in this study may not be applicable in extreme situations, such as the one tested here. Several theoretical interpretations can be suggested. Seligman and Miller (1979), in describing the phenomenon of helplessness, suggest that predictability is a more basic human need than controllability. They speculated that individuals tend to settle for predictability if control is not possible, as may have been the case with the subjects in this study.

Miller (1981) hypothesized that individuals relinquish control in situations where they believe some factor other than their own response may provide more stability. In this study, mothers who had not been able to successfully treat their children when they did have control (at home) may have tended to relinquish control to the hospital personnel once their children were hospitalized. By relinquishing control, the mothers may have perceived that the hospital personnel would institute the necessary measures to change the children's situation, thus reestablishing order and predictability. (p. 45)

Another substantive explanation focused on the need to incorporate other concepts into the theoretical model. Schepp commented:

The amount of variance that was not explained for control and anxiety suggests other variables should be included in the [theoretical] model. Although a strength of the magnitude estimation instrument strategy is the more accurate measurement of concepts, other variables such as demographic variables could not be included in the empirical test of the model since they were not measured at ratio level. Therefore, demographic variables that might have contributed significantly to the explained variance of the concepts could not be identified. The model needs to be tested with multiple indicators for the variables using other measurement strategies, i.e. [sic], Likert, which would allow greater flexibility in identifying other key variables

Also, the theoretical model may be more correctly specified with the addition of the concept of social support. Mishel and Braden (1988), in their latest research on uncertainty in illness with adult cancer clients, report social support to be an important variable in predicting client outcomes. In the theoretical model of this study, social support may be an important mediating variable. This model needs to be tested with social support as one of the key variables. (p. 45)

Competing Hypotheses. Platt (1964) maintained that every theory-testing study should include multiple competing hypotheses derived from alternative theories. He claimed that this approach eliminates errors in interpreting findings that are due to the investigator's intellectual or emotional investment in one particular theory. A test of the two most likely substantive theories about a phenomenon is called a crucial experiment. It requires the investigator "to construct, for any two competing theories, conditions in which they yield different observable results" (Popper, 1965, p. 174). A crucial experiment is a culminating experiment that follows considerable work to refine methods and techniques that narrow the question asked to an either/or situation. If research findings indicate that the hypothesis derived from one theory is not rejected but the alternative hypothesis *is* rejected, then the appropriate interpretation is that the first theory is very adequate and the second theory is false.

These experiments are common when rigid external control is possible, as in physics and chemistry laboratories, but rare in situations involving human beings in natural settings. A hypothetical example of a crucial experiment involving humans can, however, be constructed by comparing two alternative theories accounting for reduction of distress associated with a threatening event. Suppose that one theory proposes that information given prior to an event, about the procedural aspects of the event and typical sensations experienced, reduces distress associated with the event. Suppose also that the most likely alternative to the information theory is a theory postulating that the presence of a supportive person reduces distress associated with a threatening event. The information theory implies that the presence of a supportive person has an insignificant effect on reduction of distress, and the supportive person theory implies that information has an insignificant effect. If study findings demonstrate that the presence of the supportive person had no statistically significant effect on distress reduction and if information given prior to the event reduced distress at a statistically significant level, then the appropriate interpretation is that the supportive person theory is false and the information theory is the best available theory.

Although crucial experiments are not common in situations involving human beings, critical tests of two or more competing theories have been conducted by using human beings in clinical situations. For example, Braden (1990) tested three alternative explanations for the learned self-help response to arthritis and arthritis-related chronic illnesses. She developed a theoretical self-help model that included identical, complementary, and oppositional hypotheses from the theories of learned helplessness, instrumental passivity, and learned resourcefulness. The oppositional hypotheses provided the opportunity for a critical test of the three competing theories.

Although a crucial experiment or a critical test of competing theories can improve its adequacy, a theory should not be regarded as truth. Indeed, no theory should be considered final or absolute, for it is always possible that subsequent studies will yield different findings or that other theories will provide a better fit with the data. Mishel's tests of the uncertainty in illness theory serve as an example (Mishel, Padilla, Grant, & Sorenson, 1991; Mishel & Sorenson, 1991). The findings of the initial study provided empirical support for 14 hypothesized relationships between concepts. In contrast, the replication study, which used a more heterogeneous sample, revealed consistent support for just 5 of the 14 relationships (Fig. 3–1).

The aim of research, then, is not to determine the absolute truth of theories, but rather to determine the degree of confidence warranted by the best empirical evidence. Nonetheless, certain laws that may emerge are, insofar as is known, not violated under certain circumstances. For example, humans are not likely to fly unaided within the confines of earth's gravitational force.

Taken together, the requirements of the criterion of empirical adequacy stipulate that conclusions do not go beyond what was demonstrated by the data. Possible conclusions are (1) the data are inaccurate and cannot be relied upon for theory development, (2) the data are accurate but the theory is faulty and should be abandoned or must be modified, (3) the data are accurate and the theory should be regarded as empirically adequate, and (4) the data are accurate but have no relevance to the theory (Downs, 1984).

Application of the Criterion of Empirical Adequacy. In theory-generating research, the empirical adequacy criterion is once again applied to the theory as presented by the study findings. In theory-testing research, this criterion is applied to a comparison of the version of the theory that was tested and the version that was retained after testing. The

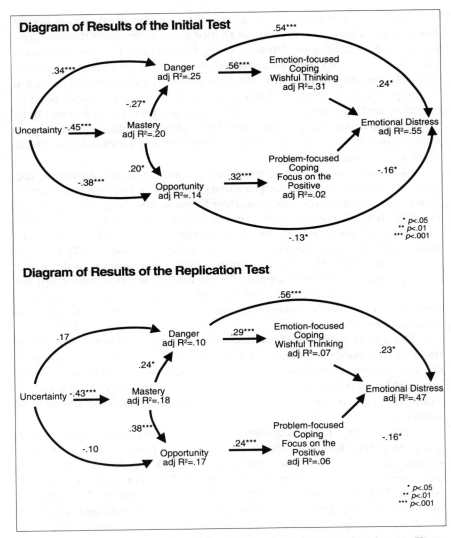

Figure 3–1. Comparison of two tests of the uncertainty in illness theory. (From Mishel, Padilla, Grant, & Sorenson, 1991, pp. 237–238, with permission.)

dual application of the criterion in the case of theory testing yields an informative judgment about what was proposed versus what was actually found.

Evaluation of Utility of Theory and Research For Practice

The fourth component of evaluation of a research report focuses on the implications of a theory and its related research findings for practice. The criterion is pragmatic adequacy.

Pragmatic Adequacy

The pragmatic adequacy criterion requires the theories of professional disciplines such as nursing, medicine, social work, education, law, and engineering to be useful in practice. Indeed, according to Kerlinger (1979), "the most important influence on practice is theory" (p. 296). Despite its importance, theory has an indirect rather than a direct influence on practice. The indirect influence is best appreciated when it is understood that theories, per se, cannot be applied in practical situations. Instead, innovative actions such as assessment formats, planning strategies, and intervention protocols are derived from the results of empirical tests of theories and used in practice.

Furthermore, the influence of theory on practice is slow to occur because a theory and its related research findings do not tell clinicians what to do. Rather, they gradually influence thinking and doing over the long periods of time required to first disseminate the research findings and then change fixed sets of beliefs (Brett, 1987; Coyle & Sokop, 1990).

The pragmatic adequacy criterion requires the research findings to be related to the particular area of practice for which a theory is sought. That means that the findings are applicable to a particular clinical specialty, particular client problems, and/or particular client ages or developmental phases. Although that may seem self-evident, it is not unusual to find that an innovative action is based on a theory that is unrelated to the relevant clinical problem and client population. For example, suppose that a clinician wants to use an intervention that will facilitate the process of bereavement in parents who have experienced the death of a child. Suppose also that the intervention protocol was based on research dealing with the process individuals experience in dealing with their own impending death. In this constructed example, the research deals not with survivor bereavement, but rather with the dying person's grief. In contrast, suppose that the protocol was based on research dealing with widow bereavement. Here, the question would be whether the process of bereavement is the same for parents as it is for wives. Furthermore, the cause of death may be an important factor that has to be taken into account. For example, survivor bereavement when death was caused by a sudden accident may be different from the bereavement associated with death due to a chronic illness.

The criterion of pragmatic adequacy further requires the implementation of an innovative action in a particular practice setting to be feasible. Feasibility is determined by an evaluation of the resources needed to establish a new way of doing things, including the time needed to learn and implement the innovation, the number, type, and expertise of personnel required for its implementation, and the cost of in-service education, salaries, equipment, and testing procedures. Furthermore, the willingness of those who control financial resources to pay for the innovation must be determined.

The pragmatic adequacy criterion also requires innovative actions to be congruent with clients' expectations of practice. If the actions do not meet existing expectations, they should be abandoned or attention should be given to helping clients to develop new expectations. Indeed, "current . . . practice is not entirely what it might become and [thus clients] might come to expect a different form of practice, given the opportunity to experience it" (Johnson, 1974, p. 376).

In addition, the pragmatic adequacy criterion requires the practitioner to have the legal ability to control the application and measure the effectiveness of theory-based actions. Such control may be problematic in that, because of the resistance of others, practitioners are not always able to carry out legally sanctioned responsibilities. Sources of resistance against implementation of nursing innovations, for example, include attempts by physicians to control nursing practice, financial barriers imposed by clinical agencies and third-party payers, and skepticism by other health professionals about the ability of nurses to carry out the proposed interventions (Edwardson, 1984). The cooperation and collaboration of others may, therefore, have to be secured. Implementation of a medication education program, for example, may be opposed by physicians who are concerned that their patients will be upset by information about side effects or may even develop certain side effects due to a self-fulfilling prophecy. Implementation of the educational program may also be opposed by hospital administrators who are concerned about the cost of the resources needed to implement the program.

Finally, this criterion requires the innovative actions to be socially meaningful, that is, to address major social problems and to lead to favorable outcomes for recipients of the action. Major social problems include universal situations, such as care of the poor, as well as more time-bound situations, such as epidemics of a disease for which a treatment has not yet been developed. Examples of favorable outcomes include reduced incidence of client complications, improved client health status, reduced rates of student attrition or staff turnover, and increased client, student, and staff satisfaction. Repeated tests of innovations in practical situations provide the evidence needed to determine whether the innovations result in favorable outcomes. Quantitative analyses of outcomes should consider not only statistical significance but also clinical or practical significance. Statistical significance is, of course, determined by the alpha or p value. Clinical significance is determined by the magnitude of the outcome, which can be calculated as an effect size (Cohen, 1977). An important point to keep in mind here is that "statistical significance does not guarantee clinical significance and, more to the point, *the magnitude of the* p *value (.05, .01, .001, .00029, or whatever) is no guide to clinical significance*" (Slakter, Wu, & Suzuki-Slakter, 1991, p. 249).

The importance of both statistical and clinical significance is exemplified by a study of the effects of an innovative nursing intervention designed to reduce environmental stress and thereby support the development of very low birth weight infants. The study findings revealed that the infants receiving the intervention were discharged from the hospital 2 weeks sooner than the infants in the control group. Although the difference was statistically significant at the somewhat unimpressive level of $p < .04$, the clinical significance was very impressive, with a cost savings of almost $12,250 per infant (Becker, Grunwald, Moorman, & Stuhr, 1991).

Outcomes of Evaluation of Pragmatic Adequacy. The outcome of evaluation of pragmatic adequacy is a thorough understanding of the research base for various clinical practices, including methods of observation, assessment, and intervention. As can be seen in Figure 3–2, the evaluation of pragmatic adequacy leads to identification of what needs to be studied as well as the efficacy of what has been studied (Hunt, 1981).

Evaluation of the findings of a descriptive or correlational study frequently leads to a recommendation for experimental studies of interventions to deal with a clinical problem. In that case, a relevant clinical practice has not yet been developed. For example, the findings of a descriptive study of the sensation of dyspnea experienced by school-age

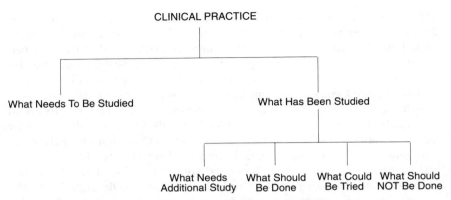

Figure 3-2.   Outcomes of evaluation of pragmatic adequacy.

children, precipitants of shortness of breath, and coping strategies used by the children led to the following recommendation regarding clinical practice: "In future research studies [sic], coping strategies should be related to precipitants so that the findings can be used clinically to target interventions to specific triggers (Carrieri, Kieckheffer, Janson-Bjerklie, & Souza, 1991, p. 85).

In contrast, when a study of clinical practices has been conducted, the findings can lead to a recommendation for additional research, adoption of a new practice, a trial of a new practice in the clinical setting, or discontinuation of a current practice (Fig. 3-2). Many reports of clinical practice research end with recommendations for additional study. Such recommendations indicate that the reported findings do not yet meet the pragmatic adequacy criterion. For example, the results of a study of three methods of monitoring blood pressure led to a recommendation for additional research prior to incorporating one particular method into clinical practice (Norman, Gadaleta, & Griffin, 1991).

Other reports of clinical intervention studies indicate that the intervention should be adopted. A study of tympanic and oral temperatures in afebrile adults who had major abdominal surgery exemplifies this situation. The investigators explained, "The study findings suggest that while the tympanic site offers some advantage, either the tympanic or oral site would provide a satisfactory index of body temperature for routine intermittent monitoring during the perioperative period" (Erickson & Yount, 1991, p. 92).

The recommendation for adoption of a clinical practice may be qualified by a further recommendation to conduct a trial of the intervention under controlled real-world clinical conditions and systematically evaluate the outcomes. Fourteen nursing practices identified by the staff of the Conduct and Utilization of Research in Nursing (CURN) Project exemplify this situation (Horsley, Crane, Crabtree, & Wood, 1983). One such practice is mutual goal setting by patient and nurse, which has been found to enhance goal achievement and increase patient and nursing staff satisfaction (Horsley, Crane, Haller, & Reynolds, 1982).

Conversely, some reports of clinical practice research end with a recommendation to discontinue a practice. The results of a test of a maternal attachment theory that specified a particular sequence of handling newborn infants supported the discontinuation of a widely used method of assessing maternal attachment. More specifically, the investigator maintained, "The results of this study cast some doubt on the validity of fingers-palms-arms-trunk as a parameter for clinically assessing maternal attachment for either vaginally or cesarean-delivered women. The continued use of the fingers-palms-arms-trunk sequence as a nursing clinical assessment tool . . . is therefore not a valid clinical practice" (Tulman, 1986, p. 299).

Selecting the Best Theory. Sometimes the actions derived from more than one equally adequate theory are found to be useful in a particular situation. In this admittedly rare case, the theory that leads to the most effective actions should be selected. Hardy (1988) offered the following guidelines for selection of the best theory.

1. Select the theory that deals most adequately with the variables of concern to the clinician.
2. Select the theory whose central variables can be altered or modified by the clinician to bring about the desired change.
3. Select the theory whose application leads to desired changes that are strong enough or significant enough to make it worthwhile to implement a plan of action based on the theory.

Application of the Criterion of Pragmatic Adequacy. In theory-generating research, the pragmatic adequacy criterion is applied to the long-range potential of the study results; in theory-testing research, it is confined to the version of the theory that was retained after analysis of the study findings.

CONCLUSION

The merit of research is frequently said to be the logical consistency among the theoretical, design, and analysis components of an investigation. The criteria for evaluation of research reports presented in this chapter direct attention to those three components of a study as well as to the study findings. An outline of the criteria in question form is given in Table 3 – 1. Use of the criteria should facilitate an understanding of the relationship between theory and research. Examples of use of the criteria for evaluation of descriptive, correlational, and experimental studies are presented in the Appendix.

TABLE 3 – 1. Criteria for Evaluation of the Relation Between Theory and Research

Is the theory that was generated or tested *significant*?
  • Does the theory address a phenomenon of interest to the discipline and to society?
  • Does the theory improve the precision with which a phenomenon can be predicted as well as the understanding of the phenomenon?
Is the theory *internally consistent*?
  • Do the concepts reflect semantic clarity and consistency?
  • Are concepts redundant?
  • Do the propositions reflect structural consistency?
  • Are there incomplete or redundant sets of propositions?
  • Do the observations substantiate the conclusions of an inductively developed theory?
  • Are the premises of a deductively developed theory valid?
Is the theory *parsimonious*?
  • Is the theory stated clearly and concisely?
Is the theory *testable*?
  • Can the concepts be empirically observed?
  • Can the propositions be measured?
  • Can the derived hypotheses be falsified?
Is *operational adequacy* evident?
  • Is the sample representative of the population of interest?
  • Are the empirical indicators valid and reliable?
  • Is the research procedure appropriate?
  • Are the procedures for data analysis appropriate?
Is *empirical adequacy* evident?
  • Are theoretical claims congruent with empirical evidence?
  • Are alternative methodologic and substantive theories considered?
Is *pragmatic adequacy* evident?
  • Are the research findings related to the problem of interest?
  • Is it feasible to implement innovative actions?
  • Are the innovative actions congruent with clients' expectations?
  • Does the practitioner have the legal ability to implement the innovation?
  • Do the innovative actions lead to favorable outcomes?

REFERENCES

Babbie, E. R. (1990). *Survey research methods* (2nd ed.). Belmont, CA: Wadsworth.

Becker, P. T., Grunwald, P. C., Moorman, J., & Stuhr, S. (1991). Outcomes of developmentally supportive nursing care for very low birth weight infants. *Nursing Research, 40,* 150–155.

Benoliel, J. Q., McCorkle, R. M., & Young, K. (1980). Development of a social dependency scale. *Research in Nursing and Health, 3,* 3–10.

Braden, C. J. (1990). Learned self-help response to chronic illness experience: A test of three alternative learning theories. *Scholarly Inquiry for Nursing Practice, 4,* 23–42.

Brett, J. L. (1987). Use of nursing practice research findings. *Nursing Research, 36,* 344–349.

Bridgman, P. W. (1927). *The logic of modern physics.* New York: Macmillan.

Carrieri, V. K., Kieckheffer, G., Janson-Bjerklie, S., & Souza, J. (1991). The sensation of dyspnea in school-age children. *Nursing Research, 40,* 81–85.

Chinn, P. L., & Kramer, M. K. (1991). *Theory and nursing: A systematic approach* (3rd ed.). St. Louis: Mosby Year Book.

Cohen, J. (1977). *Statistical power analysis for the behavioral sciences* (rev. ed.). New York: Academic Press.

Cohen, J. M., Sarill, W. J., & Vishveshwara, C. V. (1982). An example of induced centrifugal force in general relativity. *Nature, 298*(5877), 829.

Cook, T. D., & Campbell, D. T. (1979). *Quasi-experimentation: Design and analysis issues for field settings.* Boston: Houghton Mifflin.

Coyle, L. A., & Sokop, A. G. (1990). Innovation adoption behavior among nurses. *Nursing Research, 39,* 176–180.

Crossley, D. J., & Wilson, P. A. (1979). *How to argue: An introduction to logical thinking.* New York: Random House.

Donaldson, S. K., & Crowley, D. M. (1978). The discipline of nursing. *Nursing Outlook, 26,* 113–120.

Downs, F. S. (1984). *A sourcebook of nursing research* (3rd ed.). Philadelphia: F. A. Davis.

Dubin, R. (1978). *Theory building* (rev. ed.). New York: The Free Press.

Edwardson, S. R. (1984). Using research in practice: Factors associated with the adoption of a nursing innovation. *Western Journal of Nursing Research, 6,* 141–143.

Erickson, R. S., & Yount, S. T. (1991). Comparison of tympanic and oral temperatures in surgical patients. *Nursing Research, 40,* 90–93.

Fawcett, J. (1984). The metaparadigm of nursing: Current status and future refinements. *Image: Journal of Nursing Scholarship, 16,* 84–87.

Gerber, R. M., & Van Ort, S. R. (1981). Topical application of insulin to pressure sores: A questionable therapy. *American Journal of Nursing, 81,* 1159.

Goebel, J. B., Copps, T. J., & Sulayman, R. F. (1984). Infant car seat use: Effectiveness of a postpartum educational program. *Journal of Obstetric, Gynecologic, and Neonatal Nursing, 13,* 33–36.

Goodson, F. E., & Morgan, G. A. (1976). Evaluation of theory. In M. H. Marx & F. E. Goodson (Eds.), *Theories in contemporary psychology* (2nd ed., pp. 286–299). New York: Macmillan.

Gortner, S. R. (1980). Nursing science in transition. *Nursing Research, 29,* 180–183.

Hanson, N. R. (1958). *Patterns of discovery.* New York: Cambridge University Press.

Hardy, M. E. (1988). Perspectives on science. In M. E. Hardy & M. E. Conway (Eds.), *Role theory: Perspectives for health professionals* (2nd ed., pp. 1–27). Norwalk, CT: Appleton and Lange.

Horsley, J. A., Crane, J., Crabtree, M. K., & Wood, D. J. (1983). *Using research to improve nursing practice: A guide*. New York: Grune and Stratton.

Horsley, J. A., Crane, J., Haller, K. B., & Reynolds, M. A. (1982). *Mutual goal setting in patient care*. New York: Grune and Stratton.

Hunt, J. (1981). Indicators for nursing practice: The use of research findings. *Journal of Advanced Nursing, 6,* 189–194.

Hyman, R. B., Feldman, H. R., Harris, R. B., Levin, R. F., & Malloy, G. B. (1989). The effects of relaxation training on clinical symptoms: A meta-analysis. *Nursing Research, 38,* 216–220.

Johnson, D. E. (1974). Development of theory: A requisite for nursing as a primary health profession. *Nursing Research, 23,* 372–377.

Katz, S. (1983). Assessing self-maintenance: Activities of daily living, mobility, and instrumental activities of daily living. *Journal of the American Geriatric Society, 31,* 721–727.

Kerlinger, F. N. (1979). *Behavioral research: A conceptual approach*. New York: Holt, Rinehart & Winston.

Kerlinger, F. N. (1986). *Foundations of behavioral research* (3rd ed.). New York: Holt, Rinehart & Winston.

Mann, C. C. (1989). Armies of physicists struggle to discover proof of a Scot's brainchild. *Smithsonian, 19*(12), 106–117.

Marx, M. H. (1976). Formal theory. In M. H. Marx & F. E. Goodson (Eds.), *Theories in contemporary psychology* (2nd ed., pp. 234–260). New York: Macmillan.

Mishel, M. H., Padilla, G., Grant, M., & Sorenson, D. S. (1991). Uncertainty in illness theory: A replication of the mediating effects of mastery and coping. *Nursing Research, 40,* 236–240.

Mishel, M. H., & Sorenson, D. S. (1991). Coping with uncertainty in gynecological cancer: A test of the mediating functions of mastery and coping. *Nursing Research, 40,* 167–171.

Moody, L. E. (1990). *Advancing nursing science through research* (Vols. 1 and 2). Newbury Park, CA: Sage.

Norman, E., Gadaleta, D., & Griffin, C. C. (1991). An evaluation of three blood pressure methods in a stabilized acute trauma population. *Nursing Research, 40,* 86–89.

Phillips, D. C. (1987). *Philosophy, science and social inquiry: Contemporary methodological controversies in social science and related applied fields of research*. New York: Pergamon Press.

Platt, J. R. (1964). Strong inference. *Science, 146,* 347–353.

Popper, K. R. (1965). *Conjectures and refutations: The growth of scientific knowledge*. New York: Harper and Row.

Reed, P. G. (1991). Self-transcendence and mental health in oldest-old adults. *Nursing Research, 40,* 5–11.

Schepp, K. G. (1991). Factors influencing the coping effort of mothers of hospitalized children. *Nursing Research, 40,* 42–46.

Shearing, C. D. (1973). How to make theories untestable: A guide to theorists. *The American Sociologist, 8,* 33–37.

Slakter, M. J., Wu, Y-W. B., & Suzuki-Slakter, N. S. (1991). *, **, and ***: Statistical nonsense at the .00000 level. *Nursing Research, 40,* 248–249.

Tulman, L. J. (1986). Initial handling of newborn infants by vaginally and cesarean-delivered mothers. *Nursing Research, 35,* 296–299.

ADDITIONAL READINGS

Acton, G. J., Irvin, B. L., & Hopkins, B. A. (1991). Theory-testing research: Building the science. *Advances in Nursing Science, 14*(1), 52–61.

Bircumshaw, D. (1990). The utilization of research findings in clinical practice. *Journal of Advanced Nursing, 15*, 1272–1280.

Blalock, H. M., Jr. (1969). *Theory construction. From verbal to mathematical formulations.* Englewood Cliffs, NJ: Prentice-Hall.

Campbell, J. C. (1989). A test of two explanatory models of women's responses to battering. *Nursing Research, 38*, 18–24.

Diesing, P. (1971). *Patterns of discovery in the social sciences.* New York: Aldine, Atherton.

Duffy, M. E. (1988). The research appraisal checklist: Appraising nursing research reports. In O. L. Strickland & C. F. Waltz (Eds.), *Measurement of nursing outcomes. Vol. 2. Measuring nursing performance: Practice, education, and research* (pp. 420–437). New York: Springer.

Haller, K. B., Reynolds, M. A., & Horsley, J. A. (1979). Developing research-based innovation protocols: Process, criteria, and issues. *Research in Nursing and Health, 2*, 45–51.

Hinshaw, A. S. (1979). Planning for logical consistency among three research structures. *Western Journal of Nursing Research, 1*, 250–253.

Knafl, K. A., & Howard, M. J. (1984). Interpreting and reporting qualitative research. *Research in Nursing and Health, 7*, 17–24.

Kuhn, T. S. (1981). A function for thought experiments. In I. Hacking (Ed.), *Scientific revolutions* (pp. 6–27). New York: Oxford University Press.

Mahon, N. E., & Yarcheski, A. (1988). Loneliness in early adolescents: An empirical test of alternate explanations. *Nursing Research, 37*, 330–335.

Merton, R. K. (1957). *Social theory and social structure* (rev. ed.). New York: The Free Press.

Moody, L. E., Wilson, M. E., Smyth, K., Schwartz, R., Tittle, M., & Van Cott, M. L. (1988). Analysis of a decade of nursing practice research: 1977–1986. *Nursing Research, 37*, 374–379.

Murphy, E., & Freston, M. S. (1991). An analysis of theory-research linkages in published gerontologic nursing studies, 1983–1989. *Advances in Nursing Science, 13*(4), 1–13.

Nunnally, J. C. (1978). *Psychometric theory.* New York: McGraw-Hill.

O'Connell, K. (1983). Nursing practice: A decade of research. In N. L. Chaska (Ed.), *The nursing profession: A time to speak* (pp. 183–201). New York: McGraw-Hill.

Popper, K. R. (1968). *The logic of scientific discovery.* New York: Harper and Row.

Suppe, F. (1977). Afterword. In F. Suppe (Ed.), *The structure of scientific theories* (2nd ed., pp. 615–730). Chicago: University of Illinois Press.

Walker, L. O., & Avant, K. C. (1988). *Strategies for theory construction in nursing* (2nd ed.). Norwalk, CT: Appleton and Lange.

4

Integrating
Research Findings

The empirical adequacy of a theory can be determined only by evaluating the findings of the research that generated and tested it. This chapter extends the discussion of empirical adequacy begun in Chapter 3, by describing formal procedures that can be used to integrate the findings of related research and to estimate the magnitude of relationships between concepts.

PURPOSES OF INTEGRATING RESEARCH FINDINGS

When more than one study has been conducted on the same phenomenon, some procedure for integrating the results is needed so that conclusions regarding the weight of evidence for and/or against the theory that was generated or tested can be reached. Integrative reviews of research findings supply this evidence by providing crucial information about the existence, direction, and strength of relationships between concepts, as well as the magnitude of experimental effects.

Thus, the results of integrative reviews "are indispensable for theory construction" (Hunter & Schmidt, 1990, p. 40). That is because the integration of findings provides direction for the next step in theory development. Suppose, for example, that the correlation between uncertainty about the meaning of illness-related events and adjustment to the illness is found to be consistently high in several studies with heterogeneous samples. In that case, further research probably is not needed. If, on the other hand, the correlation is found to be consistently low or moderate, research must be undertaken to identify other concepts that influence the relationship between uncertainty and adjustment to illness (see Mishel, Padilla, Grant, & Sorenson, 1991).

The procedures described in this chapter can be used to evaluate the empirical adequacy of a theory, as well as when reviewing literature prior to undertaking a new study, making recommendations for future research, preparing state-of-the-art manuscripts that present a critique and synthesis of separate empirical studies, and recommending research-based public policies. In short, integrative reviews are crucial to advance knowledge and to make decisions about educational programs, nursing interventions, medical treatments, and the like.

STEPS OF INTEGRATING RESEARCH FINDINGS

The integration of research findings encompasses three steps. The first step is a comprehensive review of studies based on a particular theory, the second is the classification of studies according to the merit of research methodology and the findings, and the third is the qualitative and/or quantitative synthesis of the findings of the studies.

Review of Related Research

The pragmatics of identifying related studies are discussed in detail by Cooper (1989). In general, the review should include all reports of pertinent research published in journals, books, monographs, conference proceedings, *Dissertation Abstracts International*, and *Masters Abstracts*, as well as the uncatalogued and unpublished works of colleagues and students.

Retrieval of relevant studies is facilitated by use of indexing and abstracting services. Printed and/or on-line computer versions of these services are available at university libraries, and many services are now available via personal computers. One limitation of print or computer-based literature searches is that most data bases contain only published reports; another is the time lag between completion of a study and the appearance of the publication citation in the data base (Cooper, 1989).

Still another limitation is that an estimated 95 percent of all the empirical research actually conducted remains in investigators' file drawers (Rosenthal, 1979). That is because many scholars believe that reports of research with statistically nonsignificant (e.g., $p > .05$) results will not be accepted for publication. Thus, the inclusion of unpublished research in a review may lead to a more accurate appraisal of the empirical adequacy of a theory because the potential bias toward studies with statistically significant results that may be reflected in published research is offset.

Some research remains unpublished because it suffers from serious theoretical and/or methodologic flaws. The inclusion of such studies, whether unpublished or published, is a cause for concern because it is believed that such research yields inflated estimates of the strength of theoretical relationships. Interestingly, integrative research reviews that included a comparison of the results of more versus less flawed studies have found no difference in the strength of theoretical relationships (e.g., Smith & Glass, 1977) or have found evidence of stronger relationships in the better studies (e.g., Devine & Cook, 1983; Wampler, 1982). Furthermore, Heater, Becker, and Olson (1988) found no evidence of a statistically significant difference in effect size for published and unpublished studies.

It is recommended that all relevant studies that can be located be taken into account in initial appraisals of empirical adequacy. Access to unpublished research can be facilitated by use of data bases such as the Computer Retrieval of Information on Scientific Projects (CRISP), which contains citations of biomedical research supported by the United States Public Health Service, and the Sigma Theta Tau International Directory of Nurse Researchers, which contains citations of on-going nursing research. Techniques for comparing the weight of evidence for or against a theory from published versus unpublished studies, more flawed versus less flawed research, and studies with null findings versus those with statistically significant findings are discussed later in this chapter.

Cooper (1989) identified two threats to validity associated with the retrieval of related studies. The first is the inability to identify all relevant studies, which is reduced by including as many data bases as possible to ensure that no avoidable bias exists. For example, failure to use *Dissertation Abstracts* to locate relevant studies would introduce an avoidable bias.

The second threat to validity is that the target population may not be adequately represented. Research reviewers cannot, of course, control the selection of samples by the primary investigators, but they can describe the missing elements of the target population and draw careful and precise conclusions regarding generalization of the findings of the integrative review. For example, if a theory purports to deal with a phenomenon common to all adults with chronic illness, then the collective samples must include adults of various ages, from various socioeconomic backgrounds, and with many different chronic illnesses.

Classification of Research

The second step of research integration requires evaluation of the scientific merit of each study and assessment of the findings, which is accomplished by determining the operational adequacy of each study. As discussed in Chapter 3, the operational adequacy criterion requires the research methods to be congruent with the underlying theory. Particular attention should be given to evaluation of the rigor of the research methods in terms of threats to internal and external validity. Comprehensive discussions of threats to validity are available in Cook and Campbell (1979) and Bracht and Glass (1968).

The outcome of evaluation of the scientific merit of each study is classification as more or less flawed. The classification may be a dichotomy, such as "good" and "bad" studies, or a more elaborate continuum ranging from "few flaws" to "many flaws." The continuum could include a "no flaws" pole, although it is unlikely that such a study could ever be conducted. Cooper (1989) recommended relying on the conclusions reached by integrating the findings of good studies if overall results are different from those of bad studies. If no differences are evident, however, the bad studies may be retained because the additional data may facilitate refinement of a theory by providing clues to the theory's scope and to intervening or extraneous variables.

Assessment of findings is accomplished by classifying the results of each study as supportive or nonsupportive of the theory. If hypotheses were tested, each one can be considered separately or an overall conclusion regarding the evidence for or against the theory can be drawn. The traditional criterion for tentative acceptance or rejection of study hypotheses is the statistical significance level. The level is most frequently set at $p < .05$, although a more or less stringent one may be used. When this criterion is used, each study is classified as having statistically significant or nonsignificant results. The direction of the findings (positive or negative), if known, also should be noted.

The findings of each study may also be assessed for their magnitude; examples are the observed incidence of phenomena, the strength of relationships between variables, and the extent of difference between treatment groups. The value of the additional information obtained when magnitude is taken into account is illustrated by two studies of temperature measurement. Baker, Cerone, Gaze, and Knapp (1984) found that although the length of time an oral thermometer was inserted had a statistically significant ($p < .05$) effect on temperature reading, the magnitude of the difference was just 0.12°C. The investigators commented that because this difference is not clinically impressive, readers should consider the distinction between statistical significance and clinical relevance. Bliss-Holtz (1989) found that the mean difference between 4-minute and maximum axillary temperature readings was only 0.1°F. She commented, "Although what determines a clinically significant temperature difference in an infant population has not been determined empirically, a difference of 0.1°F does not seem to justify placement of axillary thermometers for longer periods of time" (p. 87).

Integration of the magnitude of findings of separate studies requires a common metric. The effect size, which is a standardized numerical index of the magnitude of a finding, can be used. Although investigators rarely include the effect size in their research reports, it can sometimes be calculated from the available statistical information. Formulas for the effect sizes for many statistics are given in Cohen (1977), Cooper (1989), Hunter & Schmidt (1990), and Rosenthal (1984), among others. For example, one effect size for differences between groups, the d metric, can be obtained by the formula $(M_e - M_c) \div s_x$, where M_e is the experimental group mean, M_c is the control group mean, and s_x is the within-group standard deviation. The interpretation of an effect size is relative in that it depends on the size of other effects within a particular research area. A comprehensive discussion of the interpretation of various effect sizes is presented by Glass, McGaw, and Smith (1981).

Synthesis of Findings

The third step of research integration is synthesis of the findings of the separate studies. The qualitative approach to synthesis is a narrative evaluation of related studies that leads to relatively subjective conclusions about the empirical adequacy of a theory. The quantitative approach to synthesis uses statistical techniques to combine the findings of related studies numerically and draw relatively objective conclusions about empirical adequacy.

Qualitative Synthesis of Research Findings

The typical review of research using a qualitative approach to synthesis of research findings includes a detailed narrative description of each study and its findings. Conclusions regarding the empirical adequacy of the underlying theory reflect the reviewer's subjective impressions of the evidence rather than use of formal procedures of synthesis. An example of the qualitative synthesis of research is a review of literature on cocaine abuse during pregnancy (Lindenberg, Alexander, Gendrop, Nencioli, & Williams, 1991). The synthesis of literature revealed a paucity of theoretical explanations for observed differences in the effects of prenatal cocaine use on obstetrical, neonatal, infant health, and child developmental outcomes.

The typical qualitative approach to synthesis of the findings of related studies is strengthened by use of a formal procedure to assess the empirical adequacy of a theory (Stinchcombe, 1968). This procedure is based on the assumption that the studies are of equal scientific merit. One situation in Stinchcombe's procedure is the interpretation of multiple tests of a theory that used the same empirical indicators with similar samples. If the findings for all of the tests are statistically significant in the hypothesized direction, then the appropriate interpretation is that the theory is more adequate than it would be with just one test.

The above situation is exemplified by tests of the theory of adaptation to chronic illness (Pollock, 1989). Studies that tested the theory revealed support for the relationship between health-related hardiness and components of psychosocial adaptation for samples of chronically ill adults in the three diagnostic groups of rheumatoid arthritis, insulin-dependent diabetes, and hypertension. The appropriate interpretation of the findings from those studies of chronically ill adults is that the theory is more adequate than it would be if only one diagnostic group had been included.

A second situation in Stinchcombe's procedure is the interpretation of multiple tests of a theory that used the same or similar empirical indicators with different samples or populations. If all findings are statistically significant in the hypothesized direction in the tests of the theory, the appropriate interpretation is that the theory is much more adequate.

Pollock's (1989) research using healthy adults illustrates the second situation. In this study, Pollock found that hardiness was again related to a component of psychosocial adaptation. When the findings of this study of well adults are combined with those of the studies of chronically ill adults, the appropriate interpretation is that the theory is much more adequate than it was when only chronically ill adults were used as subjects.

In contrast to situations in which findings support the theory, consider those in which findings reject the theory. A theory may be considered false when any one test yields statistically nonsignificant findings, but researchers rarely abandon a theory after just one test. Yet if additional tests of equal scientific merit reveal consistent nonsignificant findings, the appropriate interpretation is that the theory is false. This situation is exemplified by repeated empirical tests that failed to yield support for the propositions comprising a theory of similarity in wives' and husbands' pregnancy-related experiences (Fawcett, 1989).

These procedures are helpful when the findings of several studies of equal scientific merit are similar. When studies are of unequal merit and/or when findings conflict, a quantitative approach to synthesis is required.

Quantitative Synthesis of Research Findings

The Voting Method. The voting method, also referred to as the vote count or the box count, is the weakest of the quantitative procedures used for synthesis of the findings of related studies. It represents one formal procedure that can be used to resolve conflicting findings from a group of studies. It involves a simple tally of study findings as significantly positive (i.e., in the hypothesized direction), significantly negative (i.e., in the direction opposite to that hypothesized), or not statistically significant. The modal category is considered the winner and is assumed to be the best estimate of the empirical adequacy of the underlying theory (Light & Smith, 1971). Cooper (1989) recommended moving beyond reliance on the modal category to use of the sign test to determine if the tally of results indicates that one direction occurs more frequently than chance would suggest. He explained that "If the null hypothesis is true — that is, if no relation between the variables under consideration exists in the population sampled by any study — we would expect the number of findings in each direction to be equal" (p. 92). The formula for the sign test is: $Z_{vc} = [(N_p) - (\frac{1}{2} \times N_t)] \div \frac{1}{2}\sqrt{N_t}$, where Z_{vc} is the Z-score for the overall series of comparisons, N_p is the number of positive findings, and N_t is the total number of comparisons (positive plus negative findings). The significance of the Z-score can be determined by reference to a table of standard normal deviates (Cooper, 1989, p. 92).

The voting method is based on the assumption that the nonmodal categories of findings are due either to chance alone or to undetected methodologic errors. If studies differ in scientific merit, weights may be assigned to account for the differences in quality. Exactly what weight to assign each study, however, is a very complex question that is just beginning to be addressed in detail (Hunter & Schmidt, 1990). For that reason, research integration by means of the voting method usually excludes seriously flawed studies.

The voting method is illustrated by the following example that assumes equal merit of the studies. Suppose that the findings from three studies reveal that subjects who received preoperative information resumed their usual activities after discharge from the hospital sooner than subjects who did not receive the information and that two studies found no difference between the subjects who received the information and those who did not (Johnson, 1984). According to the voting method, the correct interpretation of these results is that the theory proposing that provision of preoperative information leads to earlier resumption of usual activities is empirically adequate.

Meta-Analysis. The techniques of meta-analysis are regarded as strong formal quantitative procedures. One technique combines the significance tests obtained from two or more independent studies. The other technique is the average effect size for a group of related studies.

Combining Significance Tests. The technique of combining significance tests can be accomplished in several ways, including adding logs of p levels, adding p levels, adding t's, adding Z's, adding weighted Z's, testing the mean p, and testing the mean Z (Rosenthal, 1984). This meta-analytic technique is based on the assumption that the studies are essentially replicates of each other. However, it can be used only when directional hypotheses were tested. Rosenthal outlined the advantages and limitations of each method of combining significance tests. The method of adding p levels, for example, requires exact probability levels. Furthermore, it is limited to synthesis of the results of a small number of studies because it requires that the sum of the p levels be less than or equal to 1.0.

The following hypothetical example employs the method of adding p levels. Suppose that the findings of four studies of the effects of preoperative information on length of hospital stay yield one-tailed p levels of .02, .05, .06, and .75. The formula to be used is $P = (\Sigma p)^N \div N!$, where P is the overall significance level, p is the exact probability for each study, and N is the number of studies (Rosenthal, 1984, p. 94). In this con-structed example, the overall one-tailed p level is .025.

Although the various methods of combining significance tests pro-vide procedures for resolving conflicting findings, most do not take the merit of each study into account. An exception is the method of adding weighted Z's, which requires assignment of a weight reflecting scientific merit to the Z obtained in each study. As in the case of the voting method, however, determination of weights is complicated. Rosenthal (1984) indicated that degrees of freedom for each study could be used as weights, but that approach does not take all aspects of scientific merit into account.

Furthermore, the voting method and combined significance tests have the same limitations as a single probability level: They depend on sample size and indicate only that the observed results occurred more or less by chance. Nothing is known about the magnitude of findings.

Average Effect Size. The magnitude of the findings of a group of studies can be determined by means of the meta-analytic technique of average effect size (Glass et al., 1981). The technique involves computation of the arithmetic mean for the effect sizes of two or more studies. Conflict-ing findings are resolved in that results that are in the hypothesized direction are averaged with those in the opposite direction. Furthermore, variations in study characteristics can be taken into account by comparing the average effect sizes of more versus less flawed studies, published versus unpublished studies, recent versus older studies, and any other comparisons of interest to the investigator.

Broome, Lillis, and Smith's (1989) meta-analysis of the effects of pain management interventions on behavioral responses, physiologic re-sponses, and self-report of degree of pain is an example of the technique of average effect size. Their calculations revealed a mean effect size of .41 for behavioral responses, .30 for physiologic responses, and .34 for self-report of pain, using r as the effect size metric. The investigators also explored the relationship of methodological and substantive study char-acteristics with effect size. The methodological characteristics included the quality of the research, type of statistical tests used, number and type of outcome variables, publication date, number of authors, method of assignment to treatment groups, and sample size. The substantive study characteristics included age and race of study subjects, clinical setting for treatment administration, presence or absence of a parent during the intervention, discipline of intervenor, type of pain stimulus, time of administration of the intervention, and type of pain management interventions.

The meta-analytic technique of average effect size can be combined with the technique of binomial effect size display (BESD), developed by Rosenthal and Rubin (1982), to determine the pragmatic adequacy or practical importance of experimental effects. The BESD is a measure of the rate of improvement (e.g., success rate, survival rate, cure rate, or selection rate) of a treatment, procedure, or predictor variable. It is calculated by the formula $0.50 + r \div 2$ for the experimental group and $0.50 - r \div 2$ for the control group rate, where r is the effect size expressed as a correlation coefficient. Application of the BESD formula for the average effect sizes reported by Broome and her associates (1989) revealed improvement in the success rate of pain management interventions from 30 to 70 percent for behavioral responses, from 35 to 65 percent for physiologic responses, and from 33 to 67 percent for self-reports of pain.

Uses of Meta-Analysis. Meta-analysis typically is used to determine the average effect of some experimental treatment. Indeed, most of the literature on meta-analysis focuses on experimental research, but Hunter and Schmidt (1990) presented a detailed discussion of techniques and issues associated with meta-analysis of correlational studies. Moreover, Wilke and her associates (1990) conducted a meta-analysis to determine normative values on the McGill Pain Questionnaire (MPQ). They noted that the information obtained from the meta-analysis "is crucial to help pain researchers make informed decisions about using the MPQ" (p. 36).

Computer programs for meta-analysis are given by Mullen and Rosenthal (1985) and Hunter and Schmidt (1990). Moreover, the Mullen and Rosenthal programs are available as computer software.

Comparison of Quantitative Procedures for Research Integration. A comparison of the various quantitative procedures for synthesis of the findings of related studies indicates that both the voting method and the technique of combining significance tests provide information about the statistical significance of findings. In contrast, the technique of average effect size does not deal directly with statistical significance but does yield an estimate of the magnitude of findings. The most informed judgments about the empirical adequacy of a theory would be those that would take both statistical significance and magnitude of findings into account.

Comparison of Qualitative and Quantitative Integrative Reviews. Integrative reviews of research that employ quantitative methods generally are more informative than qualitative reviews. McCain and Lynn's (1990) meta-analysis of 15 of the 29 studies of patient teaching included in Wilson-Barnett and Oborne's (1983) qualitative narrative review illustrates the increase in information obtained in a quantitative review. Wilson-Barnett and Oborne concluded that patient teaching has a beneficial effect. McCain and Lynn's meta-analysis of the 15 studies that provided sufficient data for calculation of effect sizes revealed a weighed mean effect size of $+.50$, using the d effect size metric. Their finding indicated that "there was indeed a clear benefit of patient teaching: The score of the average individual in the experimental group exceeded that of 69% of the individuals in the control group" (McCain & Lynn, 1990, p. 352).

McCain and Lynn (1990) also calculated average effect sizes for various categories of studies. The categories, which were based on the goals of teaching, and their respective average effect sizes were as follows: improving knowledge, $+.54$; improving compliance, nonsignificant effect size; improving physical well-being, $+.43$; improving psychological well-being, $+.59$; and improving self-care, $+.55$. These effect size calculations revealed that teaching was not effective in one of the goal categories, whereas the results of the narrative review indicated that teaching was effective in all five goal categories.

CONCLUSION

Investigators usually conclude their research reports by recommending that the study be replicated or that the research be extended to determine the generalizability of findings or to discover more about the nature of theoretical propositions. Although researchers tend to believe that "more is better," there are times when a research area should be abandoned because the underlying theory is false or the magnitude of findings is so small that no matter how many studies are conducted, the explanatory power and predictive precision most likely will never be practically meaningful. Use of the procedures for integrating research findings presented in this chapter should help scholars to determine the empirical adequacy of a theory and decide if more research is warranted.

REFERENCES

Baker, N. C., Cerone, S. B., Gaze, N., & Knapp, T. R. (1984). The effect of type of thermometer and length of time inserted on oral temperature measurements of afebrile subjects. *Nursing Research, 33,* 109–111.

Bliss-Holtz, J. (1989). Comparison of rectal, axillary, and inguinal temperatures in full-term newborn infants. *Nursing Research, 38,* 85–87.

Bracht, G. H., & Glass, G. V. (1968). The external validity of experiments. *American Educational Research Journal, 5,* 437–474.

Broome, M. E., Lillis, P. P., & Smith, M. C. (1989). Pain interventions with children: A meta-analysis of research. *Nursing Research, 38,* 154–158.

Cohen, J. (1977). *Statistical power analysis for the behavioral sciences* (rev. ed.). New York: Academic Press.

Cook, T. D., & Campbell, D. T. (1979). *Quasi-experimentation: Design and analysis issues for field settings.* Boston: Houghton Mifflin.

Cooper, H. M. (1989). *Integrating research: A guide for literature reviews* (2nd ed.). Newbury Park, CA: Sage.

Devine, E. C., & Cook, T. D. (1983). A meta-analytic analysis of effects of psychoeducational interventions on length of postsurgical hospital stay. *Nursing Research, 32,* 267–274.

Fawcett, J. (1989). Spouses' experiences during pregnancy and the postpartum. *Image: Journal of Nursing Scholarship, 21,* 149–152.

Glass, G. V., McGaw, B., & Smith, M. L. (1981). *Meta-analysis in social research.* Beverly Hills: Sage.

Heater, B. S., Becker, A. M., & Olson, R. K. (1988). Nursing interventions and patient outcomes: A meta-analysis of studies. *Nursing Research, 37,* 303–307.

Hunter, J. E., & Schmidt, F. L. (1990). *Methods of meta-analysis. Correcting error and bias in research findings.* Newbury Park, CA: Sage.

Johnson, J. E. (1984). Coping with elective surgery. In H. H. Werley & J. J. Fitzpatrick (Eds.), *Annual review of nursing research* (Vol. 2, pp. 107–132). New York: Springer.

Light, R. J., & Smith, P. V. (1971). Accumulating evidence: Procedures for resolving contradictions among different research studies. *Harvard Educational Review, 41,* 429–471.

Lindenberg, C. S., Alexander, E. M., Gendrop, S. C., Nencioli, M., & Williams, D. G. (1991). A review of the literature on cocaine abuse in pregnancy. *Nursing Research, 40,* 69–75.

McCain, N. L, & Lynn, M. R. (1990). Meta-analysis of a narrative review: Studies evaluating patient teaching. *Western Journal of Nursing Research, 12,* 347–358.

Mishel, M. H., Padilla, G., Grant, M., & Sorenson, D. S. (1991). Uncertainty in illness theory: A replication of the mediating effects of mastery and coping. *Nursing Research, 40,* 236–240.

Mullen, B., & Rosenthal, R. (1985). *BASIC meta-analysis: Procedures and programs.* Hillsdale, NJ: Lawrence Erlbaum.

Pollock, S. E. (1989). The hardiness characteristic: A motivating factor in adaptation. *Advances in Nursing Science, 11*(2), 53–62.

Rosenthal, R. (1979). The "file drawer problem" and tolerance for null results. *Psychological Bulletin, 86,* 638–641.

Rosenthal, R. (1984). *Meta-analytic procedures for social research.* Beverly Hills: Sage.

Rosenthal, R., & Rubin, D. B. (1982). A simple, general purpose display of magnitude of experimental effect. *Journal of Educational Psychology, 74*, 166–169.

Smith, M. L., & Glass, G. V. (1977). Meta-analysis of psychotherapy outcome studies. *American Psychologist, 32*, 752–760.

Stinchcombe, A. L. (1968). *Constructing social theories.* New York: Harcourt, Brace and World.

Wampler, K. S. (1982). Bringing the review of literature into the age of quantification: Meta-analysis as a strategy for integrating research findings in family studies. *Journal of Marriage and the Family, 44*, 1009–1023.

Wilkie, D. J., Savedra, M. C., Holzemer, W. L., Tesler, M. D., & Paul, S. M. (1990). Use of the McGill Pain Questionnaire to measure pain: A meta-analysis. *Nursing Research, 39*, 36–41.

Wilson-Barnett, J., & Oborne, J. (1983). Studies evaluating patient teaching: Implications for practice. *International Journal of Nursing Studies, 20*, 33–44.

ADDITIONAL READINGS

Cook, T. D., & Leviton, L. C. (1980). Reviewing the literature: A comparison of traditional methods with meta-analysis. *Journal of Personality, 48*, 449–472.

Engle, V. F., & Graney, M. J. (1990). Meta-analysis for the refinement of gerontological nursing research and theory. *Journal of Gerontological Nursing, 16*(9), 12–15.

Hardy, M. E. (1978). Perspectives on nursing theory. *Advances in Nursing Science, 1*(1), 37–48.

Jackson, G. B. (1980). Methods for integrative reviews. *Review of Educational Research, 50*, 438–460.

Lynn, M. R. (1989). Meta-analysis: Appropriate tool for the integration of nursing research? *Nursing Research, 38*, 302–305.

Pillemer, D. B., & Light, R. J. (1980). Synthesizing outcomes: How to use research evidence from many studies. *Harvard Educational Review, 50*, 176–195.

Stock, W. A., Okun, M. A., Haring, M. J., Miller, W., Kinney, C., & Ceurvorst, R. W. (1982). Rigor in data synthesis: A case study of reliability in meta-analysis. *Educational Researcher, 11*(6), 10–14, 20.

5

Conceptual Models, Theories, and Research

Every theory development effort is based on an implicit or explicit frame of reference for the phenomena of interest to a discipline, that is, a conceptual model. This chapter presents a discussion of conceptual models and their influence on theory and research. In addition, it presents an extension of the techniques of theory formalization discussed in Chapter 2 and the criteria for evaluation of the relation of theory and research, discussed in Chapter 3, to the linkage between conceptual models and theories.

CONCEPTUAL MODELS

A conceptual model is a set of abstract and general concepts and propositions that provides a distinctive frame of reference or perspective for phenomena within the domain of inquiry of a particular discipline. The global nature of conceptual model concepts and propositions precludes direct empirical observation and testing. Rather, a conceptual model contributes to theory development by focusing on certain things and ruling them as relevant. Other things are then ruled out because of their lesser importance. For example, one conceptual model may declare that interventions are designed to help the person adapt to environmental stressors, and another may emphasize individuals' abilities to care for themselves. In the first example, nothing is said about self-care; in the second, no mention is made of adaptation or stressors. Thus, when a concept or phenomenon is not mentioned, it is, in effect, ruled out of the domain of interest.

"Conceptual model" is synonymous with "paradigm" or "disciplinary matrix." It reflects the philosophic stance, cognitive orientation, research tradition, and practice tradition of a particular group of scholars within a discipline, rather than all members of the discipline. Most disciplines, therefore, have more than one conceptual model. Nursing, for example, has at least seven major conceptual models, including Johnson's Behavioral System Model, King's Interacting Systems Framework, Levine's Conservation Model, Neuman's Systems Model, Orem's Self-Care Framework, Rogers's Science of Unitary Human Beings, and Roy's Adaptation Model (Roy & Andrews, 1991; Barrett, 1990; Johnson, 1990; King, 1990; Neuman, 1989; Orem, 1991; Schaefer & Pond, 1991).

CONCEPTUAL MODELS AND THEORIES

The concepts and propositions of a theory "are not created out of nothing. [Indeed,] no one ever starts out with a completely clean slate to create a theory. . . . We might say that you already have a general point of view or frame of reference" (Babbie, 1989, p. 47). The frame of reference — the conceptual model — guides theory generation and testing by directing "the questions one asks and the theories one proposes and subsequently tests. It provides a network within which questions, theories, and data fit together and makes possible the identification of needed areas of theory development" (Newman, 1979, p. 6).

Conceptual models act as guides for the development of new theories by focusing attention on certain concepts and their relationships, and they place those concepts and their relationships in a distinctive context. For example, Johnson's Behavioral System Model emphasizes the person's behavior; King's Interacting Systems Framework focuses on attainment of goals; Levine's Conservation Model requires consideration of conservation of the individual's energy, structural integrity, personal integrity, and social integrity; Neuman's Systems Model highlights client system stability; Orem's Self-Care Framework emphasizes self-care abilities; Rogers's Science of Unitary Human Beings draws attention to the unity of human life; and Roy's Adaptation Model focuses on the individual's ability to adapt to a constantly changing environment.

Many theories are needed to fully describe, explain, and predict all the phenomena encompassed by a conceptual model. That is because any one theory deals only with a portion of the domain of inquiry identified by a model. Each theory is, therefore, more circumscribed than its parent conceptual model. For example, three theories have been derived from Orem's Self-Care Framework, and each one focuses on a different component of the more abstract conceptual model. The theory of self-care deficit proposes that people can benefit from nursing because they are subject to health-related or health-derived limitations that render them incapable of continuous self-care or that result in ineffective or incomplete care. The theory of self-care proposes that self-care is a learned behavior that purposely regulates human structural integrity, functioning, and human development. The theory of nursing systems proposes that nursing systems are formed when nurses use their abilities to prescribe, design, and provide nursing care.

At times it may be appropriate to link an existing theory with a conceptual model rather than develop a new theory, as when an existing theory provides the necessary specificity of conceptual model concepts and propositions needed for a particular situation. In that case, there is no need to duplicate knowledge by deriving a new theory from the conceptual model. Care must be taken, however, to ensure that the conceptual model and the theory are logically congruent. That is, the model and the theory must reflect compatible views about the nature of the phenomenon to be studied.

Suppose, for example, that a conceptual model includes the proposition that the person actively engages in interactions with the surrounding environment rather than being a passive reactor to external forces. Behavior modification theory is not compatible with the conceptual model because it proposes that the person's behavior is shaped by external conditioning stimuli. In contrast, the client-centered theory of personality is compatible with the conceptual model because it proposes that the individual is actively responsible for his or her behavior.

CONCEPTUAL MODELS AND RESEARCH

The influence of a conceptual model on research has been addressed by Batey (1971/1986), who pointed out that although two investigators may observe the same real-world situation or event, "their notions of why it occurs, their conceptual organization about the problem, [and] the knowledge base they select for studying that problem, may differ" (p. 543). In other words, each investigator views the world through a particular lens or frame of reference, which is encapsulated in a conceptual model.

More specifically, each conceptual model guides research by identifying the phenomena to be investigated, the methods to be used to investigate these phenomena, how theories about these phenomena are to be generated and tested, and how data are to be collected. A fully developed conceptual model reflects a particular research tradition that is made up of six guidelines for inquiry that encompass all phases of a study (Laudan, 1981; Schlotfeldt, 1975). The first guideline deals with the phenomena that are to be studied; the second focuses on the distinctive nature of the problems to be studied and the purposes to be fulfilled by the research; and the third focuses on the subjects who are to provide the data and the settings in which data are to be gathered. The fourth guideline deals with the research designs, instruments, and procedures that are to be employed; the fifth focuses on the methods to be employed in reducing and analyzing the data; and the sixth deals with the nature of contributions that the research will make to the advancement of knowledge.

Each guideline is derived from the distinctive substantive content and focus of the conceptual model and the model author's view of research. An overview of research guidelines derived from Neuman's Systems Model and those derived from Roy's Adaptation Model illustrate the differences in guidelines derived from different conceptual models.

The first guideline of Neuman's Systems Model states that the phenomena to be studied encompass (1) physiological, psychological, sociocultural, developmental, and spiritual variables, (2) properties of the central core of the client system, (3) properties of the flexible and normal lines of defense as well as of the lines of resistance, (4) characteristics of the internal, external, and created environments, (5) characteristics of intrapersonal, interpersonal, and extrapersonal stressors, and (6) elements of primary, secondary, and tertiary prevention interventions. In contrast, the first guideline of Roy's Adaptation Model states that the phenomena to be studied include basic life processes and how nursing enhances those processes. In particular, the Roy Adaptation Model focuses inquiry on adaptive processes in the areas of physiological responses, self-concept, role function, and interdependence behaviors.

The second guideline of Neuman's model states that the clinical problems to be studied are those that deal with the impact of stressors on client system stability. The ultimate purpose of Neuman Systems Model–based research is to predict the effects of primary, secondary, and tertiary prevention interventions on retention, attainment, and maintenance of client system stability. This focus contrasts with the second guideline of Roy's conceptual model, which directs researchers to study problems in adaptation to constantly changing environmental stimuli. The purpose of research is to describe how people adapt to environmental stimuli, explain how adaptive processes affect health, and predict the effects of nursing interventions on adaptive life processes and functioning.

In the Neuman Systems Model, the third guideline states that subjects can be individuals, families, or communities. Data may be collected in both inpatient and outpatient settings. The third guideline of Roy's model specifies that the people who might serve as study subjects may be well or have acute or chronic illnesses. Roy (1988) cited particular interest in individuals in situations in which "positive [adaptive] processes are threatened by health technologies and behaviorally induced health problems" (p. 28). Data can be gathered in any health care setting.

The fourth guideline of the Neuman Systems Model indicates that this nursing model is an appropriate base for inductive and deductive research using both qualitative and quantitative research designs and associated instrumentation. The fourth guideline of the Roy Adaptation Model indicates that research is directed toward the development of both basic and clinical science. Basic research designs involve investigation of human life processes with emphasis on adaptation that occurs as the human being interacts with the environment. Clinical research designs involve study of the effects of nursing care on adaptive life processes. Both qualitative and quantitative approaches can be used.

The fifth guideline of Neuman's conceptual model states that data analysis techniques associated with both qualitative and quantitative research designs would be appropriate. The fifth guideline of Roy's conceptual model states that data analysis techniques encompass qualitative content analysis and nonparametric and parametric statistical procedures.

The sixth guideline of the Neuman Systems Model states that research will advance our understanding of the influence of prevention interventions on the relationship between stressors and client system stability. In the Roy model, the sixth guideline indicates that research enhances understanding of the person's use of adaptive mechanisms and the role of nursing intervention in the promotion of adaptation to constantly changing environmental stimuli.

CONCEPTUAL-THEORETICAL-EMPIRICAL STRUCTURES

Conceptual models guide theory development and the selection of research methods. Three levels of abstraction are, therefore, evident in theory-generating or theory-testing research. As illustrated in Figure 5–1, conceptual models, theories, and empirical indicators are the three components of conceptual-theoretical-empirical structures. The conceptual model concepts and propositions that provide the frame of reference for the study are at the most abstract level of the structure. The concepts and propositions of the theory that was generated or tested are at the intermediate level. The empirical indicators used to collect the data, including the instruments, procedures, and/or experimental conditions that are used to observe or measure a concept, are at the most concrete level. Thus, the conceptual-theoretical-empirical structure depicted in Figure 5–1 extends the linkage between theory concepts and empirical indicators described in Chapter 2 of this book to the inclusion of a conceptual model.

As can be seen in Figure 5–1, vertical propositions link the concep-

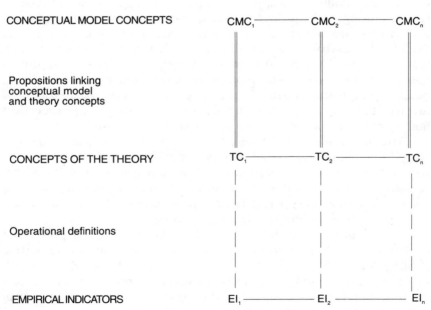

Figure 5–1. General form of a conceptual-theoretical-empirical structure.

tual model concepts to the theory concepts and the theory concepts to the empirical indicators. Vertical propositions in the form of representational statements indicate which theory concepts represent which conceptual model concepts. The representational statements typically are phrased as "Conceptual Model Concept$_n$ is represented by Theory Concept$_n$." Thus, each theory concept acts as a proxy for the more abstract conceptual model concept. These propositions are depicted by double lines ($=$). Vertical propositions in the form of operational definitions link the theory concepts to the empirical indicators. The operational definitions state exactly how the theory concepts are to be observed or measured. The operational definitions are depicted by broken lines ($- - -$). The conceptual-theoretical-empirical structure may also include horizontal relational propositions at each level of abstraction. Relational propositions, therefore, state how the conceptual model concepts are related to each other, how the theory concepts are related to one another, and how the scores on the empirical indicators are interrelated. These propositions are depicted by unbroken lines ($-$). If desired, the sign ($+ - ?$) for the direction of each relationship could be added to the diagram. Arrowheads ($\blacktriangleleft \blacktriangleright$) also could be added to depict the symmetry of the relationship.

Conceptual Models and Theory Testing

Conceptual models can guide theory testing through use of the research guidelines. In this case, the theory is derived from or linked with one or more concepts and propositions of the conceptual model and is then empirically tested by using a research design, subjects, setting, instruments, and procedures that are in keeping with the guidelines of the conceptual model. As illustrated in Figure 5–2, theory testing proceeds from the conceptual model to the theory and then to the empirical indicators. The data obtained from the empirical indicators are analyzed by following the methodological guidelines of the conceptual model, and the theory is supported or refuted. For simplicity, the horizontal propositions were not depicted in the diagram but could be added to show those linkages.

An example of theory testing from an explicit conceptual model is Tulman and associates' (1990) study of functional status following childbirth. The investigators derived a theory of correlates of postpartum functional status from the Roy Adaptation Model. The role function mode of the Roy model was represented by functional status, which was measured by the Inventory of Functional Status After Childbirth. The physio-

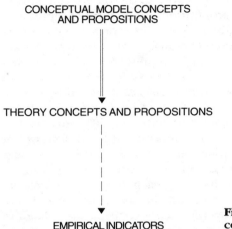

CONCEPTUAL MODEL CONCEPTS
AND PROPOSITIONS

THEORY CONCEPTS AND PROPOSITIONS

EMPIRICAL INDICATORS

Figure 5 – 2.   Theory testing from a conceptual model.

logical mode was represented by health variables, which were measured by data obtained from a Background Data Sheet. The self-concept mode was represented by individual psychosocial variables, which were measured by subscales of the Postpartum Self-Evaluation Questionnaire (PSQ). The interdependence mode was represented by family variables, which were measured by other PSQ subscales and the Infant Temperament Questionnaire. The focal stimulus was represented by childbirth, which was operationalized through a sample of women who had delivered healthy, full-term infants. The contextual stimuli were represented by demographic variables, which were obtained from information on the Background Data Sheet. The conceptual-theoretical-empirical structure for this study is diagrammed in Figure 5 – 3.

Conceptual Models and Theory Generation

Conceptual models also can guide theory generation through use of the research guidelines. In this case, the guidelines identify the phenomena to be studied and help the investigator to focus on particular problems, and they also facilitate selection of methods for the discovery of new theories. Thus, as can be seen in Figure 5 – 4, theory generation proceeds from the conceptual model directly to the empirical indicators. The data obtained from the empirical indicators are then analyzed and a new theory emerges. Figure 5 – 4 illustrates that the vertical propositions go

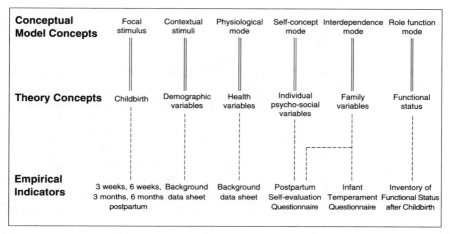

Figure 5–3. Example of theory testing from a conceptual model. (Diagram adapted from Fawcett, J., & Tulman, L. (1990). Building a programme of research from the Roy Adaptation Model of Nursing. *Journal of Advanced Nursing, 15,* 723, with permission.)

directly from the conceptual model concepts and propositions to the empirical indicators (═), and then from the empirical indicators to the concepts and propositions that make up the newly discovered theory (– – –). Once again, for simplicity, the horizontal propositions were not depicted in the diagram but could be added to show the linkages.

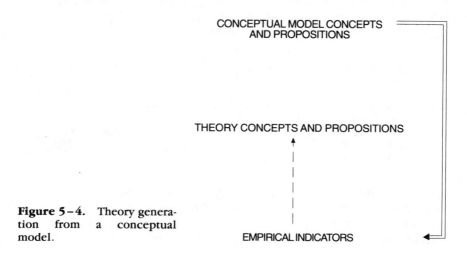

Figure 5–4. Theory generation from a conceptual model.

The proponents of such qualitative methods as grounded theory and phenomenology may not agree that a conceptual model guides theory generation. They fail, however, to take into account that the method they use, along with its underlying philosophical position, represents a frame of reference — a conceptual model. The goal of phenomenological inquiry, for example, is to identify the lived experiences of human beings, and it is reached by using such qualitative methods as open-ended interviews. The method of grounded theory also uses open-ended interviews to identify basic social psychological problems and basic social psychological processes. In both instances, the phenomena of interest (lived experiences or basic social psychological problems and processes) and the appropriate method (interviews) are specified prior to empirical theory development, and they constitute guidelines from a frame of reference that fits the definition of a conceptual model. Thus, both theory testing and theory generation are guided by conceptual models.

The use of a conceptual model to guide theory generation is exemplified by a qualitative study conducted by Blank, Clark, Longman, and Atwood (1989), who used the research guidelines of Neuman's Systems Model to identify a relevant phenomenon, a method for data collection, and categories for content analysis of data for a study of cancer patients and their caregivers. The phenomenon of interest was stressors, and the method selected was the use of two Neuman Stressors Inductive Interview guides. One of these structured interview guides was used to assess stressors experienced by patients, and the other one was used to assess stressors experienced by the patients' caregivers. In keeping with Neuman's classification schema, the stressors identified by the patients and caregivers were then categorized as intrapersonal, interpersonal, or extrapersonal. The investigators explained:

> Data from the interviews were tape-recorded and transcribed for content analysis. Consistent with the underlying [conceptual] model, the data were analyzed in relation to: intrapersonal stressors, i.e., stressors occurring within the individual; interpersonal stressors, i.e., stressors occurring between the individual and others; and extrapersonal stressors, i.e., stressors occurring between the individual and the environment. . . . The individual stressors identified by the subjects were then placed in the categories offered by Neuman. (Blank et al., 1989, p. 82)

A descriptive classification theory of patient and caregiver needs emerged from the data analysis. Needs were induced from each category of stressors. For patients, treatment uncertainty, physical restriction/role change, anger/depression, and isolation were the needs that emanated

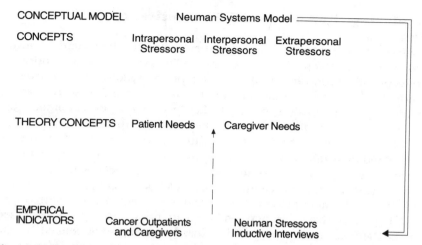

Figure 5–5. Example of theory generation from a conceptual model. (Diagram constructed from Blank, Clark, Longman, & Atwood, 1989.)

from intrapersonal stressors. Lack of support was the need emanating from interpersonal stressors, and transportation and finances were the needs emanating from extrapersonal stressors. Caregiver needs emanating from intrapersonal stressors included treatment uncertainty, role conflict/worry/added responsibilities, fear of being alone, coping with patient situation, and guilt. Needs from interpersonal stressors were lack of support, relationship with patient, activities of daily living of patient, and lack of information. Needs from extrapersonal stressors included transportation and finances. The conceptual-theoretical-empirical structure for the study conducted by Blank and her associates is illustrated in Figure 5–5.

Analysis and Evaluation of Conceptual-Theoretical-Empirical Structures

The techniques of theory formalization presented in Chapter 2 can be extended to the analysis of the entire conceptual-theoretical-empirical structure. Furthermore, the criteria for evaluation of the relation between theory and research, which were discussed in Chapter 3, also can be extended to encompass the entire conceptual-theoretical-empirical structure.

Analyzing the Conceptual-Theoretical-Empirical Structure

Analysis of the linkage of a conceptual model with a theory and empirical indicators is accomplished in two steps. The first step is to identify the concepts and propositions of the conceptual model that were used to guide the theory-generating or theory-testing research. The second step is to identify the vertical propositions that link the conceptual model concepts and propositions to the components of the theory.

The two steps of the analysis are illustrated by analyses of the studies conducted by Blank et al. (1989) and by Tulman et al. (1990) that were discussed earlier in this chapter. Blank and her associates used the concept of stressors from the Neuman Systems Model to guide the generation of a theory of cancer patients' and caregivers' needs. Furthermore, Blank et al. explained that their focus on both patients and caregivers was based on the Neuman model proposition that "stressors experienced by the patient and stressors experienced by the caregiver are not always compatible" (p. 81). As can be seen in Figure 5–5, the conceptual model concept of stressors was linked to the theory concepts of patients' and caregivers' needs through an empirical indicator, the Neuman Stressors Inductive Interviews. More specifically, the data obtained from the interviews were analyzed according to the Neuman model categories of intrapersonal, interpersonal, and extrapersonal stressors. Patients' and caregivers' needs were then induced from the identified stressors (see pages 104 and 105).

Tulman and her associates used the Roy Adaptation Model concepts of adaptive modes and stimuli to guide their theory-testing study of changes in functional status during the postpartum. The links between those concepts and the theory concepts are outlined on pages 107 to 108 and depicted in Figure 5–3. In addition, two propositions of the Roy model were linked to the relational propositions of the functional status theory. Tulman et al. (1990) explained:

According to Andrews and Roy (1986), "the four adaptive modes are interrelated. Responses in any one mode have an effect on or act as a stimulus for one or all of the other modes" (p. 43). Therefore, the associations between the adaptive modes were explored by testing the relationships of health, individual psychosocial, and family variables to functional status. Roy (1984) postulated that contextual stimuli influence adaptation. Thus, the relationship between demographic variables and functional status was also explored. (p. 70)

Evaluating the Conceptual-Theoretical-Empirical Structure

The criteria for evaluation of the linkage of a conceptual model with a theory and empirical indicators, adapted from work by Silva (1986), are listed in Table 5–1. These criteria reflect the guidelines for conceptual model–based research discussed earlier in this chapter (see page 108).

Examination of the studies by Blank et al. (1989) and Tulman et al. (1990) revealed that the criteria were met. The conceptual model was explicitly identified and summarized in both research reports. The links between the conceptual models and the theories were described clearly. A review of the methods of both studies indicated that the empirical indicators were appropriate and reflected the intent of the model in each case. In fact, the interview guide used by Blank and her associates was directly derived from the Neuman Systems Model, and the Inventory of Functional Status After Childbirth used by Tulman and her colleagues was directly derived from the role function adaptive mode of the Roy Adaptation Model. Furthermore, Tulman et al. noted that the data supported the credibility of the Roy model inasmuch as relationships between the theory concepts representing the adaptive modes and contextual stimuli were evident. Blank et al. did not address the credibility of the Neuman model in an explicit manner, but the results of their data analysis suggested that the model was sufficiently comprehensive to permit categori-

TABLE 5–1. Criteria for Evaluation of the Linkage of Conceptual Models with Theories and Empirical Indicators

- The conceptual model is explicitly identified as the underlying guide for the theory-generating or theory-testing research.
- The conceptual model is discussed in sufficient breadth and depth so that the relationship between the model and the purpose of the research is clear.
- The linkages between the conceptual model concepts and propositions and the theory concepts and propositions are stated explicitly.
- The methodology reflects the conceptual model:
  The study subjects are drawn from a population that is appropriate to the focus of the conceptual model.
  The instruments are appropriate measures of phenomena encompassed by the conceptual model.
  The study design clearly reflects the focus of the conceptual model.
  The statistical techniques are in keeping with the focus of the conceptual model.
- Discussion of research results includes conclusions regarding the empirical adequacy of the theory and the credibility of the conceptual model.

zation of all responses to the interviews according to Neuman's classification of stressors.

Credibility of Conceptual Models. The final criterion listed in Table 5–1 requires the theory to demonstrate empirical adequacy and the conceptual model to demonstrate credibility. Empirical adequacy was discussed in detail in Chapter 3. Credibility is introduced here and requires further discussion.

As noted earlier in this chapter, the abstract and general nature of a conceptual model precludes direct empirical testing. The propositions of the conceptual model are instead tested indirectly through the empirical testing of the theories that are derived from or linked with the model. If the findings of theory-testing research support the theory, it is likely that the conceptual model is credible. If, however, the research findings do not support the theory, both the empirical adequacy of the theory and the credibility of the conceptual model must be questioned. The former situation is evident in the Blank et al. (1989) and Tulman et al. (1990) studies reviewed above. It is also evident in a Neuman Systems Model-based study conducted by Ali and Khalil (1989), whereas the latter situation is evident in a study, also derived from the Neuman Systems Model, conducted by Ziemer (1983).

Ali and Khalil investigated the effect of a psychoeducational intervention on anxiety among Egyptian bladder cancer patients and found that the experimental intervention had the expected effect of anxiety reduction. Their findings supported the empirical adequacy of the theory of psychoeducational intervention. Inasmuch as their study was directly derived from Neuman's model, the findings also supported the model's credibility. In particular, the finding of a decrease in postoperative state anxiety supported Neuman's contention that nursing intervention increases resistance to stressors and strengthens the flexible line of defense.

Ziemer investigated the effect of preoperative information on use of postoperative coping behaviors and subsequent occurrence of postoperative symptoms by linking a theory of cognitive imagery with the Neuman Systems Model. She found that preoperative information did not result in the expected coping behaviors, nor did use of coping behaviors result in reduction of postoperative symptoms. These findings raise questions about the empirical adequacy of the cognitive imagery theory and the credibility of the conceptual model. More specifically, Ziemer's findings did not support Neuman's contentions that primary prevention increases resistance to stressors and that the lines of defense reduce the penetration of stressors and the development of symptoms.

CONCLUSION

Many published research reports do not mention the conceptual model on which the study was based. By failing to identify the conceptual model, the investigator does not fully inform readers of the distinctive conceptual perspective and sociohistorical context of the study (Lavee & Dollahite, 1991). The omission may lead to a critique of the research that is inappropriate because it reflects an entirely different perspective. It also has created difficulties in identifying groups of related studies and programs of research. Thus, it is recommended to those planning and reporting research that the conceptual model be explicitly identified and be clearly linked with the theoretical and empirical components of the study.

REFERENCES

Ali, N. S., & Khalil, H. Z. (1989). Effect of psychoeducational intervention on anxiety among Egyptian bladder cancer patients. *Cancer Nursing, 12*, 236–242.

Babbie, E. (1989). *The practice of social research* (5th ed.). Belmont, CA: Wadsworth.

Barrett, E. A. M. (Ed.) (1990). *Visions of Rogers' science-based nursing.* New York: National League for Nursing.

Batey, M. V. (1986). Conceptualizing the research process. In L. H. Nicoll (Ed.), *Perspectives on nursing theory* (pp. 541–548). Boston: Little, Brown. (Original work published 1971.)

Blank, J. J., Clark, L., Longman, A. J., & Atwood, J. R. (1989). Perceived home care needs of cancer patients and their caregivers. *Cancer Nursing, 12*, 78–84.

Fawcett, J., & Tulman, L. (1990). Building a programme of research from the Roy Adaptation Model of Nursing. *Journal of Advanced Nursing, 15*, 720–725.

Johnson, D. E. (1990). The behavioral system model for nursing. In M. E. Parker (Ed.), *Nursing theories in practice* (pp. 23–32). New York: National League for Nursing.

King, I. M. (1990). King's conceptual framework and theory of goal attainment. In M. E. Parker (Ed.), *Nursing theories in practice* (pp. 73–84). New York: National League for Nursing.

Laudan, L. (1981). A problem-solving approach to scientific progress. In I. Hacking (Ed.), *Scientific revolutions* (pp. 144–155). New York: Oxford University Press.

Lavee, Y., & Dollahite, D. C. (1991). The linkage between theory and research in family science. *Journal of Marriage and the Family, 53*, 361–373.

Neuman, B. (1989). *The Neuman Systems Model* (2nd ed.). Norwalk, CT: Appleton and Lange.

Newman, M. A. (1979). *Theory development in nursing.* Philadelphia: F. A. Davis.

Orem, D. E. (1991). *Nursing: Concepts of practice* (4th ed.). St. Louis: Mosby Year Book.

Roy, C., & Andrews, H. A. (1988). An explication of the philosophical assumptions of the Roy adaptation model. *Nursing Science Quarterly, 1*, 26–34.

Roy, C., & Andrews, H. A. (1991). *The Roy Adaptation Model: The definitive statement.* Norwalk, CT: Appleton and Lange.

Schaefer, K. M., & Pond, J. B. (Eds.) (1991). *Levine's Conservation Model: A framework for nursing practice.* Philadelphia: F. A. Davis.

Schlotfeldt, R. M. (1975). The need for a conceptual framework. In P. J. Verhonick (Ed.), *Nursing research I* (pp. 1–24). Boston: Little, Brown.

Silva, M. C. (1986). Research testing nursing theory: State of the art. *Advances in Nursing Science, 9*(1), 1–11.

Tulman, L., Fawcett, J., Groblewski, L., & Silverman, L. (1990). Changes in functional status after childbirth. *Nursing Research, 39,* 70–75.

Ziemer, M. M. (1983). Effects of information on postsurgical coping. *Nursing Research, 32,* 282–287.

ADDITIONAL READINGS

Acton, G. J., Irvin, B. L., & Hopkins, B. A. (1991). Theory-testing research: Building the science. *Advances in Nursing Science, 14*(1), 52–61.

Burton, A. (Ed.). (1974). *Operational theories of personality.* New York: Brunner/Mazel.

Coward, D. D. (1990). Critical multiplism: A research strategy for nursing science. *Image: Journal of Nursing Scholarship, 22,* 163–167.

Fawcett, J. (1989). *Analysis and evaluation of conceptual models of nursing* (2nd ed.). Philadelphia: F. A. Davis.

Kuhn, T. S. (1977). Second thoughts on paradigms. In F. Suppe (Ed.). *The structure of scientific theories* (2nd ed., pp. 459–482). Chicago: University of Illinois Press.

Munhall, P. L., & Oiler, C. J. (1986). *Nursing research: A qualitative perspective.* Norwalk, CT: Appleton-Century-Crofts.

Nye, F. I., & Berardo, F. N. (Eds.). (1981). *Emerging conceptual frameworks in family analysis.* New York: Praeger.

Whall, A. L. (1986). *Family therapy theory for nursing: Four approaches.* Norwalk, CT: Appleton-Century-Crofts.

Williams, C. A. (1979). The nature and development of conceptual frameworks. In F. S. Downs & J. W. Fleming (Eds.), *Issues in nursing research* (pp. 89–106). New York: Appleton-Century-Crofts.

6

Writing Research Grant Proposals and Reports

The techniques of theory formalization, the criteria for evaluation of theory and research, the methods of integrating research findings, and the process of developing conceptual-theoretical-empirical structures that were presented in Chapters 2 to 5 of this book can be used not only to analyze and evaluate previously reported studies but also to prepare research grant proposals and research reports. This chapter presents guidelines for the preparation of research documents that emphasize the close connection between theory and research. It also includes many excerpts from research documents that exemplify the guidelines.

GUIDELINES FOR RESEARCH PROPOSALS AND REPORTS

The guidelines for writing research proposals and reports are summarized in Table 6–1. Included are guidelines for the customary sections of a research document, which encompass the introduction to the research problem, methodology, results, and discussion of results. These guide-

TABLE 6 – 1.   Guidelines for Writing Research Proposals and Reports

INTRODUCTION

The introduction establishes the need for theory-generating or theory-testing research to investigate a particular physical, psychological, social, or behavioral problem. The introduction also identifies the frame of reference for the research.
- Summarize the *social significance* of the study by explaining how it addresses a research priority or social policy issue.
- Summarize the *theoretical significance* of the research by explaining how the study extends knowledge or fills in gaps in knowledge about a phenomenon of interest to a discipline.
- State the *purpose* or specific aims of the study.
- Describe the *background* for the study:
    Summarize the conceptual model or other frame of reference for the study.
    Describe the linkages between the conceptual model and the study topic or concepts and propositions.
    Provide a critical review of relevant theoretical and empirical literature, including pilot or preliminary studies conducted by the investigator.
    For theory-testing research, provide constitutive definitions for the concepts of the theory to be tested.
    For theory-testing research, provide evidence regarding any propositions that are to be tested.
    For theory-testing research, state the research hypotheses.
    For research proposals, link the proposed study to long-range goals in a program of research.

METHODS

The methods section includes a description of the sample, instruments, procedure, and data analysis plan.
- Describe the *sample*:
    Describe the study subjects.
    Provide the number of subjects and the power analysis calculations.
    Explain how subjects were recruited.
    Give refusal and attrition rates.
    Identify restrictions on the sample and relevant characteristics that set the limits on generalizability of study findings.
    Explain how informed consent was obtained.
- Identify each *instrument* used:
    Identify the theory concept that was measured by each instrument.
    Describe the psychometric properties of each instrument, including validity and reliability for the study sample.
    Describe the items on each instrument and the scale used to rate the items.
    Identify the range of possible scores and explain how the scores are interpreted.
- Describe the *procedures* used to collect the data:
    Identify the data collectors.

TABLE 6 – 1. Guidelines for Writing Research Proposals and Reports (*Continued*)

Identify the setting and time required for data collection.

For experimental studies, describe the experimental and control conditions.

State the order of administration for the instruments.

For research proposals, provide a timetable for the conduct of all phases of the study from training of personnel to preparation of the final report.

For research proposals, provide a detailed protocol for protection of human or animal subjects.

• Describe the *data analysis plan*:

Identify the strategies for data processing and statistical techniques of analysis of the data.

RESULTS

The results section presents the findings of data analysis. It is structured according to specific aims, purposes, or hypotheses.

• For theory-generating research, identify and describe the concepts and propositions that emerged from the analysis of data.

• For theory-testing research, provide descriptive statistics for study variables and the results of inferential statistical tests of hypotheses.

• For theory-testing research, draw a definitive conclusion regarding support or lack of support for each hypothesis.

DISCUSSION

The discussion section presents the investigator's interpretation of the results. This section also is structured according to specific aims, purposes, or hypotheses.

• Draw conclusions with regard to the empirical adequacy of the theory and the credibility of the conceptual model.

• Provide alternative methodological and/or substantive explanations.

• Identify implications for future research.

• Discuss pragmatic adequacy, including implications for formulation of practice guidelines and health policy.

---

lines can be used to prepare applications for research funds, journal articles, dissertations, and theses. Readers are, however, cautioned to refer to the specific directions for preparation of research documents provided by each funding agency, journal publisher, or university.

Examples taken from a funded research grant proposal and several published research reports are used to illustrate the guidelines. Complete references for the literature cited within the examples are available in the original documents.

Introduction to the Research Problem

The proposal or report begins with an introduction that provides an overview of the problem. This section establishes the need for the study and identifies the frame of reference for the research. The introduction has three major subsections: a brief description of a physical, psychological, social, or behavioral problem that requires investigation, a statement of the purpose of the research, and the background literature.

Description of the Research Problem

The research problem description should present a compelling reason for the study. It is *not* sufficient to state that no research dealing with the topic has been conducted. Rather, the social significance and the theoretical significance of the study are described. The social significance can be established by identifying the magnitude or prevalence of a problem or by explaining how the study addresses a research priority or social policy issue. The theoretical significance can be established by delineating what is already known about the problem and explaining how the proposed research will extend or fill in gaps in current knowledge about a phenomenon of interest to a discipline.

The following example was taken from a published report of a study of psychosocial predictors of maternal depressive symptoms, parenting attitudes, and child behavior. The excerpt illustrates how the social significance of a study can be described by identifying the magnitude of a social problem.

Example: Description of the Social Significance of a Study

Low-income, single mothers and their children constitute a rapidly growing population at high risk for adverse health outcomes. The mental health of these women is particularly at risk. In turn, there is evidence that parental psychological disturbance places children at increased risk for negative outcomes and may lead to abusive parenting behavior. (Hall, Gurley, Sachs, & Kryscio, 1991, p. 214)

The next example was taken from a research grant proposal. In this excerpt, the theoretical significance of the proposed investigation is established by a brief review of current knowledge and an explanation of how the proposed study would extend that knowledge.

Example: Description of the Theoretical Significance of a Study

Pregnancy and the postpartum are times of considerable transition in the life of a woman. Previous research has focused almost exclusively on the process of maternal role attainment and factors influencing transition to the maternal role (Mercer, 1986; Rubin, 1984). Other studies have explored the extent to which achievement of parenthood is regarded as a crisis (Hobbs & Cole, 1976). Still other reports have examined psychological responses to childbearing (Ahmed, 1981; Blum, 1980; Colman & Colman, 1971; Grossman, Eichler, Winickoff, Anzalone, Gofseyeff, & Sargent, 1980; Shereshefsky & Yarrow, 1973). Moreover, textbook descriptions of the postpartum tend to focus on healing of reproductive organs and the taking on of the maternal role during the first few weeks after delivery (Pritchard, MacDonald, & Gant, 1985; Reeder, & Martin, 1987). Thus, little is known of the social response to pregnancy and the postpartum in the form of alterations in the woman's performance of usual responsibilities and activities associated with roles other than that of mother. And little is known of the variables that influence alterations in performance of usual role responsibilities and activities during the childbearing period.

We have begun to explore alterations in performance of usual role responsibilities and activities associated with childbearing by retrospectively and prospectively assessing functional status during the postpartum in healthy women and identifying specific demographic, health, individual psychosocial, and family variables that are related to functional status after childbirth (Tulman & Fawcett, 1988a, 1988b). The proposed study has been designed to extend our previous and currently ongoing research to encompass both pregnancy and the postpartum. (Tulman & Fawcett, 1990–1993)

Purpose of the Study

The statement of the study purpose might come at the end of the introduction, or it could be the very first sentence of the proposal or report. The study purpose is stated precisely and concisely. Proposals for or reports of theory-generating research identify the topic to be studied and may identify the methodologic frame of reference (e.g., phenomenology, grounded theory, ethnography). In theory-testing research, the statement of the study purpose identifies the main concepts and propositions of the theory.

The purpose of the study may be stated as a list of aims, in narrative form, or in the form of research questions. The typical format for research proposals is a list of specific aims, whereas a narrative or question format is frequently seen in research reports. Examples for all three forms are given below.

Example: Purpose of the Study Stated as Aims

The proposed longitudinal study will encompass the three trimesters of pregnancy and the first six months of the postpartum. The specific aims are:

1.   To describe changes in functional status during pregnancy and the postpartum.
2.   To determine the relationship between selected health variables (physical symptoms; parity; physical energy; minor prenatal, intrapartal, postpartal, and neonatal complications; type of delivery; medical restrictions; and method of infant feeding) and functional status during pregnancy and the postpartum.
3.   To determine the relationship between selected individual psychosocial variables (psychological symptoms; acceptance of pregnancy; identification of a motherhood role; preparation for labor; fear of pain, helplessness, and loss of control during labor; concern for well-being of self and baby; gratification with labor and delivery; life satisfaction; satisfaction with the parental role; and maternal competence) and functional status during pregnancy and the postpartum.
4.   To determine the relationship between selected family variables (relationship with own mother, relationship with husband during pregnancy, social support, quality of the marital relationship after delivery, maternal perception of father's participation in child care, and infant difficultness) and functional status during pregnancy and the postpartum.
5.   To determine the relationship between selected demographic variables (age, education, occupation, employment status, maternity leave and compensation policies of the employer, job income lost due to childbearing, household income, place of residence, and household composition) and functional status during pregnancy and the postpartum.
6.   To determine the relative importance, in terms of var-

iance accounted for, of selected health, individual psychosocial, family, and demographic variables on functional status during pregnancy and the postpartum.

Selection of the proposed study variables has been guided, in part, by Roy's (1984) conceptual model of nursing. Thus, the final aim of the study is:

7.   To determine the credibility of Roy's Adaptation Model and its utility for research investigating variables associated with changes in functional status during pregnancy and the postpartum. (Tulman & Fawcett, 1990–1993)

Example: Purpose of Theory-Generating Research Stated in Narrative Form

The grounded theory method of data collection and analysis was used to explore and describe the recovery process of chemically dependent nurses. (Hutchinson, 1987, p. 339)

Example: Purpose of Theory-Testing Research Stated in Narrative Form

The primary purpose of the present study was to test the usefulness of the multivariate HPM [Health Promotion Model] in explaining the occurrence of health-promoting lifestyles among employees who had made an initial commitment to change health habits by enrolling in workplace health promotion programs yet varied greatly in their level of participation. A second purpose was to ascertain if the model was useful for predicting health-promoting lifestyles among the same employees at a later point in time. (Pender, Walker, Sechrist, & Frank-Stromborg, 1990, p. 327)

Example: Purpose of Theory-Generating Research Stated as a Research Question

The study reported here involves survivors who had recently lost a family member through suicide. The major question explored was, What do adult survivors report regarding their perceived life experience 3 to 9 months after the suicide death of a family member? (Van Dongen, 1990, p. 224)

Example: Purpose of Theory-Testing Research Stated as a Research Question

The purpose of this investigation was to test [a] structural model of stress and symptomatic experience. This model addresses the question: What is the relationship between the explanatory variables of psychosocial attributes, basic need satisfaction, perceived stress, [and] disease severity, and the dependent variable symptomatic experience in people with COPD [chronic obstructive pulmonary disease]? Also, gender differences in the levels of need satisfaction, perceived stress, and symptomatic experience and in the relationships among the variables were explored. (Leidy, 1990, p. 232)

Background

The background subsection includes a description of the conceptual model and/or theoretical perspective that guided the study, as well as a critical review of relevant theoretical and empirical literature.

Theory-Generating Research. In theory-generating research proposals or reports, the background subsection may be quite brief. Here the conceptual model or other frame of reference for the study is summarized and linked to the research problem. The typical literature review is a critical discussion of previous theoretical and empirical works that clearly underscores the lack of knowledge that supports the need for a theory-generating study.

The following example of the background subsection was taken from a theory-generating study of the process of nurses' recovery from chemical dependency. The excerpt illustrates the explicit identification of the methodologic frame of reference for the study and clearly links that frame of reference to the major concepts of the theory that was generated. Furthermore, the literature review enhances understanding of need for the study by presenting a brief review of related descriptive reports.

Example: Background for Theory-Generating Research

A goal of grounded theory is to discover a basic social psychological problem in the data and a basic social psychological process that resolves the problem. In this research the basic social psychological problem discovered was self-annihilation and the basic social psychological process was self-integration. The problem and the process were unarticulated by the participants yet fundamental to their personal experiences and social interaction.

The literature on impaired nurses' recovery and treatment programs is sparse, consisting mainly of descriptive reports in the general nursing literature. Treatment suggestions include self-exploration of the meaning of addictive behavior (Morton, 1979); client teaching (Morton); individual, family, or group therapy (Morton); inpatient and outpatient treatment (Isler, 1978); and peer assistance programs (American Nurses' Association, 1984; Green, 1984). Additional approaches include behavior modification, relaxation training, desensitization, simulation exercises, and educational programs that present new coping behaviors (Morton). Schnurr (1979) offered a self-report of her own recovery from alcoholism and drug addiction. Jaffe (1982) discussed chemically dependent nurses' feelings about themselves — rejection, shame, worthlessness, insanity — and problems in recovery. From the perspective of a nurse administrator, Kabb (1984) called chemical dependency the "primary personal problem affecting employee job performance today" (p. 23) and described employee warning signs, diagnosis, management, and treatment of the problem. Fulton (1981) proposed management strategies, and Jefferson and Ensor (1982) suggested plans for on-the-job intervention.

The nursing literature focusing on self-help groups includes descriptive articles (Newton, 1984), a book chapter (Steiger & Lipson, 1985), and reports of research (Levy, 1976; Lieberman & Bond, 1978; Rothlis, 1984). The quantitative studies demonstrated that participants found self-help groups useful. To date, there is no research on the recovery process of chemically dependent nurses. (Hutchinson, 1987, p. 339)

Theory-Testing Research. In theory-testing research proposals or reports, a concise summary of the conceptual model is presented and the conceptual model concepts and propositions are linked with the concepts and propositions of the theory that are or were to be tested. The review of literature includes statements of the theory propositions and a critical discussion of the evidence for each proposition. Typically, constitutive definitions for the theory concepts are given as each concept is introduced. The theory propositions may introduce the paragraph(s) dealing with relationships between particular concepts, or the propositions may be presented as the summary statements. The review of literature may conclude with a statement of the research hypotheses. The concepts and propositions of the theory are explicated in the narrative and may also be depicted in a diagram.

The following example illustrates how the linkage between a conceptual model and a theory can be explained. The excerpt was taken from a proposal for a longitudinal study of functional status during pregnancy and the postpartum. Although the excerpt was taken from a grant proposal, the same content could be used for a journal article reporting the study results.

Example: Background for Theory-Testing Research with Linkage of Conceptual Model to Theory Concepts and Propositions

Roy's (1984) Adaptation Model depicts people as biopsychosocial beings who adapt to environmental stimuli. Adaptation is considered to take place in one biological and three psychosocial modes. The biological mode of adaptation, called the physiological mode, is concerned with basic needs requisite to maintaining the physical and physiological integrity of the human system. The psychosocial modes of adaptation are self-concept, role function, and interdependence. The self-concept mode is concerned with the conception of the physical and personal self. The role function mode is concerned with performance of roles on the basis of position within society. The interdependence mode deals with development and maintenance of satisfying affectional relationships with significant others. Environmental stimuli are categorized as focal, which refers to the stimuli most immediately confronting the person; contextual, which refers to contributing factors in the situation; and residual, which refers to other unknown factors that may influence the situation. When the factors making up residual stimuli become known, they are considered contextual stimuli.

In the proposed study, the role function mode is represented by functional status. The physiological mode is represented indirectly by health variables, the self-concept mode by individual psychosocial variables, and the interdependence mode by family variables. The focal stimulus is represented by pregnancy and childbirth, and contextual stimuli are represented by demographic variables.

Andrews and Roy (1986) postulated that "the four adaptive modes are interrelated. Responses in any one mode have an effect on or act as a stimulus for one or all of the other modes" (p. 43). The proposed study will explore the relationships between the four adaptive modes by testing the relationships between health variables and functional status, individual psychosocial variables and functional status, and family variables and functional status. Roy (1984) also has postulated that contextual stimuli influence adaptation. The proposed study, therefore, will test the relationship between demographic variables and functional status. (Tulman & Fawcett, 1990–1993)

The next example illustrates the development of the theoretical path model for a correlational study of adaptation to multiple sclerosis. The study was designed to test a theory of the relationships among social support, functional disability, perceived uncertainty, and psychosocial adaptation. The excerpt includes a narrative explanation and a diagram of concepts and propositions. Furthermore, the excerpt clearly illustrates how constitutive definitions of concepts are woven into the narrative and how propositions are justified through review of related theory and research.

Example: Background for Theory-Testing Research with Relational Propositions

The concepts in the [theoretical] framework included *social support, functional disability, perceived uncertainty, and [psychosocial] adaptation. Social support* is defined as the degree to which the individual's needs for socialization, tangible assistance, cognitive guidance, social reinforcement, and emotional sustenance are met through interaction with the social network (Hirsch, 1980). The social network includes people whom the individual identifies as important. *Functional disability* includes physical limitations in ability to perform one's usual roles and activities (Slater, 1981). These limitations may be associated with physical pathology, but they need not always refer to an underlying disease process. The individual's perception of a situation as ambiguous constitutes *perceived uncertainty*. It involves uncertainty regarding symptoms, diagnosis, treatment, relationships with caregivers, and future plans (Mishel, 1981). The definition of *adaptation* is, according to Feldman (1974), a process of "discarding both false hope and destructive hopelessness . . . so that there is meaning and purpose to living that transcends the limitations imposed by the illness" (p. 290).

Durkheim (1951) theorized that membership within a social group fosters a sense of belonging and meaningfulness in life and that the absence of social integration may lead to despair and hopelessness. The underlying premise in Durkheimian anomie theory is that social integration directly affects psychological well-being. Social integration is one component of social support (Dimond & Jones, 1983). Some researchers

(Andrews, Tennant, Hewson, & Valliant, 1978; Berkman & Syme, 1979; Henderson, Duncan-Jones, McAuley, & Ritchie, 1979) provide evidence for a direct, positive relationship between social support and psychological well-being, while others (Fiore, Becker, & Coppel, 1983; Rook, 1984; Ruehlman & Wolchik, 1988) have documented the potentially harmful effects of negative social interactions on well-being. Taken together, these findings suggest that it is important to examine both the positive and negative components of social support. Social support, therefore, is divided into two separate dimensions in the present study, one reflecting the positive aspects of social interactions (supportiveness) and the other the negative (unsupportiveness). *Supportiveness* is defined as satisfaction with the various components of social support received during interactions with the social network, while *unsupportiveness* is dissatisfaction with those interactions. Thus, two paths were predicted, one between supportiveness and psychosocial adaptation (Figure [6 – 1], path 1) and the other between unsupportiveness and adaptation (Figure [6 – 1], path 2). Two indirect paths (Figure [6 – 1], paths 3 & 4) between

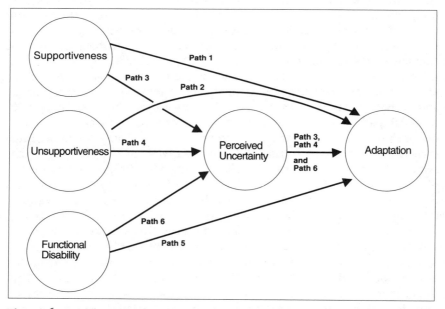

Figure 6 – 1. Theoretical path model for adaptation to multiple sclerosis. (From Wineman, 1990, p. 297, with permission.)

these social support concepts and psychosocial adaptation through perceived uncertainty were also predicted. These paths (3 & 4) were predicted because social support may facilitate the individual's ability to clarify uncertain situations (Mishel & Braden, 1988) and because the uncertainty about one's illness may influence psychological outcomes (Mishel & Braden, 1987).

Because there is general agreement in the literature that people with more severe MS [multiple sclerosis] have less favorable psychosocial outcomes (Dalos, Rabins, Brooks, & O'Donnell, 1983; McIvor et al., 1984; Zedlow & Pavlou, 1984), a direct path (Figure [6–1], path 5) between functional disability and adaptation was predicted, suggesting that more extensive functional disability would be related to less successful adaptation. This relationship, however, may be mediated by the individual's illness, in that MS creates an unusually ambiguous situation, which is likely to lead to high levels of perceived uncertainty, particularly for the person with relapsing-remitting MS (Mishel & Braden, 1988). The model also purports, therefore, that functional disability is indirectly related to adaptation through the concept of perceived uncertainty (Figure [6–1], path 6). (Wineman, 1990, pp. 294–295)

The following example illustrates the theoretical justification for hypotheses in an experimental study of medical regimen compliance after myocardial infarction. The experimental group received a nursing intervention derived from the theory of reasoned action 30 days after discharge from the hospital. The control group did not receive the nursing intervention. Data on intention to comply with the medical regimen prescriptions were collected prior to hospital discharge, and actual compliance data were collected at 1 and 2 years posthospitalization.

Example: Background for Theory-Testing Research with Hypotheses

The Fishbein Model of Reasoned Action (Ajzen & Fishbein, 1980) guided development of tools and the nursing intervention used in this study. Attitudes, perceived beliefs of others, and intentions have been found to be related to behavior by Ajzen and Fishbein. Their definitions of variables were used in this study. Attitudes were defined as the values of the individual of certain behaviors and were reported as favorable or unfavorable.

Intentions were a function of two determinants: attitudinal and normative. The attitudinal component was identified as favorableness or unfavorableness toward a behavior in question; the normative component was identified as actions the individual believed others thought he or she should perform (perceived beliefs of others) and the motivation to comply with their beliefs. In the Fishbein model, attitudes, the perceived beliefs of others, and the motivation to comply with others' beliefs are predictive of the person's intentions to perform a behavior. Intentions, in turn, are the immediate predictors of the person's behavior. In this study, data on attitudes, perceived beliefs of others, intentions, and behaviors as defined in the Fishbein model were part of the nursing intervention.

Hypotheses

I.   Medical regimen compliance of MI [myocardial infarction] patients 2 years after hospitalization will be greater for the experimental group who received a nursing intervention than for a control group.

II.   Compliance at 2 years will not change from that at 1 year for either the experimental or control group.

III.   Attitudes and perceived beliefs of others at 2 years and intentions during hospitalization are significantly related to regimen compliance for MI patients 2 years after hospitalization.

(Miller, Wikoff, Garrett, McMahon, & Smith, 1990, p. 333)

Preliminary Studies and Long-Range Goals. The literature review for both theory-generating and theory-testing studies may include discussion of pilot studies or preliminary research conducted by the investigator. Furthermore, the background section of research proposals frequently ends by linking the proposed study to long-range goals in a program of research.

The next two examples were taken from a research proposal for a study of functional status during pregnancy and the postpartum. The first example is an excerpt from the description of preliminary studies undertaken by the investigators in preparation for the proposed study. A concise summary of these studies could be included in the background subsection of a journal article reporting the study findings. In the second example, the proposed study is linked to the long-range goals of the research program, including the development of nursing interventions and the formulation of maternity leave policies.

Example: Description of Preliminary Studies in a Research Proposal

Our research related to the proposed study began with a retrospective study designed to determine the likely times of changes in functional status of women After delivery (Tulman & Fawcett, 1988a). Seventy women who had delivered a living child within the past five years were surveyed on their recall of their recovery of functional status following their last delivery. An early version of the Inventory of Functional Status After Childbirth, then called the Childbirth Impact Profile-Form MQ, was used to collect data. Analysis of the data indicated that there were significant differences in women's retrospective recollections of their recovery times according to the type of delivery, with cesarean delivered women ($N = 40$) reporting a longer recovery than women who had had vaginal deliveries ($N = 30$).

Our research continued with the development and assessment of the psychometric properties of the Inventory of Functional Status After Childbirth (IFSAC) (Fawcett, Tulman, & Myers, 1988). The IFSAC was found to have satisfactory content validity, internal consistency reliability, and test-retest reliability. Furthermore, the multidimensional nature of the concept of functional status after childbirth was supported by empirical evidence of independence of the subscales.

In our current study, subjects are being followed for the first 6 months after delivery. Data are being collected at 3 weeks, 6 weeks, 3 months, and 6 months postpartum. The sample includes 100 married English-speaking women over 18 years of age who had delivered healthy term infants and had no major prenatal obstetrical complications with carryover effects to the postpartum (e.g., severe eclampsia) or underlying medical problems (e.g., diabetes, chronic renal or cardiac disease). Questionnaires being used include the IFSAC, the Postpartum Self-Evaluation Questionnaire, the Infant Characteristics Questionnaire, and Background Data Sheets, all of which will be used in the proposed study.

Preliminary analysis of data from our first 50 subjects revealed that functional status increased steadily over the first 6 months postpartum ($F(3,38) = 58.49$, $p = < .001$). Post hoc analysis by Scheffé tests revealed a statistically significant increase in functional status between 3 weeks and 6 weeks ($p < .001$), 6 weeks and 3 months ($p = .03$), and 3 months and 6 months ($p < .001$) after delivery. (Tulman & Fawcett, 1990–1993)

Example: Description of Long-Range Goals in a Research Proposal

The proposed study will provide normative data from healthy women on the within-subject changes in functional status from the end of the first trimester of pregnancy until 6 months postpartum. In addition, factors affecting functional status during pregnancy and after childbirth will be delineated. Furthermore, the findings of the proposed study will provide data that may be used to develop interventions that may facilitate optimal functional status during pregnancy and the postpartum period.

Socioeconomically, the results of this study would supply data that could help shape legislation concerning state and national maternity leave/compensation policies. Currently, experts in the field of social policy have limited research data on functional status during pregnancy and after childbirth on which to base various proposed lengths of maternity leave (Kamerman, Kahn, & Kingston, 1983; Zigler & Frank, 1988). This critical information would place current discussions on length of maternity leave on a firm empirical basis. (Tulman & Fawcett, 1990–1993)

Methods

The methods section includes a description of the sample, instruments, procedure, and data analysis plan. Within the limits of space, the information given should be sufficient so that the study could be replicated.

Sample

The sample subsection presents a description of the study subjects, how the subjects were recruited, the sample size, restrictions on the sample (e.g., an age range, language spoken, or medical condition), and relevant sample characteristics that set the limits on generalizability of study findings (e.g., age, education, occupation). The subsection also gives the response rate or the number of invited subjects who actually agreed to participate in the study, as well as the attrition rate. It may also include the informed consent procedure, or that information may be given in the subsection on data collection procedures. The characteristics of the sample may be presented in the narrative of the final research report or in a table.

A proposal for research includes the power analysis calculations to justify the number of subjects to be included. The final report may include a power analysis stating the obtained power, given the actual sample size and the effect size of the study findings.

The first example of the sample subsection was taken from a proposal for a longitudinal study of functional status during pregnancy and the postpartum. The excerpt includes the typical content of the sample subsection as well as a justification for the longitudinal study design.

Example: Sample Description in a Research Proposal

The proposed study is a prospective panel study designed to explore functional status during pregnancy and the first six months following childbirth. Subjects will be followed longitudinally, and data will be collected at the end of each trimester of pregnancy: at 12 to 14 weeks, 25 to 27 weeks, and 36 to 37 weeks of gestation; and at four points after delivery: 3 weeks, 6 weeks, 3 months, and 6 months postpartum. The pregnancy intervals were based on the traditional divisions of the prenatal period noted in the literature. The postpartum intervals were based on data from our retrospective study (Tulman & Fawcett, 1988a) and the preliminary findings from our current study (Tulman & Fawcett, 1988b), which indicate these are the times when changes in functional status occur after childbirth. Data for the end of the third trimester will be collected at 36 to 37 weeks of gestation rather than at 38–40 weeks of gestation to avoid losing third trimester data on women who deliver at term but up to two weeks before their due dates. This longitudinal panel design was selected in preference to a cross-sectional/short-term longitudinal design because the number of subjects required for the mixed design would be prohibitive from a budgetary viewpoint as well as would preclude examination of within-subject changes over an extended period of time.

Subject recruitment will continue until 291 women are enrolled in the study. It is anticipated that there will be a 20% voluntary attrition rate, allowing for a doubling of the rate over our current study's attrition rate of 10% because women in the proposed study will be followed for 12 months rather than 6 months. Of the anticipated remaining 233 women who will complete the study, we estimate that approximately 10% will develop a major complication during pregnancy, delivery, or the postpartum (e.g., premature delivery, infant with a life-threatening birth defect, eclampsia, pulmonary embolus), or have a multiple birth, even though they were categorized as low-risk at the time of recruitment. The women who experience a major complication but deliver a viable infant will continue to be followed, although their data will not be included with the other subjects' in the data analysis. Women who experience an intrauterine or neonatal death will not continue to be followed for this study. Given that type of delivery is a variable, cesarean delivery, per se, will not preclude continuation in the main study. The resulting remaining sample of 210 subjects is sufficient to allow an alpha level of .05, a power of .80, and a medium effect size for the multiple regression analyses to be done for the proposed study (Cohen, 1977). Of course, during data collection, should it become apparent that our attrition rate is either higher or lower than our estimates, we will increase or decrease our initial recruitment estimates accordingly.

The sample will be limited to married English-speaking women over 18 years of age who have no underlying medical problems (e.g., diabetes, chronic renal or cardiac disease) or preexisting factors in their obstetrical histories (e.g., previous premature delivery, history of incompetent cervix) that would classify them as high-risk at the time of recruitment during the first trimester of pregnancy. Even given these sampling criteria, we do recognize that some of our sample will develop complications during pregnancy or after delivery and/or deliver infants who are either premature and/or ill. This small group of high-risk subjects (approximately 23) will continue to be followed in the study, and their data will be analyzed separately as pilot data for a future study of functional status during pregnancy and postpartum among high-risk women.

Subjects will be recruited by trained research assistants from large obstetrical and nurse-midwifery practices. (See Appendix for letters of access.) Informed consent will be obtained when subjects are recruited. A copy of the consent form is in the Appendix. Subjects will be compensated for their time by a payment of $10 at the end of each of the first six sessions and a payment of $25 at the end of the last session (total payment = $85 per subject). (Tulman & Fawcett, 1990–1993)

The next example was taken from a report published in a journal. The study was designed to determine the relationship of psychosocial variables to maternal depressive symptoms and parenting attitudes, as well as the relationships of psychosocial variables, depressive symptoms, and parenting attitudes to children's behavior.

Example: Narrative Sample Description in a Research Report

Mothers were recruited in clinics of a county health department. Inclusion criteria were: (a) at least 18 years of age; (b) never married, widowed, divorced, or separated at least 6 months; (c) family income at or below 185% of poverty level; and (d) at least one child between one and four years of age. Of the women approached, 89% agreed to participate. The final sample consisted of 225 mothers. At the time of recruitment, one child for each mother was identified as the index child.

The mean age of the mothers was 25.8 years (SD = 4.9), with a range of 18 to 48 years. More than 90% of the sample reported an annual household income under $10,000. The majority had never married (63.6%) and were unemployed (66.7%). The mothers had a mean of 11.4 years of education (SD = 2.0), but more than half (54.6%) had at least a high school education. The mothers had a mean of 2.4 children (SD = 1.2, range 1 – 7). The majority of the index children were females (57%). (Hall et al., 1991, p. 215)

The following example illustrates how the sample characteristics can be presented in a table. The excerpt was taken from a study of the social support needs of family caregivers of severely mentally ill patients.

Example: Sample Description in Narrative and Table Forms in a Research Report

The sample consisted of 60 family members who were identified as the primary caregiver for their relative, lived in the patient's household, were not financially reimbursed for the care they provided, and had been providing care for a minimum of six weeks. Three groups of 20 family caregivers were obtained from three age groups of patients who met standard diagnostic criteria (American Psychiatric Association, 1987) for the following diagnoses: (a) children with pervasive developmental disorders; (b) adults with schizophrenic or bipolar disorders; and (c) elderly persons with Alzheimer's-type dementias. Patients who had chronic physical illnesses that required special caregiving were not included in the study.

Subjects were recruited from public and private mental health agencies and through family volunteer organizations. Demographic characteristics of the three groups are shown in Table [6 – 2]. The age differences

TABLE 6-2. Sample Characteristics Presented in a Table

Demographic Characteristics of the Groups (N = 60)

	Total	Child	Adult	Elderly
CAREGIVERS				
Mean age	55.8	48.3	56.7	62.4
Age range	27–85	27–65	33–79	29–85
Mean years educ.	14.6	14.8	15.0	13.9
Educ. range	6–26	6–26	9–21	6–21
Percent female	80.0	95.0	75.0	70.0
Percent married	76.7	70.0	70.0	90.0
Percent white	83.3	95.0	70.0	85.0
Percent employed	46.7	65.0	60.0	15.0
PATIENTS				
Mean age	41.9	17.2*	32.3	76.1
Age range	7–88	7–28	20–56	55–88
Mean years educ.†	12.0	9.3	12.6	13.8
Educ. range	2–20	2–18	2–20	6–20
Percent female	45.0	25.0	35.0	75.0
Percent married	21.7	0	10.0	55.0

The high mean age of these children reflects the fact that some subjects had cared for their child since an initial psychiatric diagnosis many years ago.

†*Includes special education classes.*

Source: From Norbeck, Chaftez, Skodol-Wilson, & Weiss, 1991, p. 209, with permission.

among groups are consistent with the generational stage of life of the caregivers. (Norbeck, Chaftez, Skodol-Wilson, & Weiss, 1991, p. 208)

The final example of the sample subsection illustrates how a power analysis can be presented in a research report. The study was designed to determine the effect of six different interventions on pain reduction during neonatal circumcision. The sample included 121 full-term neonates. Using a random procedure, 20 neonates were assigned to each of the five experimental intervention groups and 21 neonates were assigned to the control group. A special feature of the description of this power analysis is the inclusion of the analysis to calculate sample size prior to conduct of the study and the obtained power based on the study results.

Example: Power Analysis in a Research Report

A power analysis was done to estimate sample size which demonstrated that 20 participants per group, alpha = .05, effect size = .35, would yield ANOVA power of .88 (Cohen, 1988). The power analysis was repeated, calculating the effect size for each ANOVA with this study's means and standard deviations. The power was at least .88 in each analysis. (Marchette, Main, Redick, Bagg, & Leatherland, 1991, p. 242)

Instruments

The instruments subsection includes the name and psychometric properties of each instrument. A statement linking the instrument with the concept that it measures is included. Evidence of validity and reliability also is included. Final reports present reliability coefficients for the study sample. A brief description of the items for each questionnaire and the scale used to rate the items are given. The range of possible scores is noted, and interpretation of scores is explained.

The example features a description of an instrument developed by the first author of the study. As the investigators explained, the instrument was used to measure chronic stressors in their study of psychosocial predictors of maternal depressive symptoms, parenting attitudes, and child behavior in single-parent families.

Example: Description of an Instrument

The 20-item Everyday Stressors Index (ESI; Hall, 1983) measures chronic daily stressors faced by mothers with young children. Mothers rated how much each problem worried, upset, or bothered them from day to day on a 4-point scale ranging from *not at all bothered* (0) to *bothered a great deal* (3). Item values were summed for a total score ranging from 0 to 60. Construct validity of the index was supported by discrimination of everyday stressors from maternal depressive and psychosomatic symptoms (Hall, 1983; Hall, 1987). Cronbach's alpha in this sample was 0.82, comparing favorably to previous alphas of 0.80 to 0.85 (Hall et al., 1985; Hall, 1987). (Hall et al., 1991, p. 215)

Procedure

The procedure subsection provides a concise but detailed description of the data collection procedures. The procedure used to recruit subjects is explained if it has not been noted in the sample subsection. Data collectors are identified, and any special training required for data collection is explained. The setting for data collection is identified and, if more than one instrument is used, the order of administration is noted. The time required for data collection also is noted, as is any financial compensation given to subjects. Furthermore, the procedure for obtaining informed consent is explained in this subsection if it has not been described in the sample subsection. In experimental studies, the procedure subsection presents a description of the experimental and control conditions.

This subsection usually is shorter in a journal article than it is in a proposal or unpublished report, such as a dissertation. Regardless of space limitations, however, the essential information about the procedures used to collect the data is required.

The first example is the procedure subsection of a proposal for a longitudinal study of functional status during pregnancy and the postpartum. Here the procedures are not only explained but also justified by a citation of a related study.

Example: Description of Procedures in a Research Proposal

Subjects will be recruited from obstetrical and nurse-midwifery practices. The obstetricians and nurse-midwives will identify potential subjects who meet the sampling criteria for the proposed study. Potential subjects will be approached by the research assistants, and informed consent will be obtained from those agreeing to participate in the study.

Data will be collected by trained research assistants, who will be graduate students in nursing, in the subjects' homes at the end of the second and third trimesters of pregnancy and at 3 weeks, 6 weeks, 3 months, and 6 months following delivery. Preliminary findings from our ongoing study (Tulman & Fawcett, 1988b) have revealed that home visits enhance retention of subjects and the quality of the data obtained. Data collection for the first trimester will be done either at the time of subject recruitment or at a later scheduled home visit. The data collectors will be trained in clinical interviewing techniques and eliciting health histories. Each subject will be followed by the same data collector to allow a building of rapport (and thereby decrease attrition) as well as to follow up on topics raised by the subjects. Each home visit will be scheduled in advance by telephone at a mutually convenient time. A Background Data Sheet, the Inventory of Functional Status-Antepartum Period, the Symptoms Checklist, and the Prenatal Self-Evaluation Questionnaire will be administered at each prenatal visit. A Background Data Sheet, the Inventory of Functional Status After Childbirth, the Infant Characteristics Questionnaire and the Postpartum Self-Evaluation Questionnaire will be administered at each postpartum visit. These instruments will be administered in random order at each visit for each subject to control for order effects. In addition, the Open-Ended Questionnaire will be administered as the last instrument at the last home visit. Subjects' responses to the Open-Ended Questionnaire will be audiotaped. It is anticipated that each visit will take no more than one hour. At the conclusion of each visit, the subject will be financially compensated for her participation in the study. (Tulman & Fawcett, 1990–1993)

The next example was taken from a journal article. The excerpt is from a study that used grounded theory methodology to generate a descriptive theory of adults' life experiences following the suicide of a family member. The investigator referred to the study subjects as survivors.

Example: Description of Procedures for Theory-Generating Research in a Journal Article

In-depth interviews, averaging 90 minutes in length, were conducted an average of 5.8 months after the suicide. Interviews were held in survivors' homes or the researcher's office. Written informed consent was secured from all subjects. Written consent to audiotape interviews also was obtained from all but two subjects. In the latter situations, the interviews were documented through extensive field notes. An interview guide consisting of open-ended questions and associated probes was used to facilitate the interview process with each subject. The guide was not used as a structured questionnaire, rather it served only as a reminder to the researcher to explore various issues with the subjects if they were not spontaneously addressed during the interview.

Descriptive field notes were kept to document information related to details of individual interviews (i.e., nonverbal behaviors and other contextual information). Reflective field notes, documenting the researcher's own responses to the interviews and the overall research process, were also recorded in a field journal. (Van Dongen, 1990, p. 225)

The following example also was taken from a journal article. The excerpt is from a study that tested a theoretical path model of adaptation in a sample of patients with multiple sclerosis.

Example: Description of Procedures for Theory-Testing Research in a Journal Article

Most subjects were screened by the researcher during their outpatient clinic visit. In a few cases, the researcher was unable to screen the potential subject in clinic because of time constraints. These subjects were called within 48 hours of their clinic visit and screened by telephone. Informed consent was obtained both orally and in writing. Of the individuals who met sampling criteria, only 6 (4.8%) declined to participate. Data were collected during a 2-hour interview using a combination of standardized instruments and a semi-structured format. Ninety-seven of the 118 interviews were conducted in the subjects' homes. Seven of the interviews were done while the person was receiving cytoxan, six as inpatients and one as an outpatient. Data were collected in the clinic for 11 people and at the individual's place of work for 3 subjects. (Wineman, 1990, p. 296)

The next example of the procedure subsection illustrates the description of experimental and control conditions in an experimental study. The excerpt was taken from a study of interventions designed to reduce pain during neonatal circumcision. One control and five experimental interventions were tested. The control condition was no nurses present and no pain reduction interventions used. The experimental conditions were classical music, intrauterine sounds, pacifier, music and pacifier, and intrauterine sounds and pacifier.

Example: Description of Experimental and Control Conditions

The 121 neonates were randomly assigned to six groups as follows. The 21 control group neonates received the usual care: no nurses present and no pain reduction interventions used. Neonates in the treatment groups received the treatments from the time they were placed on the restraint board until the time they were removed from the board.

The 20 neonates in the Music Group (M) heard a tape recording of classical music selected for [the] relaxing effect on neonates (Bonnytapes, Salina, KS). The 20 neonates in the Intrauterine Sounds Group (I) heard a commercially prepared tape of intrauterine heartbeat and circulation

sounds (Rock-a-Bye Bear, Dakin & Co, San Francisco, CA). The 20 neonates in the Pacifier Group (P) were encouraged to suck on a pacifier by
gentle nudging of the tongue whenever sucking did not occur for more
than 30 seconds (Hushmaster Soother model, Binky-Griptight, Walling-
ton, NJ). The 20 neonates in the Music Plus Pacifier Group (MP) listened
to the neonatal relaxing classical music while also sucking on a pacifier.
The 20 neonates in the Intrauterine Sounds Plus Pacifier Group (IP)
listened to the intrauterine sounds tape while also sucking on a pacifier.
(Marchette et al., 1991, p. 242)

Study Timetable. The procedure section of a proposal for research may
also include a timetable for the study. The timetable indicates how long
each phase of the study is expected to take, including training of research
assistants, subject recruitment, data collection, data analysis, and preparation of the research report. An example of a timetable was taken from a
longitudinal study of functional status, with data collection encompassing each trimester of pregnancy and the first 6 months postpartum.

Example: Study Timetable in a Research Proposal

The proposed study will take 36 months to complete. The timetable
is presented in Table [6–3]. (Tulman & Fawcett, 1990–1993)

TABLE 6–3. Example of a Study Timetable

Timetable for Study of Functional Status during Pregnancy and the Postpartum

Prefunding phase	Pilot Inventory of Functional Status — Antepartum Period
Months 1–2	Recruit and train research assistants
Months 3–20	Begin recruitment of subjects
	Begin data collection
	Begin data entry on computer
Month 21	Complete subject recruitment
Months 22–32	Continue data collection
	Continue data entry
	Begin preliminary data analysis
Month 33	Complete data collection
	Complete data entry
	Complete preliminary data analysis
Months 34–36	Complete final data analysis
	Prepare research reports

Source: From Tulman & Fawcett, 1990–1993.

Human Subjects Protocol. Research proposals frequently include a detailed discussion of the protocol for obtaining informed consent and protection of human subjects. When a study involves animals rather than or in addition to human beings as subjects, procedures for the care of the animals are included. The example was taken from a proposal for a study of functional status that used a sample of pregnant and postpartal women.

Example: Human Subjects Protocol in a Research Proposal

Characteristics of the Subject Population
Subjects recruited will be married English-speaking women over 18 years of age who are in the first trimester of pregnancy and who have no underlying medical problems (e.g., diabetes, chronic renal or cardiac disease). Each subject will be followed from the end of the first trimester of pregnancy through 6 months postpartum. Pregnant women are necessary subjects because the study is an investigation of functional status during pregnancy and after childbirth.

Sources of Research Material
Subjects will be identified only by code numbers. No reference to individuals will be made in any published reports of the proposed study. Data will be obtained only for research purposes.

Recruitment of Subjects and Consent Procedures
Potential subjects will be approached while having a prenatal visit with their obstetrician or nurse-midwife. The proposed study will be explained to potential subjects by a trained research assistant. Potential subjects will be asked to review the consent form with the research assistant and sign the consent form if they wish to participate in the study. Potential subjects will be told that willingness to participate or not participate in the study will in no way affect their medical or nursing care. Subjects will be compensated a modest sum ($85) for their time spent during the seven one-hour data collection sessions. Letters confirming access to the subject recruitment sites are in the Appendix. A copy of the consent form is in the Appendix.

Potential Risks
There is minimal risk involved.

Protection of Subjects
Confidentiality will be safeguarded through a system of coding on all research instruments. Subjects will be identified only by code numbers

on research instruments. A master list will contain the names, addresses, and telephone numbers of subjects and their corresponding code numbers. This list will be kept in a locked file and be made available only to the investigators and research assistants. The master list will be destroyed at the earliest possible time after all data are collected and a summary of the study results is mailed to subjects who have requested them. No reference to individuals will be made in any published reports of the proposed study. Data will be obtained and used only for research purposes.

Risk/Benefit Ratio
There are no specific direct benefits, other than a modest sum of money for study participation, to be gained by individual subjects. Societal benefits would include objective data upon which to base maternity leave/compensation policies and legislation and interventions to facilitate improved functional status during pregnancy and after delivery. The potential benefits of the proposed study to society far outweigh the potential of minimal risk for individual subjects. (Tulman & Fawcett, 1990–1993)

Data Analysis Plan

The subsection for the data analysis plan includes an explanation of how the data are to be or were processed. When qualitative data are collected, the data analysis plan specifies the specific content analysis techniques used. When the data are quantitative, the plan usually includes measures of central tendency and variability, a correlation matrix of all major research variables, and the inferential statistical test for each relationship being examined.

The data analysis plan from a proposal for a longitudinal study of functional status during pregnancy and the postpartum exemplifies this subsection for a theory-testing study that included collection of both quantitative and qualitative data.

Example: Plan for Analysis of Quantitative and Qualitative Data in a Research Proposal

Quantitative data will be coded and entered into a computer for analysis using a statistical package. Wherever possible, data will be analyzed on a personal computer using SPSS/PC+. If necessary, the data can be uploaded onto a mainframe and SPSS-X used for data analysis. Internal consistency reliabilities will be calculated for the Inventory of Functional Status-Antepartum Period (IFSAP), the Inventory of Functional Status After Childbirth (IFSAC), the Symptoms Checklist, the Prenatal Self-Evaluation Questionnaire, the Postpartum Self-Evaluation Questionnaire, and the Infant Characteristics Questionnaire for the study subjects. Interrater reliability will be established for the Open-Ended Questionnaire. Frequency distributions and measures of central tendency and variability will be calculated for all variables. Normality and equality of variances will be assessed in the relevant continuous variables, and normalizing transformations will be considered where appropriate. Correlation matrices will be constructed for all variables. The determinant of the correlation matrix of the independent variables will be examined for evidence of multicollinearity (Pedhazur, 1982).

Data related to the FIRST AIM of the proposed study will be subjected to two separate repeated measures analyses of variance: the first repeated measures analysis of variance will examine the changes in functional status over the three data collection points of pregnancy, i.e., the IFSAP scores obtained at the end of the first, second, and third trimesters; the second repeated measures analysis of variance will examine the changes in postpartum functional status over the four data collection points after delivery, i.e., the IFSAC scores obtained at 3 weeks, 6 weeks, 3 months, and 6 months postpartum. Post hoc Scheffé tests will be used in both analyses if an F ratio is significant at the .05 level to determine when the changes in functional status occurred.

Because of the number of variables involved, data related to the SECOND, THIRD, FOURTH, and FIFTH AIMS of the proposed study will first be subjected to correlational analysis to determine which of the independent variables at each point in time correlate with functional status at that timepoint. Second, those variables that demonstrate statistically significant correlations ($p<.05$) and at least medium effect sizes ($r = .30$) with functional status will be then subjected to multivariate analyses of variance (MANOVA). Two separate MANOVAs with functional status over time as the dependent variables will be done for each set of independent variables (i.e., health, individual psychosocial, family, and demographic variable sets) — one for the three time intervals of pregnancy; the second for the four time intervals of the postpartum. Each MANOVA procedure will be further tested by multiple regression analyses for each time interval (i.e., the three trimesters of pregnancy and the four data collection periods of the postpartum) if the overall MANOVA F test is significant at the .05 level.

For the analysis of data to answer the SIXTH AIM, the health, individual psychosocial, family and demographic variables that were found to be statistically significantly related to functional status will be entered as sets (i.e., health, individual psychosocial, family, and demographic) into separate stepwise multiple regressions to analyze the relative importance, in terms of variance accounted for, of functional status for each time interval of pregnancy and the postpartum.

The order of entry of variables for all multiple regression analyses will be selected by the computer program because the literature does not reveal any a priori hierarchical order. The Bonferroni adjustment (alpha/ number of tests) will be used to set the maximum probability of a Type I error among all multiple regressions at alpha = .05.

Qualitative data from the Open-Ended Questionnaire will be analyzed by means of content analysis to categorize subjects' audiotaped and transcribed responses to the questions.

The overall study results will provide evidence related to the SEVENTH AIM of the proposed study. More specifically, the study findings will provide evidence of the credibility of Roy's (1984) Adaptation Model of Nursing. If relationships between study variables are established (e.g., between health variables and functional status), it may be concluded that the model is credible. If, however, relationships are not found, the credibility of the model will be questioned. Furthermore, the findings from the content analysis of responses to the Open-Ended Questionnaire, as well as subjects' additional comments on the IFSAP and IFSAC, will provide evidence of the utility of Roy's conceptual model for research investigating variables associated with changes in functional status during pregnancy and the postpartum. (Tulman & Fawcett, 1990–1993)

The next example was taken from a journal article. The excerpt exemplifies the data analysis plan for theory-generating research using grounded theory methodology. The study was designed to describe the life experiences of adults following the suicide death of a family member. A special feature of this example is the investigator's discussion of efforts to limit bias in the data analysis phase of the study.

Example: Plan for Analysis of Qualitative Data in a Journal Article

Interview transcripts were coded using Glaser's (1978) process of "open substantive" coding in which the data were examined, line by line, to identify the substance of what the data actually represent. For example, subjects often described experiences involving anger. Accordingly, such data were coded or labeled as *anger* and descriptive comments made on the transcripts. The process of coding overlapped with the process of concept formation in which data were continually coded, compared, and recoded until patterns or categories began to emerge. The initial level concepts that emerged from the substantive coding were transferred to a computer-based word processing program with sort capabilities. Similar initial level concepts from multiple transcripts were then grouped together and/or combined with other concepts. Patterns and categories emerged as the coded data and concepts were found to cluster in meaningful ways. Concurrent with the process of identifying conceptual categories and linkages, emerging theoretical ideas were preserved through written memos. These theoretical memos were critical in refining conceptual relationships and in eventually developing an integrated theoretical framework.

Efforts to limit potential bias included recognition of the researcher's responses in the field journal and periodic evaluation of transcripts and data analysis sheets by several research colleagues for leading interview behaviors and/or biased interpretations of data by the researcher. This process of peer review or "member check" has been suggested by Guba and Lincoln (1981) as a means of ensuring the credibility of the data. The researcher also used the validity check, "phenomenon recognition" (Guba & Lincoln), whereby 4 subjects review the theoretical description of SOS [survivors of suicide] reported life experiences. The subjects agreed that the researcher's conceptualization of their overall experience was accurate. (Van Dongen, 1990, p. 225)

The following example of a data analysis plan was taken from a journal article reporting the results of theory-testing research. The study was a replication of a test of the influence of mediating variables on the relationship between uncertainty in illness and emotional distress. The plan provides the detail needed to facilitate the reader's understanding of a complex statistical technique.

Example: Plan for Analysis of Quantitative Data in a Journal Article

Regression analysis was used to test the mediating effects of mastery and coping following the procedure described by Baron and Kenny

(1986) and applied in the initial test of the [theoretical] model (Mishel & Sorenson, 1991). To test for mediating effects of each mediator, three regression equations were run. The mediator was regressed on the independent variable, the dependent variable was regressed on the independent variable, and the dependent variable was regressed on both the independent variable and the mediators. In order to have the appropriate conditions to test the mediation effect of a variable, the independent variable must have a significant relationship with the mediating variable and with the dependent variable, plus the mediator must significantly account for variation in the dependent variable. When both the independent variable and mediating variable are entered on the dependent variable, the strength of the relationship between the independent and dependent variable should decrease. The ideal case is a reduction in the magnitude of the beta so that the path is insignificant. (Mishel, Padilla, Grant, & Sorenson, 1991, p. 238)

Results

The results section is structured according to specific aims or hypotheses. The results section of theory-generating research reports presents the concepts and propositions that emerged from the data analysis. In theory-testing research, this section starts with descriptive statistics for the major concepts of the theory, including measures of central tendency and variability. Statistical procedures used to test each hypothesis or analyze the data related to each specific aim are identified if a separate data analysis plan is not included in the report. The findings for each statistical test are presented, and a definitive conclusion is drawn with regard to the support or lack of support for each hypothesis that was tested.

Tables and figures can be used to supplement the narrative research results. Regardless of the format(s) used for presentation of the results, sufficient data should be presented to permit calculation of effect sizes for power analysis and future meta-analysis.

Presentation of Theory-Generating Research Results

The following example was taken from a theory-generating study of the life experiences of adults 3 to 9 months after the suicide death of a family member. The study was guided by grounded theory methodology. In this narrative excerpt, the investigator identified the main concept (the core variable) that emerged from the data, along with the dimensions of the main concept (the conceptual categories).

Example: Narrative Presentation of Theory-Generating Research Results

Agonizing questioning was identified as the *core variable* or process that represented the core or heart of the phenomenon under study (Glaser & Strauss, 1967; Stern, 1980). A repetitive theme of questioning why the suicide occurred, as well as questioning the implications of the death for the personal lives of the subject and other survivors, was apparent in survivors' reports of their experiences both immediately after the death and for months later.

Upon identification of the core variable, meaningful relationships among conceptual categories soon became apparent. Data were found to fit into a concise theoretical description. Evidence of persistent questioning in the lives of survivors was apparent in subjects' descriptions of emotional turmoil, cognitive dissonance, physical disturbances, and altered socialization. It was also found that searching for answers to these questions was a major survival strategy or effort by survivors to cope with the impact of the suicide on their lives. Although all subjects reported having some questions related to the suicide, there appeared to be definite differences in the survivors' perceptions of the suicide victim before the death. (Van Dongen, 1990, p. 225)

The next example demonstrates how the narrative presentation of theory-generating research results can be supplemented by a diagram. Figure 6–2 was taken from the report of a grounded theory study of recovery from chemical dependency. The diagram depicts the major concepts of the theory of recovery. In the published report, the presentation of the diagram was followed by a detailed narrative description of each concept and its categories.

Example: Diagram of Theory-Generating Research Results

The stages and phases of the basic social psychological process of self-integration are depicted in Figure [6–2]. (Hutchinson, 1987, p. 340)

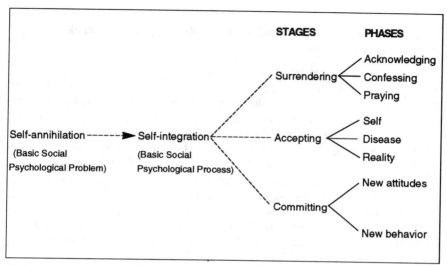

Figure 6–2.   Diagram of results of a theory-generating study. (From Hutchinson, 1987, p. 340, with permission.)

Presentation of Theory-Testing Research Results
Theory-testing research reports present descriptive statistics for the study concepts as well as the results of inferential statistical tests.

Descriptive Statistics. The following excerpt exemplifies the presentation of descriptive statistics in narrative form. In this example, the measures of central tendency and variability are given for the three dependent variables of maternal depressive symptoms, parenting attitudes, and children's behavior. The investigators not only gave the means, standard deviations, and ranges for the entire sample but also presented data for comparisons of subsamples based on various demographic characteristics.

Example: Narrative Presentation of Measures of Central Tendency and Variability

The mean CES-D [Center for Epidemiological Studies – Depression Scale] score of the mothers was 19.2 (SD = 10.3; range 0 – 52); 59.6% of the mothers scored in the high range (CES-D ≥ 16). Employed mothers reported lower CES-D scores than unemployed mothers (16.1 versus 20.7; $t(223) = 3.23, p = 0.001$). There were no significant differences in depressive symptoms by race. Mean scores on the CES-D were higher for separated mothers than for divorced mothers (20.8 versus 14.6; $p = .04$). There were no differences among other marital status categories.

The mean score for parenting attitudes was 66.2 (SD = 8.8; range 34 – 80). Employed mothers reported more positive parenting attitudes than unemployed mothers [$t(223) = -2.51, p = .01$]. There were no differences in parenting attitudes by mothers' race or marital status, or by gender of the index child.

The mean PBQ [Preschool Behavior Questionnaire] score was 19.5 (SD = 8.1; range 3 – 42). PBQ scores did not differ by the mothers' employment status, race, or marital status, nor did they differ by gender of the index child. (Hall et al., 1991, pp. 216 – 217)

The example given below illustrates the presentation of descriptive statistics for the dependent variable in a table. Table 6 – 4 was taken from an experimental study of the effects of a nursing intervention based on the theory of reasoned action on medical regimen compliance. Measures of intention to comply with five regimen prescriptions were obtained during hospitalization, and actual compliance with the prescriptions was measured at 1 and 2 years following hospital discharge.

Example: Presentation of Measures of Central Tendency and Variability in a Table

A separate analysis was run for each of the five regimen prescriptions: diet, smoking, activity, stress, and medication. The means and standard deviations are shown in Table [6 – 4]. (Miller et al., 1990, p. 335)

The next excerpt exemplifies the narrative presentation of descriptive statistics associated with correlational analyses, including the matrix of correlations between independent variables and data regarding analy-

TABLE 6–4. Measures of Central Tendency and Variability Presented in a Table

Means and Standard Deviations of Intention and Compliance Scores by Group, Prescription, and Time

| | HOSPITAL INTENTIONS | | HOME COMPLIANCE | | | |
| | | | 1 YEAR | | 2 YEARS | |
	M	(SD)	M	(SD)	M	(SD)
	CONTROL GROUP					
Prescriptions	N = 57		N = 42		N = 22	
Diet	17.21	(2.82)	14.47	(4.07)	12.00	(3.42)
Smoking	16.86	(3.98)	17.14	(3.67)	13.44	(3.74)
Activity	18.67	(1.65)	14.81	(3.93)	12.57	(4.41)
Stress	16.81	(2.66)	15.33	(3.65)	13.24	(4.57)
Medicines	19.63	(.76)	18.95	(1.78)	19.21	(2.99)
	EXPERIMENTAL GROUP					
	N = 58		N = 39		N = 29	
Diet	17.00	(2.66)	14.32	(4.29)	15.00	(4.08)
Smoking	18.00	(2.19)	10.17	(7.39)	10.00	(6.07)
Activity	18.44	(1.90)	15.09	(3.59)	14.17	(4.43)
Stress	17.54	(2.21)	15.42	(3.96)	15.42	(3.81)
Medicines	18.87	(1.79)	18.65	(2.23)	18.69	(3.69)

Note: Intention and compliance score = 20.

Source: From Miller, Wikoff, Garrett, McMahon, & Smith, 1990, p. 335, with permission.

sis of residuals. The excerpt is taken from a study designed to test the theory of uncertainty in illness.

Example: Narrative Presentation of Descriptive Statistics for a Correlational Analysis

Inspection of the correlation matrix ruled out multicollinearity. Residuals were checked and met the assumptions of the statistical and causal model (Fertetich & Veran, 1984). (Mishel & Sorenson, 1991, p. 169)

The next example illustrates presentation of descriptive statistics associated with correlational analysis in tables. In the accompanying narrative, the investigator explained how subsequent inferential statistical tests were influenced by the correlations obtained. The excerpt was taken from a study that tested a theoretical path model of adaptation to multiple sclerosis. Adaptation was represented by two concepts: depression and purpose in life. The instrument measuring supportive and unsupportive types of social support included subscales for socialization, tangible assistance, advice and guidance, social reinforcement, and emotional sustenance. One table contains the correlations between the subscales for each type of social support and the two concepts representing adaptation. The other table contains a correlation matrix of the main study concepts.

Example: Presentation of Descriptive Statistics for a Correlational Analysis in Tables

Based on the relationships between the types of social support and psychosocial adaptation reported in Table [6–5], two decisions were made about the subsequent strategy for the path analysis. The first decision involved computing two separate paths, one using depression as the outcome variable and one using purpose in life. Although depression and purpose in life were related, $r = -.69$, $p < .001$ (Table [6–6]), keeping them statistically separate could facilitate theoretical understanding of the different pathways through which the perception of supportive and unsupportive encounters operate to influence different aspects of psychosocial adaptation. The second decision involved using only the overall measures of supportiveness and unsupportiveness in the path analyses,

TABLE 6–5.   Correlations Presented in a Table

Simple Correlation Coefficients: Types of Support and Adaptation

	PSYCHOSOCIAL ADAPTATION	
Type of Supportiveness	Depression	Purpose in Life
Socialization	−.18*	.22†
Tangible assistance	−.01	.02
Advice and guidance	−.02	.21†
Social reinforcement	−.13	.27‡
Emotional sustenance	−.02	.23†
Type of Unsupportiveness		
Socialization	.26†	−.24†
Tangible assistance	.40‡	−.35‡
Advice and guidance	.36‡	−.31‡
Social reinforcement	.26†	−.20*
Emotional sustenance	.31‡	−.26†

Note: N = 118.

*p ≤ .05.

†p ≤ .01.

‡p ≤ .001.

Source: From Wineman, 1990, p. 296, with permission.

because the different types of supportive and unsupportive interactions were consistently related to either depression or purpose in life, or both (Table [6–5]). (Wineman, 1990, p. 297)

Results of Statistical Tests. Three examples are given to illustrate various ways to present the results of inferential statistical tests for correlational and experimental studies. The first example illustrates the narrative and pictorial presentation of the results of hypothesis testing from a correlational study. The study was designed to test a theoretical model of relationships between predictability of events, control, anxiety, and coping effort in a sample of mothers of hospitalized acutely ill children.

TABLE 6–6. A Correlation Matrix

Intercorrelation Matrix for Study Variables

Variable	1	2	3	4	5	6	7	8
1. SEX								
2. AGE	.03							
3. SOCST	-.13	-.01						
4. PU	.01	-.13	.05					
5. FD	-.05	.27‡	-.26†	.05				
6. SUP	-.17*	-.20†	.07	-.01	-.08			
7. UNSUP	-.07	-.05	.06	.29‡	.06	-.09		
8. DEP	-.08	-.11	-.06	.47‡	.25†	-.09	.38‡	
9. PIL	.07	.04	.13	-.36‡	-.31‡	.25‡	-.34†	-.69‡

Note. $N = 118$. SEX = sex; AGE = age; SOCST = social status; PU = perceived uncertainty; FD = functional disability; SUP = supportiveness; UNSUP = unsupportiveness; DEP = depression; PIL = purpose in life.

*$p < .05$.

†$p < .01$.

‡$p < .001$.

Source: From Wineman, 1990, p. 297, with permission.

Example: Narrative and Pictorial Presentation of Results of Statistical Tests for a Correlational Study

The results of the regression analysis are shown in Figure [6 – 3]. The first hypothesis, that predictability of events would have a direct positive impact on control and a subsequent negative impact on anxiety, was not supported. However, in accordance with the second hypothesis, predictability of events did have a direct negative impact on anxiety ($\beta = -.667$, $R^2 = .347$) and an indirect negative impact on coping effort when mediated by anxiety.

The third hypothesis was not supported: control did not have an indirect negative impact on coping effort when mediated by anxiety. Finally, the fourth hypothesis was supported: anxiety had a strong positive impact on the outcome variable, coping effort ($\beta = .987$, $R^2 = .973$). (Schepp, 1991, p. 44)

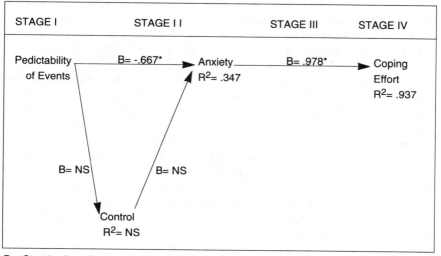

B = Standardized Regression Coefficient
NS = Not Significant
*$p < .05$

Figure 6 – 3. Diagram of the results of a theory-testing study. (Diagram adapted from Schepp, 1991, p. 45, with permission.)

The second example is an excerpt illustrating presentation of the findings for one hypothesis from an experimental study that tested the theory of reasoned action. The investigators hypothesized that "medical regimen compliance of MI [myocardial infarction] patients 2 years after hospitalization will be greater for the experimental group who received a nursing intervention than for a control group" (Miller et al., 1990, p. 333). Medical regimen compliance was measured by a questionnaire made up of subscales for five regimen prescriptions, including following diet, taking medications, performing activity, stopping smoking, and modifying responses to stress in home, work, sports, and social environments.

Example: Narrative Presentation of Results of Statistical Tests for an Experimental Study

Mean compliance scores at Year 2 for the experimental group were not significantly different from those of the control group for activity, stress, or medication prescriptions. There was a significant difference for diet, $F(1,49) = 15.88$, $p = .024$. There was a significant difference for smoking, also, but in the wrong direction, that is, there was less compliance for the experimental group at 2 years than for the control group. Therefore, Hypothesis I was not supported. (Miller et al., 1990, p. 335)

The third example, which was taken from an experimental study of interventions designed to reduce pain during neonatal circumcision, illustrates use of a table to augment the narrative presentation of statistical results. Six interventions were tested. The excerpt presents findings for heart rate, which was one outcome studied. Repeated measurements of outcomes were taken during the 14 steps of the circumcision procedure, which started with restraint of the infant and ended with application of gauze with petroleum jelly. Nine steps were considered invasive (e.g., apply Gomco clamp, Gomco clamp removed), and five steps were classified as noninvasive (e.g., restrain neonate on circumcision board, waiting for hemostasis).

Example: Presentation of Statistical Results for an Experimental Study in a Table

Mean heart rates of neonates in all six groups were above normal limits (110–180) during 6 to 9 of the 9 invasive steps; one neonate had heart rates as high as 295. No significant difference was found in the heart rates of the six groups using a repeated measures ANOVA during any

TABLE 6-7. Results of Analysis of Variance Presented in a Table

Repeated Measures Analysis of Variance of Heart Rate over 14 Steps of Neonatal Circumcision

Source	df	Sum of Squares	Mean Squares	F Ratio	p
HEART RATE					
Within cells	702	650529.17	926.68		
Steps	13	106740.44	8210.80	8.86	.0001
Groups by steps	65	50883.69	782.83	0.84	.8010
Within cells	54	359344.42	6654.53		
Groups	5	12286.37	2457.27	0.37	.8670

Source: Adapted from Marchette, Main, Redick, Bagg, & Leatherland, 1991, p. 243, with permission.

single step (Table [6-7]). There was a significant difference between the heart rates comparing the 14 steps, $p < .0001$. Heart rates increased as circumcision progressed, peaked during use of the clamp, and returned to original level by the end of the circumcision. (Marchette et al., 1991, p. 242)

Discussion

The discussion section also is structured according to specific aims or hypotheses. Results are not repeated in the discussion section, although they may be summarized for clarity in the narrative discussion. Rather, conclusions are drawn with regard to the empirical adequacy of the theory and the credibility of the conceptual model.

This section of a research report frequently includes a comparison of the study findings with results from related research. In theory-generating research, a comparison of the theory that was generated with extant theories may be included. The discussion section also may include alternative methodologic and/or substantive explanations for the study findings.

The discussion section frequently ends with the investigator's recommendations for future research. Reports of intervention studies typically present conclusions regarding the pragmatic adequacy of the theory that was tested. More specifically, a recommendation is offered regarding the implications of the study findings for clinical practice, such as formulation of practice guidelines or health policies.

Discussion of Empirical Adequacy

The following excerpt exemplifies discussion of the empirical adequacy of a theory of changes in functional status during the postpartum and the credibility of the Roy Adaptation Model, which guided the conduct of the study. Data for this longitudinal study were collected at 3 weeks, 6 weeks, 3 months, and 6 months postpartum. The instrument used to measure functional status included subscales for household activities, social and community activities, self-care activities, occupational activities, and infant care responsibilities.

Example: Discussion of Empirical Adequacy of a Theory and Credibility of a Conceptual Model

The results support the expectation derived from role theory that functional status in various aspects of life changes as the maternal role is taken on. The gradual resumption of usual role activities may reflect the adjustments required by the addition of a newborn to the family. Although these adjustments are understandable in the areas of household, social and community, and occupational activities, the finding that only a small percentage of women reported full resumption of self-care activities by 6 months postpartum was surprising. Inspection of the item scores revealed that the finding was largely due to women's reports of sitting more during the day and taking less frequent walks since the infant's birth.

Canonical analysis yielded a relatively parsimonious set of correlates of functional status and lends some credibility to the propositions of Roy's (1984) Adaptation Model inasmuch as several variables representing the physiologic, self-concept, and interdependence adaptive modes and contextual stimuli were correlated with the role function mode, represented by functional status. However, these relationships were not consistent over time. An important conclusion to be drawn from the canonical analysis is, therefore, that careful attention must be given to the specific time intervals when data are collected to examine functional status following childbirth. (Tulman, Fawcett, Groblewski, & Silverman, 1990, p. 74)

The next excerpt was taken from a report of the development of a theory of caring based on the findings of three phenomenological studies. The samples were of childbearing families. Here the investigator summarized the theory, compared it with another theory of caring, and contrasted the concept of caring as defined in the study with a similar concept: social support. This excerpt exemplifies the discussion section for theory-generating research.

Example: Discussion of Theory-Generating Research Results

Through three phenomenological studies, the five caring processes: knowing, being with, doing for, enabling, and maintaining belief were empirically identified and described. Ultimately, the following definition of caring was inductively derived: *Caring is a nurturing way of relating to a valued other toward whom one feels a personal sense of commitment and responsibility.*

Caring as defined through these three perinatal studies is very compatible with Gaut's philosophical analysis of caring. Gaut (1983) has stated that caring, at its very least, involves individual attention to and concern for another, individual responsibility for or providing for at some level, and individual regard, fondness, or attachment.

Although caring is most likely an aspect of all socially supportive relationships, not all caring relationships are experienced as social support. The proposed definition of caring may be contrasted with Cobb's (1976) definition of social support: "Information that one is cared for and loved; that one is valued and esteemed; and that one belongs to a network of mutual obligation" (pp. 300–301). The caveat between caring, as defined through these investigations, and social support, as defined by Cobb, is at the point of mutual obligation. (Swanson, 1991, p. 165)

The next example is taken from a study that tested a theory of psychosocial predictors of maternal depressive symptoms, parenting attitudes, and child behavior. The excerpt focuses on the findings for the test of the proposition that demographic variables, depressive symptoms, social resources including functional support, tangible support, the quality of family relationships and the quality of primary intimate relationships, coping strategies, and chronic stressors were related to parenting attitudes. Here the investigators summarized the results of the test of the proposition and introduced the possibility of another concept, contextual influence, as an alternative explanation for parenting attitudes.

Example: Discussion of Theory-Testing Research Results and an Alternative Substantive Explanation

Only depressive symptoms and the quality of the primary intimate relationship predicted parenting attitudes. These two factors plus controls [demographic variables] explained relatively little of the variance in parenting attitudes. Other explanatory variables, untapped by the measures used in this study, apparently were operating. Panaccione and Wahler (1986) emphasized the importance of the contextual influence of maternal depression and adult social relationships on parenting behavior. This contention is supported by the study findings. Further exploration of the predictors of parenting attitudes is warranted. (Hall et al., p. 218)

Methodologic explanations for study findings are exemplified by the following two excerpts. The first excerpt, which illustrates discussion of the sample, was taken from a study of the prevalence of substance abuse among nurses. The sample included 143 registered nurses and 1410 nonnurses who served as the comparison control group.

Example: Methodologic Explanation Related to the Sample

Due to the small sample size on which the prevalence rates for specific substances used by nurses were based ($n = 113$), caution should be used in interpreting the nurses' prevalence rates. This is because a difference of one percentage point in prevalence could occur as a result of the inclusion or exclusion of only one nurse. However, the conclusion suggested by the specific substance data — that prevalence among nurses is less than or equal to prevalence among controls — is supported by the overall drug and alcohol abuse prevalence rates. (Trinkoff, Eaton, & Anthony, 1991, p. 174)

The next excerpt illustrates an instrument-based explanation taken from a test of the mediating functions of mastery and coping in the uncertainty in illness theory. The focus is on reliability of the instrument used to measure mastery, which was .63. The two aspects of mastery that were studied were "mastery as either situationally specific or global in relation to uncertainty, and mastery as a mediator in the relationship between uncertainty and the appraisals of danger and opportunity" (Mishel & Sorenson, 1991, p. 167).

Example: Methodologic Explanation Related to the Instrument

Although the mastery scale performed adequately related to situational specificity versus global disposition and mastery as a mediator, the reliability of the mastery scale was slightly below the acceptable limit. According to Baron and Kenny (1986), measurement error in the mediator tends to produce an overestimate in the effect of the independent variable on the dependent variable. Such an effect was not found in the mediation of uncertainty and danger, but might explain the findings for the mediation of uncertainty and opportunity. Yet, others have reported that uncertainty is significantly related to a reduced sense of personal control such as enabling skill (Braden, 1990). Only further study can completely answer this question. (Mishel & Sorenson, 1991, p. 171)

Discussion of Pragmatic Adequacy

An example of a discussion of pragmatic adequacy is evident in the following excerpt from an experimental study of an intervention designed to reduce environmental stressors and thereby enhance the development of very low birth weight infants.

Example: Discussion of Pragmatic Adequacy

The findings extend those of Als et al. (1986; 1988) by demonstrating that the beneficial effects of developmental care can be achieved with the resources available in most nurseries. Of special note is the finding that the hospital stay for the study group was 2 weeks shorter than that for the control group, a difference that represents a cost savings of approximately $12,250 in base hospital rate per infant (excluding charges for items such as medications, treatments, and consultation fees), pointing to significant benefits to society as well as for the families of these infants. Most important, however, the results suggest that the developmental approach to the nursing care of very low birth weight infants holds great promise for reducing the continuing morbidity experienced by these infants. (Becker, Grunwald, Moorman, & Stuhr, 1991, p. 155).

CONCLUSION

The guidelines for writing research proposals and reports presented in this chapter continue the emphasis in this book on the relationship between theory and research. The guidelines were illustrated with examples drawn from both theory-generating and theory-testing research. The application of these guidelines should facilitate communication of what investigators plan to do and what they have actually done, always within the context of the relationship between theory and research.

REFERENCES

Becker, P. T., Grunwald, P. C., Moorman, J., & Stuhr, S. (1991). Outcomes of developmentally supportive nursing care for very low birth weight infants. *Nursing Research*, *40*, 150–155.

Hall, L. A., Gurley, D. N., Sachs, B., & Kryscio, R. J. (1991). Psychosocial predictors of maternal depressive symptoms, parenting attitudes, and child behavior in single-parent families. *Nursing Research*, *40*, 214–220.

Hutchinson, S. A. (1987). Toward self-integration: The recovery process of chemically dependent nurses. *Nursing Research*, *36*, 339–343.

Leidy, N. K. (1990). A structural model of stress, psychosocial resources, and symptomatic experience in chronic physical illness. *Nursing Research*, *39*, 230–236.

Marchette, L., Main, R., Redick, E., Bagg, A., & Leatherland, J. (1991). Pain reduction interventions during neonatal circumcision. *Nursing Research*, *40*, 241–244.

Miller, P., Wikoff, R., Garrett, M. J., McMahon, M., & Smith, T. (1990). Regimen compliance two years after myocardial infarction. *Nursing Research*, *39*, 333–336.

Mishel, M. H., Padilla, G., Grant, M., & Sorenson, D. S. (1991). Uncertainty in illness theory: A replication of the mediating effects of mastery and coping. *Nursing Research*, *40*, 236–240.

Mishel, M. H., & Sorenson, D. S. (1991). Uncertainty in gynecological cancer: A test of the mediating functions of mastery and coping. *Nursing Research*, *40*, 167–171.

Norbeck, J. S., Chaftez, L., Skodol-Wilson, H., & Weiss, S. J. (1991). Social support needs of family caregivers of psychiatric patients from three age groups. *Nursing Research*, *40*, 208–213.

Pender, N. J., Walker, S. N., Sechrist, K. R., & Frank-Stromborg, M. (1990). Predicting health-promoting lifestyles in the workplace. *Nursing Research*, *39*, 326–332.

Schepp, K. G. (1991). Factors influencing the coping effort of mothers of hospitalized children. *Nursing Research*, *40*, 42–46.

Swanson, K. M. (1991). Empirical development of a middle range theory of caring. *Nursing Research*, *40*, 161–166.

Trinkoff, A. M., Eaton, W. W., & Anthony, J. C. (1991). The prevalence of substance abuse among registered nurses. *Nursing Research*, *40*, 172–175.

Tulman, L., & Fawcett, J. (1990–1993). *Functional status during pregnancy and the postpartum*. Research grant proposal funded by the National Institutes of Health, National Center for Nursing Research, Grant No. 1 R01-NR02340.

Tulman, L., Fawcett, J., Groblewski, L., & Silverman, L. (1990). Changes in functional status after childbirth. *Nursing Research, 39*, 70–75.

Van Dongen, C. J. (1990). Agonizing questioning: Experiences of survivors of suicide victims. *Nursing Research, 39*, 224–229.

Wineman, N. M. (1990). Adaptation to multiple sclerosis: The role of social support, functional disability, and perceived uncertainty. *Nursing Research, 39*, 294–299.

ADDITIONAL READINGS

American Psychological Association (1983). *Publication manual of the American Psychological Association* (3rd ed.). Washington, DC: The Association.

Blenner, J. L. (1990). Writing the qualitative grant proposal while meeting quantitative criteria: Walking on eggshells. *Florida Nursing Review, 4*(3), 5–9.

Brooks-Brunn, J. A. (1991). Tips on writing a research-based manuscript: The review of literature. *Nurse Author & Editor, 1*(2), 1–3.

Hunter, J. E., & Schmidt, F. L. (1990). *Methods of meta-analysis: Correcting error and bias in research findings.* Newbury Park, CA: Sage.

Kerlinger, F. N. (1986). *Foundations of behavioral research* (3rd ed.). New York: Holt, Rinehart & Winston.

Knafl, K. A., & Howard, M. J. (1984). Interpreting and reporting qualitative research. *Research in Nursing and Health, 7*, 17–24.

Polit, D. F., & Sherman, R. E. (1990). Statistical power in nursing research. *Nursing Research, 39*, 365–369.

Tornquist, E. (1986). *From proposal to publication: An informal guide to writing about nursing research.* Menlo Park, CA: Addison-Wesley.

Appendix

Introduction

Throughout the text, examples drawn from various publications have been used to illustrate the process of analysis and evaluation of the conceptual, theoretical, and methodologic elements of research reports. This appendix pulls together the text material by presenting complete analyses and evaluations of the contents of six published research reports.

- Two *descriptive studies*, "Transcending options: Creating a milieu for practicing high-level wellness" (Duffy, 1984), and "Themes of grief" (Carter, 1989) exemplify descriptive theory-generating research.
- The *correlational studies*, "The relationship between social support and self-care practices" (Hubbard, Muhlenkamp, & Brown, 1984) and "Uncertainty and adjustment during radiotherapy" (Christman, 1990), are examples of explanatory theory-testing research.
- The *experimental studies*, "Promoting awareness: The mother and her baby" (Riesch & Munns, 1984) and "Effects of aerobic interval training on cancer patients' functional capacity" (MacVicar, Winningham, & Nickel, 1989), are examples of predictive theory-testing research.

A reprint of each study is followed by an analysis of the study's theoretical elements. The analysis is based on the format for theory formalization described in Chapter 2. Each report was reviewed and concepts and propositions were identified and classified. In addition, hierarchies of propositions were developed and diagrams drawn to illustrate concepts and their connections. When warranted by the content of the report, a conceptual-theoretical-empirical structure was constructed, following the format given in Chapter 5. The criteria for evaluation of the relation between theory and research discussed in Chapter 3 were then applied to determine the significance, internal consistency, parsimony, and testability of the theory that was generated or tested, the operational adequacy of the research design and the empirical adequacy and pragmatic adequacy of the theory. In addition, when the influence of the conceptual model or other frame of reference on the research was evident, it was evaluated by using the criteria presented in Chapter 5. Two of the research reports included findings from two tests of the theory (Hubbard et al., 1984; Riesch & Munns, 1984), thereby affording an opportunity to illustrate use of the technique of meta-analysis described in Chapter 4.

Tables A–1 and A–2 summarize the components of analysis and evaluation of research reports and cite the relevant chapters and pages for ready reference to the text material.

It is suggested that the reader first review the reprinted study and carry out an analysis and evaluation of its content. The results may then be compared to those included in this appendix.

REFERENCES

Carter, S. L. (1989). Themes of grief. *Nursing Research, 38,* 354–358.

Christman, N. L. (1990). Uncertainty and adjustment during radiotherapy. *Nursing Research, 39,* 17–20, 47.

Duffy, M. E. (1984). Transcending options: Creating a milieu for practicing high-level wellness. *Health Care for Women International, 5,* 145–161.

Hubbard, P., Muhlenkamp, A. F., & Brown, N. (1984). The relationship between social support and self-care practices. *Nursing Research, 33,* 266–270.

MacVicar, M. G., Winningham, M. L., & Nickel, J. L. (1989). Effects of aerobic interval training on cancer patients' functional capacity. *Nursing Research, 38,* 348–351.

Riesch, S. K., & Munns, S. K. (1984). Promoting awareness: The mother and her baby. *Nursing Research, 33,* 271–276.

TABLE A – 1. Components of Theory Analysis

Component	Text Discussion
CONCEPTS	Chapter 2, p. 19
• Pragmatics of concept identification	p. 19
• Classification by variability	p. 19
• Classification by observability	p. 20
• Classification by measurement characteristics	p. 22
• Pragmatics of concept classification	p. 24
PROPOSITIONS	Chapter 2, p. 25
• Nonrelational propositions	p. 25
Existence propositions	p. 25
Definitional propositions	p. 25
Constitutive definitions	p. 26
Operational definitions	p. 26
Empirical indicators	p. 27
• Relational propositions	p. 27
• The hypothesis	p. 36
• Pragmatics of proposition identification and classification	p. 36
HIERARCHIES OF PROPOSITIONS	Chapter 2, p. 37
• Level of abstraction	p. 38
• Inductive reasoning	p. 38
• Deductive reasoning	p. 39
• Sign of a relationship	p. 41
• Pragmatics of hierarchical ordering of propositions	p. 42
CONCEPTUAL-THEORETICAL-EMPIRICAL STRUCTURES	Chapter 5, p. 106
• Analyzing the conceptual-theoretical-empirical structure	p. 112
• Diagramming conventions	pp. 44, 45, 47, 48
• Inventories of concepts and propositions	p. 47
• Pragmatics of diagramming	p. 54
• Conceptual-theoretical-empirical structure	p. 106

TABLE A – 2.   Summary of Criteria for Evaluation of the Relation Between Theory and Research

Criterion	Text Discussion
SIGNIFICANCE	Chapter 3, p. 60
• The theory should address a phenomenon of theoretical and social significance. • The theory should improve the precision with which a phenomenon can be predicted. • The theory should improve understanding of the phenomenon.	
INTERNAL CONSISTENCY	Chapter 3, p. 63
• The theory concepts should be defined clearly, and the same concept names and definitions should be used throughout the theory. • The theory should not contain redundant concepts. • The propositions sets of the theory should be complete and free from redundancies, and they should follow the canons of inductive or deductive logic.	
PARSIMONY	Chapter 3, p. 66
• The theory should be stated clearly and concisely.	
TESTABILITY	Chapter 3, p. 67
• The concepts of the theory should be empirically observable. • The propositions should be measurable. • The hypotheses should be falsifiable.	
OPERATIONAL ADEQUACY	Chapter 3, p. 69
• The sample should be representative of the population of interest. • The empirical indicators should be valid and reliable. • The research procedure should be appropriate. • The data analysis procedures should be appropriate.	
EMPIRICAL ADEQUACY	Chapter 3, p. 71
• Theoretical claims should be congruent with empirical evidence. • Alternative methodologic and substantive explanations should be considered.	
PRAGMATIC ADEQUACY	Chapter 3, p. 77
• Research findings should be related to the practical problem of interest.	

TABLE A–2.   Summary of Criteria for Evaluation of the Relation Between Theory and Research (*Continued*)

Criterion	Text Discussion

PRAGMATIC ADEQUACY (Continued)

- Implementation of innovative actions should be feasible.
- Innovative actions should be congruent with clients' expectations.
- The practitioner should have the legal ability to implement the innovation.
- The innovative actions should lead to favorable outcomes.

CONCEPTUAL-THEORETICAL-EMPIRICAL STRUCTURE   Chapter 5, p. 106

- The conceptual model should be linked to the theory and empirical indicators
- The credibility of the conceptual model should be discussed.

Analysis and Evaluation of Two Descriptive Studies

TRANSCENDING OPTIONS: CREATING A MILIEU FOR PRACTICING HIGH-LEVEL WELLNESS

Mary E. Duffy, RN, PhD[*]

The purpose of this study was to investigate the relationship between living in a female-headed one-parent family and the family's practice of prevention behaviors. The participants included 59 female-headed, one-parent families as well as other data sources that provided a societal perspective on the phenomenon. Interviews, observations, a healthy diary, and a card sort were used for data collection.

This study was carried out according to the tenets of grounded theory. The major finding was the emergence of the theory of transcending options. This theory describes the family's practice of prevention behaviors as a subset of the family's life circumstances. The family's behaviors (health and nonhealth) were a response to the societal options that the woman perceived were available to the female-headed, one-parent family.

The theory of transcending options describes this process on a continuum. There are three major points on the continuum: choosing options, seeking options, and transcending options. The interface between the family's life circumstances and their practice of prevention behaviors is evident at each of these points.

The family is the basic unit of health care management and thus a critical determinate of the health status and practices of its individual members. The family's responsibility for its health care management lies within the three levels of prevention described by Leavell and Clark (1965, p. 21): primary, secondary, and tertiary. This study focused on primary prevention; that is, the promotion of health and the prevention of disease as

---

[*]From Brigham Young University, College of Nursing, Salt Lake City, Utah, reprinted from *Health Care for Women International*, 5, 145–161 1984.

defined by Leavell and Clark. These behaviors include those the family members practice to improve their overall well being and those behaviors aimed at reducing the risks of specific diseases.

Nursing seeks to enhance the family's abilities to nurture and promote the health of its members. To assist the family, nurses rely on empirical knowledge of family health to guide their practice. However, according to Friedman (1981, p. 3), a dearth of this knowledge exists because "too little research has been devoted to examining the relationships between the family—its structure and functions—and the health and development of its individual members."

The female-headed, one-parent family, the focus of this investigation, represents one structural form of the family. There are two characteristics of this family type, suggesting that the experiences of living in a female-headed, one-parent family differ from those in other family forms (Duffy, 1982). First, the family has available the resources of only one, not two, adult members. Second, several authors have reported that the sources of stress in the female-headed, one-parent family differ both qualitatively and quantitively from those found in other family types. Economics, time, interpersonal relationships, parenting, social supports, and feelings of loss of control plague the female-headed, one-parent family (Berman & Turk, 1981; Herman, 1977; Horowitz & Purdue, 1977; Norbeck & Sheiner, 1982; Patton, Harvill, & Michal, 1981; Smith, 1980; Weltner, 1982). The female head of the family has been described by Weltner (1982, p. 205) as being "overworked, overstressed, and often so depressed."

Qualitative data were used to develop a grounded theory that described the relationship between living in a one-parent family headed by a woman and the family's practice of primary prevention behaviors. For several reasons, this study was restricted to the female-headed, one-parent family. First, according to the U.S. Bureau of the Census (1981), 5.3 million (83%) one-parent families are headed by women. Second, the experiences of women as heads of households differ from those of men (Benston, 1971; Eisenstein, 1979; Farel & Dobelstein, 1982; Oakley, 1981; Smith, 1980). The "feminization of poverty" has been recognized as an increasing phenomenon, in which families headed by women are falling below the poverty level at greater percentages than all other family types. Third, the myths associated with the desirability of the male-headed, traditional family structure persist and influence the female-headed, one-parent family (Boulding, 1981; Smith, 1980).

The emerging legitimacy of the one-parent family headed by a woman (Brown, Feldberg, Fox, & Kohen, 1976; Rexford, 1976) remains secondary to the prevailing attitude that the one-parent family is a transitional family structure best resolved by marriage (Collison & Futrell, 1982; Herman, 1977; Horowitz & Purdue, 1977; Pearlin & Johnson, 1977; Schorr & Moen, 1980; Smith, 1980). The peril of this attitude is its influence on public policy, thwarting attempts to develop social programs to help the one-parent family (Brandwein, Brown, & Fox, 1974; Herman, 1977; Schorr & Moen, 1980).

METHODOLOGY

Study Design

The dearth of literature on the management of prevention behaviors in female-headed, one-parent families led to the selection of an inductive methodology, grounded theory (Glaser, 1978; Glaser & Strauss, 1967). This approach is a type of factor-searching study (Diers, 1979), in which concepts and their interrelationships emerge to describe a social process. Qualitative data were collected to holistically analyze the multiplicity of variables present within the context of the families.

The design of a grounded theory study is flexible and determined by the phenomenon under study. Data collecting, coding, and analyzing occur jointly.

Population

The sampling technique for a grounded theory study is theoretical sampling. Theoretical sampling is the joint collecting, coding, and analyzing of the data to determine what and where to sample next (Glaser & Strauss, 1967, p. 45). Data collection is directed by the emerging theory and not by the principles of statistical sampling. The goal of theoretical sampling is to develop a well-integrated theory from the data collected.

To facilitate this process, this study was conducted in two segments. The initial investigation was interviewing 17 women who headed one-parent families. These 17 women were selected by convenience from a nonclinical population of women. Community service agencies were used throughout the study to identify the study participants. This approach allowed the researcher to select the participants from a broader base of demographic characteristics.

The initial study familiarized the researcher with the problem area, and identified the sensitizing concepts of the phenomenon. These sensitizing concepts included women, family, health, adaptation, and decision-making. These concepts were the initial categories that guided the family interviews and the literature search. The initial study also determined the bases of the theoretical sampling when the major study began. For example, income was initially identified as a potential explanation for the variability in prevention behaviors among female-headed, one-parent families. Therefore, families of various socioeconomic levels were sampled. This explanation alone proved insufficient, and the variability seemed better explained by the women's reported feelings of self-esteem. This later category appeared to be related to occupational status and the source of income. Women in various occupational categories were then interviewed.

This process, theoretical sampling, continued until the categories of the emerging theory were developed sufficiently to explain the phenomenon being studied. The completed study included 59 female-headed, one-parent families.

The theoretical sampling was not restricted to the families. Other sources of data were felt to be essential to understanding this phenomenon. These sources were (a) a support group for women heads of households, (b) professionals who work with one-parent families, and (c) the media that portray women and one-parent families.

The support group consisted of 11 women. The group convened voluntarily and met for 10 weeks. The focus of the group was on issues of immediate concern to the women in their roles as single women and parents. The researcher was a nonparticipant observer.

The 21 professionals who were interviewed represented legal, social, and health services. The purpose of these interviews was to understand the perceptions of these caregivers toward one-parent families headed by women. These interviews became necessary when several women indicated a conflict between their perceptions of the female-headed, one-parent family and those of their counselor, lawyer, health professional, or child care provider. Previous research has indicated that mental health professionals describe perceptions that are incompatible for being both female and a healthy adult (Broverman, Broverman, Clarkson, Rosenkrantz, & Vogel, 1970).

Last, an extensive review of the media was conducted. These data were analyzed to understand the portrayal of women by the mass media.

Instruments

The instruments used were open-ended interview guides, a health diary, and a card sort. The family interview guide focused on three areas:

1. Demographic data
2. Development of and understanding the meaning of being a female-headed, one-parent family
3. The family's health status and practices.

Sample questions from sections 2 and 3 are depicted in Table 1.

Each woman was asked to keep a health diary for her family during a 2-week period. The diary, also an open-ended instrument, asked the woman to report family illnesses and health practices, as well as motivators and deterrents to health behaviors. The diary was included after a woman in the pilot study suggested it as a method of overcoming memory lapses that occurred during the interviews.

The card sort consisted of 53 health behaviors, either health-promotion or disease-prevention activities. Each woman sorted the cards into three categories according to the frequency with which the family practiced the behavior: regularly, sometimes, and not practiced or applicable. These terms were defined according to the women's perceptions of their definitions, rather than measuring the family against predetermined criteria. In addition, there was a card sort of barriers — time, money, was not allowed to, need information, do not feel good about doing, need someone's support, never thought about it, and lazy — which the women used

TABLE 1. Interview Questions for the Family

Meaning of One-Parent Family Status	Health Practices
1. What has your experience been like being the head of your family?	1. What kinds of things do you do to keep yourself and your children healthy?
2. How do you feel about being a single parent?	2. What motivates you to take care of your health and your children's the way you do?
3. What effect has this experience had on the children?	3. What are some things you would like to do for health but either cannot or do not do?

TABLE 2.   Interview Questions for Professionals

1. What do you see are the major problems faced by the female-headed, one-parent family?
2. How do you feel these problems should be handled?
3. What resources are needed by these families?
4. What are the alternatives for long-term care of the female-headed, one-parent family?
5. How well adjusted do you feel the family members are?
6. What do you see are the differences between the family that adjusts to their situation and those that have difficulties?
7. What do you see as the pattern of adjustment?
8. How do you feel about one-parent families headed by women?
9. What do you think is missing from the family that does not have a man in the home?

to describe the factor(s) preventing her family from regularly practicing health behaviors that she desired.

The fourth instrument was an interview guide for professionals. This guide was also open-ended and included the questions in Table 2.

Procedure

A pilot study was conducted from July through September 1981 in which 17 female heads of one-parent families were interviewed. The purpose of the pilot study was to map out the dimensions of the phenomenon to guide the research process. As a result of this preliminary study, the interview schedule was modified, the interview populations were defined, and the initial sensitizing concepts were identified. The major study was conducted from July 1982 until March 1983.

FAMILY

The families were contacted through several social service agencies. When permission was obtained, an appointment was made to conduct the first interview in the client's home. On completion of the first interview, the woman was asked to complete a health diary over a 2-week period. The second interview was conducted once the health diary was completed. The card sort was administered at the completion of the second interview.

PROFESSIONALS

The interviews of the professionals emerged as a potential data source from the analysis of the family interviews. Professionals who were working with various families were selected by convenience. These professionals were each interviewed once.

SUPPORT GROUP

The support group occurred during 10 weeks of the study. The researcher was a nonparticipant observer in the group and recorded observations and themes at the conclusion of each session.

MEDIA

The media, printed and audiovisual, were the last source of data. The analysis centered on determining the dominant themes related to the portrayal of women and the one-parent family. The media were considered to be influential in the formation and continuation of either stereotypical or alternative attitudes toward the female-headed, one-parent family. The media were reviewed throughout the study.

Data Analysis

In a grounded theory study, data analysis commences with the data collection. Each incoming datum is analyzed to determine its relevance to the emerging theory and its implications for the evolving study design.

The qualitative data collected in this study were organized by Schatzman and Strauss' (1973) notation scheme. Methodological, observational, and theoretical notes were kept.

Methodological notes guided the emerging study design. For example, the data indicated that the problems experienced by the women and their families were not unique to families who were divorced. Therefore, one-parent families created by separation, death, and never being married were interviewed. Second, the women expressed concern that the one-parent family headed by a woman was stigmatized through the mass media. Therefore, the analysis of the mass media was undertaken. Third, the data indicated a grieving period of 12–18 months. Families were selected to represent various periods during and after this time frame. The study design was continually adjusted to respond to impending questions.

Observational notes were made immediately after each interview and each support group meeting. Family interaction patterns, the home environment, the mass media, and group behavior were among the data collected.

The observational notes were analyzed in conjunction with the qualitative data collected by the interviews, the health diary, and card sort, and the support group discussions. These data were studied by constant comparative analysis. Units of analysis—families or support group participants—were compared with each other first on an individual basis and later by groups. The families were grouped for analysis according to several characteristics. These characteristics included income, number of children, occupation, years as a one-parent family, and health practices.

These comparisons were done in steps. First, significant empirical indicators were identified from the data. Examples are as follows:

- I never had to depend on myself.
- I think it is really unfair that some people in that situation have a choice whether they want to stay or leave. Other people kind of get left with it all.
- I won't ever depend on a man. Now I can say I am totally responsible and mature. There are a lot of women who aren't self-reliant.

The empirical indicators were recorded on index cards. The cards were analyzed to develop substantive codes, first-level conceptualizations. Control was the code that described the preceding empirical indicators. This process of conceptualizing continued until the core category emerged. "Transcending options" was the core category describing the process that occurred as the female-headed, one-parent family adjusted to their situation and assumed control over their life circumstances. This process became a prerequisite for the family in their ability to practice health-promoting and disease-preventing behaviors. The other concepts of the theory described phases in the process of transcending options.

FINDINGS

The theory of transcending options is the substantive grounded theory that emerged from the data. This theory is an integration of the societal factors impinging in the female-headed, one-parent family and the family's perceptions of their situation. Health-promoting and disease-preventing behaviors, primary prevention, emerged as a subset of the life circumstances of the families. Women who are able to totally accept their role as heads of the households also engaged themselves and their children in the practice of health-promoting as well as disease-preventing behaviors. The practice of health-promoting behaviors is synonymous with the practice of high-level wellness (Dunn, 1959; Pender, 1982). The theory explained the process of attaining this level of health practices.

The theory of transcending options is a response to the societal norms or expectations that sculpt out the options typically available to the women heads of one-parent families. The norms that emerged from the data and are perceived by the study participants are as follows:

1. A woman is the primary homemaker in a family.
2. If employed, the woman's job is typically a low-paying occupation.
3. One-parent families are "less than" the two-parent ideal. A woman and her children are incomplete without a man in the home.
4. Families remain in poverty by choice or through a character flaw of the adult member.
5. Remarriage is the solution.

Although an ideological erosion of these norms has occurred, concrete evidence of their existence persists. Transcending options is a theory of the process of going beyond these norms, this typical range of options.

The theory of transcending options is on a continuum and is cumulative. Conceptually there are three distinguishing points on the continuum; but in reality, the continuum is amorphous, fluid, and bidirectional. The three delineated points are *choosing options*, *seeking options*, and *transcending options*.

Table 3 depicts the categories and their properties.

TABLE 3.   Concepts of Options

Choosing Options	Seeking Options	Transcending Options
Securing	Redefining	Creating
Escaping	Risking	Optimizing
Reserving energy	Expanding energy	

Choosing Options

Choosing options is the process of making a conscious selection from a perceived set of restricted choices. For example, the sociopolitical environment has created barriers to adequate salaries for women and affordable, quality day care. The woman may perceive her choices to be either remaining at home on Aid to Dependent Families or seeking low-paying employment. Overcoming these two options is not a perceived choice for this woman. The contextual factors of her situation, coupled with her personal resources, restrict her sense of control over her life circumstances. Her behavior is reduced to choosing from among the options perceived to be given to her. This pattern of choosing options is characterized as habitual behaviors in which the woman secures a static and predictable environment for herself and her children. Prevention behaviors include only long-standing health habits, usually learned in childhood by the woman. These behaviors are described by the woman as "common sense" and are not perceived as conscious health actions. An excerpt that describes the health practices in this category is: "I cannot think of anything I set out to do. I do not set out to do something healthy that day."

The properties of "choosing options" explain more fully the behaviors associated with that category. *Securing, escaping,* and *reserving energy* are the properties of this category.

Securing is the establishment of a safe and predictable environment. Life styles are designed around well-established routines, with little variation or conscious thought. A secure environment permits a woman to feel a sense of control in her life and safety from an external environment that seems impenetrable. One woman expressed this experience: "I stick to what is comfortable. I don't venture out."

Escaping provides a single avenue into which the woman channels her energy; in return, she receives satisfaction, warmth, and reassurance as a temporary stress relief. Avenues for escaping include children, sex, substance abuse, and dreaming. Each of these escapes provides comfort from a situation perceived to be intolerable and uncontrollable and, at the same time, decreases the burden of decision-making. The empirical evidence describing this property emerged from the following excerpts:

> They do not have anything else. That is the easiest thing to do at the time. It takes less commitment in it but it is temporary fulfillment. Temporary ease of their pain, discomfort or whatever.

The third property is reserving energy. Fatigue prevails. Food, vitamins, sleep, and smoking are examples of supports associated with behaviors undertaken to restore or conserve energy. The struggle is to retain an adequate energy level to survive the day. One woman succinctly summarized this property:

> When I get everything else straightened out then I can try to stop smoking. Right now, smoking is the only time I sit down and relax. It is something I do for myself.

Seeking Options

Seeking options is the next point on the continuum. This category describes the woman's attempt to overcome barriers to enjoy new opportunities for herself and her children. This stage is characterized by the continuation of habits but these habits are interspersed with the trial of new behaviors, including health-promoting and disease-preventing behaviors. The range of perceived options is expanded with the woman's sense of increasing control over her life circumstances. For example, redefining her role as a woman and mother can enhance a woman's options as she abandons traditional role perceptions based on gender rather than individual preference or ability. Seeking options is a vulnerable stage where the woman needs a great deal of support to sustain herself at this level. She is engaging in a series of "experiments," social, vocational, and psychological. The family, through the woman's direction, reaches beyond their secure environment. The societal response to these experiments can either sustain the seeking-out process or terminate it.

The properties of this category are *redefining*, *risking*, and *expanding energy*. Empirical evidence from the data describe the dimensions of these properties.

Redefining is the process of substituting expanded role definitions for traditionally held ones. Traditional role perceptions and her own and her family's capabilities to try new role definitions are evaluated by the woman. This process is also influenced by the societal acceptance of these redefinitions. The following two excerpts from the data highlight this dual process. The first woman has overcome the traditional woman's role and has experienced personal growth and satisfaction. In the second excerpt, the woman perceives societal expectations to be restricting her development.

> I used to be a real weak person. When I got married, I went from being Tom and Lorraine's daughter to being Barry's wife. I never had to depend ever on myself. I have kind of been forced into depending on myself and having to make decisions. Now I really like it. I like being my own person and making my own decisions.
>
> I think it is really the negative things that people bring down on you to affect you emotionally and mentally. They do not project their mind far enough ahead to see what your potential could be.

Redefining unfolds into risking. During this process, the woman begins to extend beyond her secure environment and tries out new role definitions and their behaviors. These behaviors include moving her family to their own apartment, starting or changing employment, and trying new health behaviors. An enhanced sense of self-worth is expressed. A woman described the relationship between her feelings about herself and her health practices.

> For me, my weight is a protection from men. As I get feeling better about me and where I am going, I will probably get to a place where I can do that. I am feeling good about myself and I have started eating healthy.

Her improved eating habits included an improvement in her children's eating.

A support system is usually instrumental in initiating and sustaining the risking process. This support system was described as "motivating" by the women and was equally effective in this function by providing or withdrawing support. The first excerpt is from a woman, now an honors student, who had never been to college or even felt she was capable of being admitted. Prior to her divorce, she was a full-time homemaker and mother of four children.

> This fellow that I was dating said: "You can do it." He brought me up here and literally held my hand, walked me around campus and showed me things and took me to admissions and I admitted myself. I started real slowly.

The withdrawal of physical support contributed to the second woman's growth. This woman, the mother of three children, held a college degree and was employed full time.

> We moved in with my parents after the separation. After three months, my parents felt I should really move out on my own. That encouraged my independence and I was ready.

The success of risking is described as the process of expanding energy, the accumulation of energy from the expenditure of energy. Enthusiasm, encouragement, motivation, and feeling good are among the words used to describe this process. This heightened energy level is transferred to the children and often is expressed by higher-level health behaviors. The contrast in energy levels and health practices are evident in the next two excerpts. The first excerpt is from a woman who is at home full time with two children. She expressed a desire to seek employment but felt incapable of doing so. She remains in the choosing options stage:

> I feel so lazy. I get really bored staying home. I feel yucky. I feel like a fat slob. He (physician) said that what he thinks I should do is try to go out and try to do something to improve myself. I just do not do it because I never find the time to do anything that I want to do.

A woman who had three children, was a full-time student at the university, and was employed full time, said:

> I care about how I look so I try to stay healthy. Before, I just did not care. I watch what I eat, exercise, and keep myself neat and clean.

Redefining, risking, and expanding energy compose the process of seeking options. During this pattern of growth, family members are exploring their alternatives and experimenting with their choices. Positive reinforcement in this endeavor enhances the family members' chances of transcending options.

Transcending Options

Transcending options is the culmination of this process and is the integration of new behaviors into the woman's life-style. The women at this stage have overcome the sociopolitical barriers inhibiting their assumption of the role of household head and are in control of their family's life circumstances. These women are no longer attempting to relinquish their responsibilities as heads of households to men, the state, family members, friends, or children. Only 8 of the 59 participants in the study had reached this point, although 63% of the women had been household heads for more than 2 years.

Transcending options is a culmination, but not an end. The possibilities for change and growth are infinite if personal or societal factors do not impede the process. This pinnacle of personal growth was expressed by one woman: "For the first time in my life I found it was not necessary to define myself in terms of a man. I am complete in myself."

During the process of reaching this phase of personal development, each woman was able to identify a support system that motivated her, enhanced her feelings of self-worth, and helped launch her into new beginnings. This support system, social or professional, was credited with helping her to overcome the impeding barriers she encountered.

There are two properties of this category, and the two characterized the woman's behaviors in health and nonhealth practices. These properties are *optimizing* and *creating*.

Optimizing is the ability to make the most out of a favorable condition, establishing an advantageous milieu. This process is facilitated by the woman's enhanced perception of the range of available choices in a situation. An example of this process came from a woman who felt that a persistence of both overt and subtle discrimination existed toward the single mother. She used her single-parent status to facilitate her educational opportunities.

> I think it is a great time to be a single woman because I am getting a lot of breaks. I just applied for my grant yesterday and they did not seem to think I would have any problems because I am a divorced mother. I guess many do not use it but I have to. You have got to take advantage of every option you have.

The women in this category emphasized the importance of optimizing and protecting their own and their family's health. The parent's mental health was perceived as pivotal to the family's stability and growth: "If I am not mentally and emotionally at peace, the whole family goes." Physical as well as mental health was valued. Exercise, nutrition, stress reduction, reading health literature, and safety were among the behaviors practiced by the women and their children. The expressed goal of these behaviors was to capitalize or optimize on their good health.

Optimizing frequently depends on creative problem solving. The second property of transcending options is creating. This property is the process of developing an environment in which the family feels in control. Societal expectations and conventional patterns of behavior do not restrict the woman's choices made for herself and her children. Overcoming guilt and role expectations associated with being a single parent challenged one woman to create a parental role with which she was comfortable:

> When you are a single parent, you are not half a parent, neither do you have to be both parents, but you are yourself. The child has to learn to accept you as you are.

The creating is equally important in health behaviors as well as other life-style behaviors. The following excerpt describes this approach to life:

> I am a person who is involved in problem solving. I have been able to see a problem and cure it where it has been cured to my satisfaction. If a child has a problem, change his diet, put him in an exercise program, help him to feel like he is a special person. Let him see that you are changing his diet. Say, "Let us try this for a while; maybe this will make you feel good." With things, you just can not loiter in them.

Transcending options is a theory that explains the life-style behavior patterns in the female-headed, one-parent family. The family's prevention practices are a reflection of their life-style pattern: choosing options, seeking options, or transcending options. Long-standing habits characterize the health practices of choosing options. These habits are continued during the seeking-options stage, but they are complemented by experimentations with health-promoting and disease-preventing behaviors. Transcending options is the process of creating a milieu that sustains the practice of health-promoting or high-level wellness behaviors.

DISCUSSION

The conservative approach to the findings of this research is to generate hypotheses for further testing. This approach will test the validity of this theory as well as its generalizability. Future studies should focus on controlling the variables identified in the theory and statistically measuring them with diverse populations of female-headed, one-parent families. Income, ages of children, years of marriage, years as a one-parent family, the woman's educational preparation and occupation, and the family's health status are among the variables to consider in further testing.

A significant hypothesis that emerged is that women who have a motivating support system are able to progress along the continuum to the point of transcending options. A longitudinal study of one-parent families from their inception would test this proposition.

This theory's applicability to other populations experiencing constraints to personal development should likewise be explored. This substantive theory could be developed into a formal theory.

Whereas the researcher pursues the validity of a theory and continues to generate knowledge, the practitioner seeks knowledge that can be applied in clinical practice. The application of this theory in practice is one means of testing its validity. The theory of transcending options describes a problem faced by female-headed, one-parent families and suggests points of intervention.

Working with individual families, the nurse can assess the family according to the theory's categories and properties. Table 4 identifies

TABLE 4.   Sample Criteria for Assessing the Female-headed, One-parent Family

Categories and Properties	Assessment Criteria
1. Choosing options (securing)	1. Established routines/habits
	2. Traditional role perceptions
	3. Reluctance to try new behaviors
	4. Withdrawing
2. Seeking options (risking)	1. Support systems that are motivating
	2. Extending the environment
	3. Increasing feelings of self-worth
	4. Trying new behaviors
3. Transcending options (creating)	1. Problem-solving
	2. Resourcefulness
	3. Independence
	4. Originating

sample criteria. This framework can aid the nurse in understanding the family's life-style pattern and health practices. Interventions can then be designed to enhance the family's strengths.

The nurse can also use this theory as a basis for social and political action. The findings of this study verify previous studies and theoretical writings reporting that women, as a group, are neither expected nor prepared to be household heads. Old myths about the roles of women and mothers need to be dispelled. The mass media are often responsible for reinforcing traditional stereotypes about women. Nurses can respond to the media through letter-writing campaigns and other social action. Women, beginning with girls, need to feel capable of preparing themselves for roles that extend beyond being homemakers or being employed in traditionally female positions. These roles contribute to the poverty experienced by women and their children.

Legislative changes could facilitate the transition for families to a one-parent family. Day care and employment training programs are two examples.

These types of social and political action are slow processes. If nurses wait for research to provide definitive answers, families headed by women will continue to suffer from social injustices.

REFERENCES

Benston, M. (1971). The political economy of women's liberation. In M. H. Garskof (Ed.), *Roles women play: Readings toward women's liberation*. Belmont, CA: Brooks/Cole.

Berman, W. H., & Turk, D. C. (1981). Adaptation to divorce: Problems and coping strategies. *Journal of Marriage and the Family, 43*(1), 179–189.

Boulding, E. (1981). Familial constraints on women's work roles. In M. Blaxall & B. Reagan (Eds.), *Women and the workplace* (3rd ed.). Chicago: The University of Chicago Press.

Brandwein, R. A., Brown, C. A., & Fox, E. M. (1974). Women and children last: The social situation of divorced mothers and their families. *Journal of Marriage and Family, 36*(3), 498–514.

Broverman, I. K., Broverman, D. M., Clarkson, F. E., Rosenkrantz, P., & Vogel, S. R. (1970). Sex-role stereotypes and clinical judgments of mental health. *Journal of Consulting Psychology, 34*, 1–7.

Brown, C. A., Feldberg, R., Fox, E. M., & Kohen, J. (1976). Divorce: A chance of a new lifetime. *Journal of Social Issues, 32*, 119–133.

Collison, C. R., & Futrell, J. (1982). Family therapy for the single-parent family system. *Journal of Psychiatric Nursing and Mental Health Services, 20*(7), 16–20.

Diers, D. (1979). *Research in nursing practice*. New York: Lippincott.

Duffy, M. E. (1982). When a woman heads a household. *Nursing Outlook, 30*(8), 468–473.

Dunn, H. L. (1959). What high-level wellness means. *Canadian Journal of Public Health*, *50*(11), 447–457.

Eisenstein, Z. (1979). Developing a theory of capitalistic patriarchy and socialist feminism. In Z. Eisenstein (Ed.), *Capitalist patriarchy and the case for socialist feminism*. New York: Monthly Review Press.

Farel, A. M. & Dobelstein, A. W. (1982). Supports and deterrents for mothers working outside the home. *Family Relations*, *31*(2), 281–286.

Freidman, M. M. (1981). *Family nursing theory and assessment*. New York: Appleton-Century-Crofts.

Glaser, B. (1978). *Theoretical sensitivity*. Mill Valley, CA: The Sociology Press.

Glaser, B. G., & Strauss, A. L. (1967). *The discovery of grounded theory: Strategies for qualitative research*. New York: Aldine.

Herman, S. J. (1977). Woman, divorce, and suicide. *Journal of Divorce*, *1*(2), 107–117.

Horowitz, J. A., & Purdue, B. H. (1977). Single-parent families. *Nursing Clinics of North America*, *12*(3), 503–511.

Leavell, H. R., & Clark, E. G. (1965). *Preventive medicine for the doctor in his community: An epidemiologic approach* (3rd ed.). New York: McGraw-Hill.

Norbeck, J., & Sheiner, M. (1982). Sources of social support related to single-parent functioning. *Research in Nursing and Health*, *5*, 3–12.

Oakley, A. (1981). *Subject women*. New York: Pantheon Books.

Patton, R. D., Harvill, L. M., & Michal, M. L. (1981). Attitudes of single parents toward health issues. *Journal of the American Medical Women's Association*, *36*(11), 340–348.

Pearlin, L. I., & Johnson, J. S. (1977). Marital status, life strains and depression. *American Sociological Review*, *42*(5), 704–715.

Pender, N. J., (1982). *Health promotion in nursing practice*. Norwalk, CT: Appleton-Century-Crofts.

Rexford, M. T. (1976). Single mothers by choice: An exploratory study. *Dissertation Abstracts International*, *37*, 984B. (University Microfilms No. 76–18, 122.)

Schatzman, L., & Strauss, A. L. (1973). *Field research*. Englewood Cliffs, NJ: Prentice-Hall, Inc.

Schorr, A. L., & Moen, P. (1980).The single parent and public policy. In A. Skolnick & J. H. Skolnick (Eds.), *Family in transition* (3rd ed.). Boston: Little, Brown.

Smith, M. J. (1980). The social consequences of single parenthood: A longitudinal perspective. *Family Relations*, *29*(1), 75–81.

U.S. Bureau of the Census. (1981). *Statistical abstracts of the United States: 1981* (102nd ed.). Washington, DC: U.S. Government Printing Office.

Weltner, J. S. (1982). A structural approach to the single-parent family. *Family Process*, *21*, 203–210.

Analysis of Theory

The stated purpose of Duffy's (1984) study was to investigate the relationship between living in a one-parent family headed by a female and the family's practice of primary prevention behaviors. Although the investigator claimed that the study purpose was to investigate a relationship, she explicitly classified the work as a factor-searching study, which is another term for descriptive research (Diers, 1979). The study did not develop explanatory theory, nor did it employ a correlational design. Therefore, it may be classified as descriptive research designed to generate descriptive theory.

CONCEPT IDENTIFICATION AND CLASSIFICATION

The study used the inductive mode of grounded theory to generate a theory of transcending options, which may be categorized as a descriptive classification theory. Analysis of the study findings revealed that the theory encompasses two concepts: female-headed one-parent family and options. The concept, female-headed one-parent family, is a nonvariable because it takes just one form in this study. It may be classified as directly observable in Kaplan's (1964) schema and as observable in Willer and Webster's (1970) schema because it was determined through the women's reports of their family structure. It may be classified as enumerative in Dubin's (1978) schema because the study is limited to one type of family structure.

Options is a variable because it has three dimensions (referred to as "categories" in the report): choosing options, seeking options, and transcending options. Each of the three categories, in turn, has two or more dimensions (referred to as "properties" in the report). The properties of choosing options are securing, escaping, and reserving energy. Those of seeking options are redefining, risking, and expanding energy. And the properties of transcending options are creating and optimizing. The concept, its categories, and their properties represent a typology of options for women who head one-parent families.

The concept, options, may be classified as a construct in the Kaplan and Willer and Webster schemas because it is not observable and appears to have been invented to describe the findings of this study. At this point in the development of the theory of transcending options, the categories and properties of options can be observed only through responses to open-ended interviews and other qualitative measures. Classification of the concept according to Dubin's schema is difficult with the information given in the research report. The investigator's statement that choosing options, seeking options, and transcending options make up a process of going beyond normative options for women heads of one-parent families suggests that the concept is an associative unit. That is, it is not present for all women heads of one-parent families. Further justification for this classification comes from the fact that very few of the women in the study demonstrated the category of transcending options. The study report did not indicate how many of the women demonstrated the other two categories. If all of the study subjects demonstrated at least one of the categories of options, then options would be an enumerative unit in this study.

The two concepts of the theory of transcending options are listed in Table A-3, along with the categories of options and their properties.

PROPOSITION IDENTIFICATION AND CLASSIFICATION

A series of statements pertaining to the theory of transcending options that are given in the study report are listed:

- The theory of transcending options is on a continuum and is cumulative.
- Conceptually, there are three distinguishing points on the continuum, but in reality, the continuum is amorphous, fluid, and bidirectional.
- The three delineated points are choosing options, seeking options, and transcending options.

The statements may be formalized into two nonrelational existence propositions. The first proposition asserts the existence of the phenomenon of options; the second describes the interrelationships among the three dimensions of the phenomenon of options. The latter is not classified as relational because it does not describe the relationship between two or more concepts. Rather, it describes the interrelationships between dimensions of one concept (options). The propositions are as follows:

1. There is a phenomenon known as options.
2. The phenomenon of options has three categories — choosing options, seeking options, and transcending options — that form an amorphous, fluid, and bidirectional continuum.

All other propositions making up the theory of transcending options are listed in Table A–3 as constitutive definitions. These are classified as nonrelational definitional propositions.

TABLE A – 3.   Concepts and Constitutive Definitions for the Theory of Transcending Options

Concept	Constitutive Definition
Female-headed one-parent family	This type of family has available the resources of only one, not two, adult members. Its sources of stress differ both qualitatively and quantitatively from those found in other family types.
Options	No definition given in the study report. *Categories* are choosing options, seeking options, and transcending options.
Choosing options	The process of making a conscious selection from a perceived set of restricted choices. The pattern of choosing options is characterized by habitual behaviors in which the woman secures a static and predictable environment for herself and her children. Prevention behaviors include only long-standing health habits, usually learned in childhood by the woman. *Properties* of this category are securing, escaping, and reserving energy.
Securing	The establishment of a safe and predictable environment.
Escaping	A single avenue into which the woman channels her energy; in return, she receives satisfaction, warmth, and reassurance as a temporary stress relief.
Reserving energy	Behaviors undertaken to restore or conserve energy.
Seeking options	The woman's attempt to overcome barriers to enjoy new opportunities for herself and her children. This state is characterized by the continuation of habits, but these habits are interspersed with the trial of new behaviors, including health-promoting and disease-preventing behaviors. The range of perceived options is expanded with the woman's sense of increasing control over her life circumstances. *Properties* of this category are redefining, risking, and expanding energy.
Redefining	The process of substituting expanded role definitions for traditionally held ones.
Risking	The woman begins to extend beyond her secure environment and tries out new role definitions and their behaviors.
Expanding energy	The accumulation of energy from the expenditure of energy.
Transcending options	The process of creating a milieu that sustains the practice of health-promoting or high-level wellness behaviors, with integration of new behaviors into the woman's life-style. *Properties* of this category are optimizing and creating.
Optimizing	The ability to make the most out of a favorable condition, establishing an advantageous milieu.
Creating	The process of developing an environment in which the family feels in control.

Definitions for the concepts are evident in the research report. Female-headed one-parent family is constitutively defined by means of a description of this type of family structure. Options, per se, is not constitutively defined, although the categories of choosing options, seeking options, and transcending options are constitutively defined, as are the properties of each category of options.

Operational definitions and empirical indicators for the concepts can be extracted from the report. "Female-headed one-parent family" is operationally defined as those one-parent families created by separation, death, and never being married that were contacted through social service agencies. The empirical indicator is the actual study subjects, that is, women who head one-parent families.

The concept, options, is operationally defined as follows: Categories of options (choosing options, seeking options, transcending options) were induced through empirical data gathered by means of open-ended interview guides for family members and professionals, a health diary, a card sort of health behaviors, observations of families and support groups, and analysis of printed and audiovisual media. The empirical indicators are the actual data collected, that is, the responses to questions in the interview guides, notations in the health diaries, results of the card sorts, observational notes, and media content.

The findings of this theory-generating study suggested one hypothesis, which was stated with concept names rather than with empirical indicators. The hypothesis is: Women who have a motivating support system are able to progress along the continuum to the point of transcending options.

HIERARCHY OF PROPOSITIONS

The use of the grounded theory strategy for this study indicates that a hierarchy of propositions would be inductive. Journal space limitations most likely prevented inclusion of enough examples of data to develop an inductive hierarchy of observations and conclusions. The conclusions are represented by the concept, options, and its categories and their properties. These conclusions form a typology that appears to be hierarchical in nature. The hierarchy progresses from the abstract concept, options, to the somewhat less abstract categories of choosing options, seeking options, and transcending options, to the still less abstract properties of the categories, including securing, escaping, reserving energy, redefining, risking, expanding energy, creating, and optimizing.

CONCEPTUAL-THEORETICAL-EMPIRICAL STRUCTURE

No explicit conceptual model is evident in the study report. However, the investigator's statements about the family as the basic unit of health care management, levels of prevention, and primary prevention constitute assumptions that are at the abstract and general level of a conceptual model. These notions have been added to the diagram of theory concepts and empirical indicators to complete the conceptual-theoretical-empirical structure of the study illustrated in Figure A–1. A proposition linking the conceptual model level concept of family to the theory level concept, female-headed one-parent family, is evident in the study report. This proposition states: The female-headed, one-parent family, the focus of this investigation, represents one structural form of the family. Linkage of the conceptual model level concept of primary prevention to the theory level concept, options, is less direct but is evident in the report. The linkage is achieved through the following series of propositions:

- Health-promoting and disease-preventing behaviors, primary prevention, emerged as a subset of the life circumstances of families.
- Women who are able to totally accept their role as heads of the households also engaged themselves and their children in the practice of health-promoting as well as disease-preventing behaviors.
- The practice of health-promoting behaviors is synonymous with the practice of high-level wellness.
- The theory [of transcending options] explained the process of attaining this level of health practices.

The operational definitions linking the concepts of the theory and the empirical indicators are given on page 193.

DIAGRAM

A diagram of the conceptual-theoretical-empirical structure for Duffy's (1984) study is presented in Figure A–1.

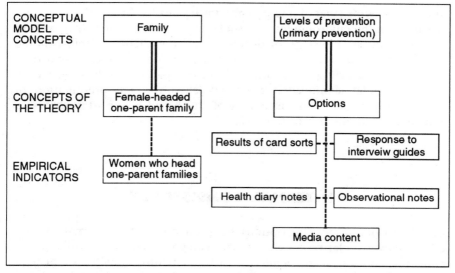

Figure A-1. Conceptual-theoretical-empirical structure for Duffy's study (1984).

EVALUATION OF THE RELATION BETWEEN THEORY AND RESEARCH

The stated intent of this study was to describe the practice of primary prevention (health-promoting and disease-preventing) behaviors in one-parent families headed by females. The outcome of the research was generation of a theory of transcending options. This theory describes the life-style behavior patterns in one-parent families headed by females. Primary prevention behaviors emerged as just one aspect of life-style.

SIGNIFICANCE

The theory of transcending options meets the criterion of significance. Theoretical significance was established by indicating how little is known about health-related behaviors of female-headed one-parent families. Furthermore, the theory deals with a phenomenon that is of interest to the discipline of nursing. In particular, it deals with the patterning of

human behavior (that of one-parent families headed by females) in interaction with the environment (the social milieu of such families). As is to
be expected at this stage of development, the theory of transcending
options does not predict with any precision. It does, however, contribute
to our understanding of the life style of one-parent families headed by
females. Social significance was established through presentation of
census bureau data and discussion of the broad scope of stressors in
female-headed one-parent families.

INTERNAL CONSISTENCY

The theory of transcending options meets the criterion of internal consistency. Semantic clarity is evident. The categories and properties of the
concept, options, were defined clearly. Semantic consistency also is
evident. Concepts retained their initial definitions throughout the report.
Furthermore, no redundancies in concepts are apparent.

The propositions of the theory appear to reflect structural consistency. Although it is not possible to construct an inductive hierarchy of
observations and conclusions, the data available in the report suggest that
the conclusions were induced from the empirical evidence. The propositions inherent in the typology of options followed a logical structure
such that each definition of a property of a category of options was more
specific than the definition of the category itself.

PARSIMONY

Formalization of the theory of transcending options indicates that the
theory meets the criterion of parsimony. The description of the phenomenon of options does not seem oversimplified, or excessively verbose.
However, repeated readings of the study report were needed to determine the major concepts of the theory. Initially, it appeared that the
categories of options (choosing, seeking, transcending) and the properties of the categories (securing, escaping, and so on) were concepts,
rather than dimensions of the concept, options.

TESTABILITY

The theory of transcending options meets the criterion of testability in that it should be possible to test the theory by replicating the study with the methods used by the investigator, although more information about actual measures would be needed. Furthermore, because empirical indicators are available in the form of qualitative measures, the propositions could be measured by stating them as hypotheses in a replication study. Moreover, the hypothesis generated from the study appears to be falsifiable.

OPERATIONAL ADEQUACY

The research design used to generate the theory of transcending options meets the criterion of operational adequacy. The theory dealt with one-parent families headed by females. As is to be expected in a grounded theory approach, theoretical sampling was employed. The investigator indicated that the sample included the women who headed one-parent families, as well as professionals who worked with one-parent families, a support group for women heads of households, and media dealing with women and one-parent families.

The empirical indicators used in the study are appropriate qualitative measures for a grounded theory study. Each of the several measures appears to be appropriate for the data it was used to collect.

The study report indicates that research and data analysis procedures typically associated with grounded theory methodology were followed throughout the investigation. The limits of generalizability of the theory would have been enhanced if numbers or percentages of the women who demonstrated the categories of choosing options and seeking options had been reported, as were the number who demonstrated the category of transcending options.

EMPIRICAL ADEQUACY

The theory of transcending options appears to meet the criterion of empirical adequacy. The data included in the study report support the conclusions.

The investigator did not question the validity or reliability of the study findings, although she did note that testing the hypotheses generated by the study with diverse samples of one-parent families headed by females would also test the validity and generalizability of the theory. An alternative substantive explanation for the study findings was not offered, nor were the study findings compared with the results of related research.

PRAGMATIC ADEQUACY

The theory of transcending options meets the initial requirement of pragmatic adequacy. The findings are applicable to women who head one-parent families. The investigator indicated that study findings could be used to develop criteria for assessment of one-parent families headed by females and presented sample criteria. The theory is not yet sufficiently developed, however, to serve as the basis for innovative nursing interventions.

CONCEPTUAL-THEORETICAL-EMPIRICAL STRUCTURE

A rudimentary conceptual model was extracted from the research report. The concepts making up this implicit frame of reference for the study were identified, as were vertical propositions that linked the conceptual model concepts to the theory concepts. The methodologic frame of reference was provided by the grounded theory approach. The study methods were in keeping with this approach to theory generation. The conceptual and methodologic frames of reference were not, however, part of a coherent research tradition. The credibility of the conceptual model was not addressed in the report.

REFERENCES

Diers, D. (1979). *Research in nursing practice*. Philadelphia: Lippincott.

Dubin, R. (1978). *Theory building* (rev. ed.). New York: The Free Press.

Duffy, M. E. (1984). Transcending options: Creating a milieu for practicing high-level wellness. *Health Care for Women International*, 5, 145–161.

Kaplan, A. (1964). *The conduct of inquiry*. San Francisco: Chandler.

Willer, D., & Webster, M., Jr. (1970). Theoretical concepts and observables. *American Sociological Review, 35*, 748–757.

THEMES OF GRIEF

Susan L. Carter

A thematic analysis of 30 narrative accounts of bereavement revealed nine themes that included five core themes in bereavement—being stopped, hurting, missing, holding, and seeking; three meta-themes *about* bereavement—change, expectations, and inexpressibility; and a contextual theme—personal history. The themes were compared with three theoretical perspectives on bereavement by Freud, Kübler–Ross, and one defined as existential–phenomenological. Features of bereavement that are dissimilar or unaddressed by the theoretical perspectives were: (a) the quality of grief's changing character, including "waves" and intense pain which may be triggered years after the death; (b) holding, an individual process of preserving the fact and meaning of the loved one's existence; (c) expectations, both social and personal, as to how the bereaved should be overlaying the experience; and (d) the critical importance of personal history in affecting the quality and meaning of individual bereavement.

Although no single, general, universally accepted theoretical perspective on the phenomenon of bereavement exists, three perspectives have been popular in the nursing literature: Freud, Kübler–Ross, and existential–phenomenological, which has been associated with humanistic psychology. The purpose of this study was to identify themes associated with bereavement in narrative accounts of those who had experienced the death of a loved one and to compare the themes disclosed by these persons with three theoretical perspectives common in the nursing literature.

Susan L. Carter, EdD, RN, is an associate professor of nursing at the School of Nursing, Indiana State University, Terre Haute.

Reprinted from *Nursing Research*, *38*, 354–358, 1989.

THEORETICAL PERSPECTIVE

The psychoanalytic perspective on the understanding of bereavement may be traced to Freud's treatise, "Mourning and Melancholia" (1957). In this work, Freud aimed to arrive at a better understanding of melancholia through a comparison of that condition with the "normal emotions of grief, and its expression in mourning" (p. 124). Freud observed that mourning has a typical general appearance, involves "painful dejection," a "loss of ability to love," a transformation of the appearance of the world ("the world becomes poor and empty") (p. 127); requires "grave departures from the normal attitude to life" (p. 125) whereby the mind performs an "inner labor" or "work of mourning" involving a transfer of libidinal energy which must be transferred to a new love object (p. 131); and is a nonpathological condition that normally reaches a state of completion (p. 139).

Kübler–Ross's (1972) five-stage model of dying has been widely used to explain the process of grief. Her model includes a predictable step-by-step sequence: (a) denial and isolation, (b) anger, (c) bargaining, (d) depression, and (e) acceptance. The stages are said to vary in length of time and to "replace each other or exist at times side-by-side" (p. 138).

A third perspective on bereavement is more descriptive than explanatory. The features include (among many others) an emphasis on the bereaved's sense of alienation from the world or loss of anchorage, the unique quality of each individual's experience, the continuity and fluidity of experience through time, and the importance of, even accentuated urgency for, creating meaning during bereavement. A select list of writers expressing this view includes Arendt (1974), Buber (1965), Frankl (1963), Needleman (1973), and Tillich (1965).

METHOD

Sample

Thirty adults who had experienced the death of a loved one were interviewed by the researcher using an open-ended, nondirective style to encourage candid self-expression. This was followed by a structured set of questions derived from the three theoretical perspectives. Interviews were tape-recorded and notes taken. In some cases, the researcher was given materials (poetry, notes, photos) to supplement the accounts.

Participants were identified through word of mouth, and all but two were solicited indirectly. All expressed appreciation for the opportunity to share their experience, as well as hope that it would ultimately benefit others. Measures were taken to protect the participants from exploitation and/or possible harm resulting from the interviews. Among these were four types of prearranged counseling resources for ready referrals, if necessary. Participants also selected the interview settings.

Participant ages ranged from 20 to 72 years; 21 were female. There were eight mothers, seven daughters, three fathers, three sons, two husbands, two wives, two in-laws, one granddaughter, and two friends of deceased persons. There were multiple causes of death. Elapsed time since the deaths ranged from 3½ weeks to 23 years. Most of the participants can be described as well-functioning individuals who were fulfilling their social responsibilities, reported no use of psychotropic medications, related thoughts clearly, and displayed affective states commensurate with the topics discussed.

Procedure

When the 30 interviews were completed, the narrative accounts of bereavement, as represented in the researcher's notes, were analyzed by theme. The framework for conducting the analysis was derived from van Kaam (1966, ch. 10), supplemented by recommendations from Taylor and Bogdan (1984, pp. 19–23), and van Manen (1984, pp. 60–61). Each thought and idea (termed elements) recorded from the narrative accounts was transferred to an index card. A preliminary grouping of the elements produced 41 broad, general categories.

Each narrative account was then examined as a whole and each element reexamined separately to illuminate particularly significant words, meanings, or themes that seemed especially revealing of bereavement (van Manen, 1984, pp. 60–61). A random set of tape-recordings was replayed. Finally, operations described by van Kaam (1966) as "reduction" and "element elimination" (p. 316), essential for separating individual or particular aspects of bereavement from features held in common, were undertaken. This included reevaluation of the preliminary categorization of elements. These operations resulted in a preliminary hypothetical explication of the bereavement phenomenon consisting of nine general themes.

Validation of findings was supported by feedback from five of the original participants and use of two uncoached second readers to criticize element allocation into categories. The second reader's agreement with the researcher on themes ranged from 62.25% to 88.88%.

Once the nine themes were finalized and fully described in narrative form, each theoretical perspective was compared with the nine themes. Points of agreement and compatibility as well as points of disagreement and incompatibility were identified.

RESULTS

Core Themes

Being stopped is the theme of bereavement that describes the interruption of life's usual flow following the death of a loved one and is characterized by varying types and degrees of inability, frequently stated in terms of "I can't." Although a few participants reported a mild cessation of usual life activities and personal functioning, an experience which might be characterized as a "pause," most reported greater disruption with expressions of "being at a loss" or being "unable." One person reported a permanent cessation, stating she felt "stuck in time" and noting that "it's like the people around us are going on and we're not."

Being "unable" extends into many domains of functioning and varies individually. Many noted the inability to believe the reality of the death, even when the deaths had been long anticipated. The fact was not denied, but the truth that the loved one was forever gone seemed unreal. The absolute inalterability of the death seemed the most difficult fact to acknowledge and induced feelings of having been overpowered and a helplessness to which some responded with protest and some, despair. One person noted, "I remember screaming 'NO! NO! NO!'" Another commented, "The strongest feeling is that I'm not in control of my life — the best laid plans — all for nothing." Perceiving oneself unable to think, feel, eat, sleep, and/or act was also conveyed. Some entertained thoughts of suicide, feeling "unable to go on."

A combination of being unable to feel, as though numb, and unable to believe was conveyed by expressions such as "I am just going through the motions," "I wasn't really there — I had a feeling that half of me was not there — like being half in the world," "I feel like a journalist or reporter," "For a day nothing affected me, I just sat there."

Frequent expressions of the total experience of sensing oneself unable included "falling to pieces," "falling apart," "unable to hold myself together," and "being at loose ends." Of greatest intensity were reports of awareness of the stark discontinuity between the world of before and the present world, and the harsh contrast between the intimate, personal world of devastation and the social natural world ("How can the sun be shining?" "How can they still be having Christmas this year?"). A metaphor used by one young participant whose first love, only a teen, had died suddenly of heart failure captures this theme: "The floor seemed to disappear."

Perhaps related to the high percentage of first-time bereaved, most participants expressed a sense of surprise of unpreparedness for the quality and duration of the experience, unmediated by length of time in preparation for the death or preparatory studies (such as reading Kübler–Ross or attending "grief" workshops). As one stated, "I had time to be prepared, but was never *really* ready." Another said, "I knew it was coming, but you're never ready, never really ready."

The participant relating the greatest duration and intensity of being stopped conveyed a sense of being frozen in time. Neither she nor her family had been able to eat together at the kitchen table since the death of her teenaged son 2½ years previously. Her sense of how completely her family's life had been stopped became poignantly evident in her simple, sorrowful revelation: "We buried him between us."

Hurting is a theme of bereavement characterized by a cluster of intensely painful emotions. Feelings of sorrow or sadness, usually accompanied by tearfulness and crying, are of such severity that they were referred to by most as "pain." The sense of having something severely hurtful done to one was revealed in expressions such as having been hit, wounded, stabbed, shattered, or crushed, and, sometimes, having been burdened as in carrying a great heaviness or weight. From this core of psychic pain (sometimes physically perceived as well) radiated variations of other painful emotions commensurate with personal experience. Painful guilt, burning anger, even to the point of hatred, or sorrowful wishing about how some aspect of the past might have been (regret) was reported by some participants.

Typical expressions of hurting included: "Pain, I can't stand it," "There is no relief — hurt, hurt, hurt," "It really hit me," "I want to lick my wounds," and "God is a gigantic practical joker who does things to people." A young mother whose memories included tying a scarf around her young daughter's bald (chemotherapy) head so she could wear the barrettes she so desparately wanted, said of her child's death, "That great sadness did something to me. . . . Nothing could hurt more. I don't think *anything could hurt more*."

It is important to note that although each participant reported some form of hurting, not all experienced the same emotions. Several, for example, reported absolutely no anger associated with bereavement and none was detected in their accounts. The only unanimously reported emotion was sadness. The most frequently used metaphors were those of physical injury, as in having been "wounded," metaphors that were extended through expressions of the need for "healing," and the existence of a permanent "scar."

Missing is a theme of bereavement that describes the acute awareness of all that has been lost. Most frequently, missing includes the wishing or yearning for the loved one's presence in the face of the irreversible, permanent nature of the absence. The loss of the loved one was perceived as a kind of emptiness, sometimes described as a "hole," "void," or "vacuum." The bereaved one was left with a sense of desolation, deprivation, or abandonment, sometimes described as utter loneliness or aloneness. But missing also included a sense of other deprivations as well, feelings of loss of one's past or future, of one's "home," dreams, social role, or personal characteristics such as "lost innocence." As one person stated, "more dies than just the person." One expression illustrating the intersection of missing with hurting was "It is like a part of me has been amputated."

Expressions of missing the loved one tended to be simple and direct, with repeated statements such as "I miss him so much." One middle-aged man, with a young family of his own, repeatedly mentioned missing his mother. Though not devastated by her death, having anticipated it for years, he noted how he caught himself thinking "I ought to be able to call her." How that since her death he felt, "I just need to reach out and say 'Hello, Mom, I love you' — so I do. . . . I wish I could hold her one more time."

Holding is a theme of selective preservation encompassing the bereaved one's desire to maintain all, particularly that which was good, from the loved one's lost existence. Or in some cases, to leave what one could behind. Ways of holding included preserving the lost relationship by "doing for him," "honoring his wishes," carrying on his legacy, valued characteristics, responsibilities, or name. Mourning rituals provided another way of *doing for* the loved one.

Holding was accomplished by many through maintaining the reality that the loved one once lived. For even the youngest deceased, with the shortest history (a newborn), the importance of accurate recording and telling of the facts of life was of utmost importance. The slightest errors in newspaper obituaries were a source of great distress. Memorials and shrines were sometimes constructed, and photographs and personal items saved.

To some extent, holding was a sorting process. Certain objects were selected as particularly significant, collected, and saved; happy, "good" memories were recalled and related, while painful ones were "pushed back." (The persistence of painful memories, such as the final gasps for breath, were reported as particularly distressing by some, along with deliberate efforts to make them fade.) For one mother, whose deceased son's history had included many "troubles," such as conflicts with the law, holding through memories was referred to as a "cleansing process where you keep the good and throw out the bad."

Holding also involved continuing the loved one's "presence" through ways such as "praying or talking aloud to him," "writing to him in a journal," or "feeling him present" from time to time. A few reported permitting themselves to pretend, momentarily, that a stranger observed to look like the deceased (such as when out shopping or driving) *was* the deceased, for a fleeting moment. A source of disappointment for several people was the reluctance of relatives and friends to mention the deceased "for fear of upsetting me." Thus, the desire to hold by talking about the loved one, keeping the memory alive, was interfered with. For some, holding was accomplished through "holding onto" the grief or the anger. For example, "I don't want to feel better really. If I give up the grief then he'll really be gone."

For two participants, both widowers, the theme of holding was partly expressed in the form of struggling to purposefully hold as little as possible. There was a desire to "put it behind me," to eradicate physical reminders from the household, particularly sentimental items, to move to new houses, and to "try not to think about her." At the same time, however, both spoke at length about their wives. One led me through the house pointing out meaning-laden items. The other performed a therapeutic treatment on my feet during which he related that he was continuing to provide such treatments to comfort others "in her (deceased wife's) honor." Thus people "held" and "let go" in highly individual ways.

Colorful statements illustrating holding included the following: "We named our first child after him"; "I want to get to a good memory"; "She'd be pleased that I'm making something come from her death" [participation in MADD]; "I enjoy wearing her clothes"; "Being a mother, I wanted to do *everything* for her — I wanted to dig the grave"; "I wrote him letters then took them to the physical plant and watched the ashes drift up to the sky!"; "I almost felt I was living for both of us."

Seeking is a theme of bereavement that describes a search for help. Expressions of "what helps" and "what doesn't help" are frequent. The search for help takes the form of seeking comfort and meaning. Comfort was sought through the conduct of rituals, prayer, staying busy, writing and reading about bereavement, and seeking out others who really understand. "Someone, somewhere must be able to help." In some cases, comfort was sought through attempts to avoid pain by using alcohol or staying frantically busy. As one person noted, "I threw myself into my work, never gave myself a chance to think about it."

For some, the search for meaning overlapped the search for comfort. Questions of "Why?" were asked and ways of creating some kind of positive meaning sought. Illustrative statements included: "I'm searching. I'm on a real quest for the meaning of life," and "I want to use the experience to help others — make it meaningful."

The value to the bereaved of caring *for* others was mentioned by 18 of the participants and illustrates a search for meaning through "making the death count for something." It may also have meaning as a way of seeking comfort for oneself by comforting others.

The ability of others to provide the comfort sought was described both positively and negatively. Most were exceptionally appreciative of the "caring presence of others." For example, one woman stated, "I felt all 50 people in the church were suffering with me. It helped." But some mentioned anger with others' inept attempts at consolation, annoyed by clichés and platitudes: "You'll have your memories"; "It was God's will."

Meta-Themes

Change is a theme about bereavement that describes its dynamic, change-inducing character. Bereavement changes in quality and intensity, and alters the life of the bereaved. That bereavement itself changes was conveyed both directly, "The ache isn't as bad now," and implicitly through the use of past verb tenses, "I *was* devastated." Nineteen participants referred to a wave like quality to bereavement, noting "mountains and valleys," "like a roller coaster," "a soft curtain seemed to come down over the whole experience," occasionally punctuated by acute, unexpected "breaks" when something triggered the grief response. Such acute, brief grief attacks were reported to occur even many years after the death. Most participants concluded that while the quality of bereavement changes and softens, some elements remain permanent. "It'll never be *over*." "If you forget, it would end, but you can't forget." "A scar remains."

The changes that bereavement brings about were varied and of a catalytic quality. Relationships with living loved ones were altered. Sometimes previously satisfying relationships were enhanced and unsatisfying ones worsened. An impetus to take actions previously only contemplated, such as returning to school or changing jobs, was also reported. Self-esteem was reported to have changed, usually for the better. Finally, the world itself was said to have changed. Places, things, and natural and social events took on a new significance relevant to the bereaved's experience with the deceased. For one bereaved, rain, once responsible for the lethal mudslide, is now permanently different and the old homestead, now achingly empty, both attracts and hurts in an unfamiliar way.

Expectations is the theme that describes a sense of "rightness" or "oughtness" that hovers over bereavement. That there is a right way to grieve, mourn, feel, honor, and conduct oneself while bereaved is a meta-dimension layered over the ongoing "natural" experience. "Correct" or "proper" bereavement was sometimes perceived as a vague awareness of "wanting to do it right," sometimes to the point of prescriptive self-impositions that one *must* be angry, go through specific stages, act in a certain way, not feel as one feels, and not grieve as long as one grieves (or should grieve longer). In general, the sense of "oughtness" tended to be a burden that led to a need to pretend either grief or recovery, a reluctance to talk openly, and a state of aloneness.

Examples of expectations included: "I wondered if I'd done a good enough job with the funeral arrangements"; "I cover it at work—the depression, dullness. It takes a lot of energy"; "Maybe I *shouldn't* laugh again."

Inexpressibility refers to the felt inadequacy of words to describe the experience of personal bereavement. Repeatedly, people spoke of how difficult it was, even impossible, to find the words to truly convey their experience. Recurring statements indicated that only comparable confrontations with death were felt to provide a shared understanding. Those who have experienced similar losses (such as death of children) were said, by some, to form "a secret society," a society into which only the same experience provides entry.

Contextual Theme

Personal history is the theme within which the five core themes (being stopped, hurting, missing, holding, seeking) are embedded and is essential for understanding bereavement's quality. Understanding the bereaved's history; who the loved one was; what that person meant to the survivor; how they were together; what their hopes, dreams, shared experiences were; and the nature of the events surrounding the death are critical for understanding bereavement.

The importance of understanding what the deceased meant to the bereaved, the quality of the lost relationship, and the circumstances surrounding the death for understanding bereavement was at first elusive. No one expressed this directly, yet participants often began their discussions with a lengthy history filled with personal details about the deceased. It was as though the participants were saying, "Before I can help you understand my bereavement, you must understand who this loved one was and what happened."

DISCUSSION

The Freudian perspective on bereavement, as expressed in "Mourning and Melancholia" (1957), was found to have points of both convergence and divergence from the bereavement themes. Areas of greatest similarity to the themes were the Freudian descriptions of bereavement's painfulness, its slow and gradual change, and the rarity in occurrence of diminished self-esteem. The greatest discrepancies pertained to the concept of bereavement's final endpoint (generally denied by participants) and the psychoanalytic mental process of replacement, whereby the bereaved are thought to replace the lost loved one with someone or something else (also denied by participants). Freud himself noted the difficulty in explaining bereavement: "Why this process . . . should be extraordinarily painful is not at all easy to explain in terms of mental economics" (p. 126). Themes especially unaccounted for by Freud were "seeking," "change," "expectations," and "inexpressibility."

Areas of agreement between the Kübler–Ross stages of dying and the bereavement themes included the sense of interruption in the normal flow of life (being stopped), a sense of loss and sadness or depression (hurting and missing), and, in some cases, an enhanced state of reflectiveness (seeking). Yet, essential features of the five core themes of bereavement were generally unaddressed, as were the three meta-themes. The Kübler–Ross stage of bargaining is irrelevant and has no counterpart in the nine bereavement themes. In addition, the Kübler–Ross model suggests an orderliness and segmentation to a life experience which was rarely noted by participants as consistent with their experience. Two participants who were members of helping professions related experiencing "going through stages." Most did not; a few, however, noted that they were told they *would* or *should* go through stages, which was at times a source of worry.

Omissions in the Kübler–Ross perspective included the sense of pain and burden in hurting, the emptiness in missing, all but the interruption of life's flow in being stopped, all but the enhancement of reflectiveness sometimes accompanying seeking, the predominant characteristics of change, and the entire content of holding.

Though expressed in different words and varying in intensity and scope, agreement was found between the themes of bereavement and an existential–phenomenological perspective with reference to being stopped, hurting, missing, and seeking. Only two-thirds of the participants, however, described themselves as experiencing a renewed interest in seeking meaning, the consequence of the loss of anchorage so stressed within the existential–phenomenological description. Most of the features of holding, a core theme, were found unaddressed as were those of expectations, a meta-theme.

None of the three theoretical perspectives on bereavement examined in this study were found to provide a wholly adequate base for nursing care. The nine themes which emerged from the analysis, though nonprescriptive, suggest appropriate responses for the care of the bereaved. Using the themes as a guide, nurses could anticipate a broad range of unique responses from the bereaved. For example, not every patient can be expected to be equally devastated or compelled to pass through a stage of anger. The nurse should understand and be patient with the need for holding, for sharing memories, for taking a photo of a dead infant in the nursery, for clipping a piece of the loved one's hair. The significance of the patient's stories about the past, about who the deceased loved ones had been and how they had died, need to be recognized. Sudden recurrences of grief in the patient whose loved one died years ago need to be understood and accepted as part of the bereavement process.

REFERENCES

Arendt, H. (1974). *The human condition*. Chicago: University of Chicago.

Buber, M. (1965). *The knowledge of man: Selected essays*. (M. Friedman & R. Smith, trans.). New York: Harper & Row Publishers.

Frankl, J. F. (1963). *Man's search for meaning: An introduction to logotherapy*. New York: Pocket Books.

Freud, S. (1957). Mourning and melancholia. (J. Riviere, trans.). In J. Rickman (Ed.), *A general selection from the works of Sigmund Freud* (pp. 124–140). New York: Liveright Publishing Corp. (Originally published 1917).

Kübler–Ross, E. (1972). *On death and dying*. New York: Macmillan Publishing Co.

Needleman, J. (1973). The moment of grief. In E. Wyschogrod (Ed.), *The phenomenon of death: Faces of mortality*. New York: Harper & Row Publishers.

Taylor, S. & Bogdan, R. (1984). *Introduction to qualitative research methods: The search for meanings* (2nd ed.). New York: John Wiley & Sons.

Tillich, P. (1965). The eternal now. In H. Feifel (Ed.). *The meaning of death*. New York: McGraw–Hill Book Co.

van Kaam, A. (1966). *Existential foundations of psychology*. Pittsburgh: Duquesne University Press.

van Manen, M. (1984). Practicing phenomenological writing. *Phenomenology and Pedagogy, 2*(1), 36–69.

Analysis of Theory

The stated purpose of Carter's (1989) study was to identify themes associated with bereavement obtained from individuals who had experienced the death of a loved one and to compare those themes with three existing theoretical perspectives of bereavement. The study may be classified as descriptive research designed to generate a descriptive theory.

CONCEPT IDENTIFICATION AND CLASSIFICATION

The investigator used a qualitative approach to collect and analyze the data, from which a descriptive classification theory of bereavement was generated. Analysis of the study findings reveals that the theory includes one concept: bereavement. This concept has nine dimensions, which are referred to as themes in the report. The dimensions are being stopped, hurting, missing, holding, seeking, change, expectations, inexpressibility, and personal history.

Its multidimensional nature indicates that bereavement may be classified as a variable. It may be classified as a theoretical term in Kaplan's (1964) schema because it is such a complex, global property; it may be classified as a construct in Willer and Webster's (1970) schema because it is so abstract; and it may be classified as a summative unit in Dubin's (1978) schema because of its complexity.

The designation of the theory of bereavement as a descriptive classification theory is based on the investigator's categorization of three types of themes, that is, concept dimensions. Being stopped, hurting, missing, holding, and seeking are categorized as core themes. Change, expectations, and inexpressibility are categorized as meta-themes. Personal history is considered the contextual theme in which the five core themes are embedded.

PROPOSITION IDENTIFICATION AND CLASSIFICATION

Statements about the concept bereavement and its nine dimensions may be classified as nonrelational propositions. The one statement pertaining to the concept of bereavement in the theory that was generated is:

> [The data analysis] resulted in a preliminary hypothetical explication of the bereavement phenomenon consisting of nine general themes.

This statement can be formalized into the following nonrelational existence proposition:

> The phenomenon of bereavement encompasses nine dimensions — being stopped, hurting, missing, holding, seeking, change, expectations, inexpressibility, and personal history.

Nine additional statements pertain to the dimensions of the concept of bereavement. These statements, which are listed in Table A–4, may be classified as nonrelational definitional propositions because they are constitutive definitions.

The operational definition for the concept bereavement can be extracted from the report. Bereavement is operationally defined as follows: Themes of bereavement (being stopped, hurting, missing, holding, seeking, change, expectations, inexpressibility, and personal history) were induced from responses to an interview consisting of open-ended, nondirective questions and structured questions, as well as supplementary materials provided by the study participants, including poetry, notes, and photos. The actual empirical indicators are taperecordings, researcher notes, and participants' documents (poems, notes, photographs).

HIERARCHY OF PROPOSITIONS

The use of a qualitative approach for collection and analysis of the data indicates that hierarchies of propositions would be inductive. In fact, the investigator included enough examples of verbatim responses from the

TABLE A – 4.   Constitutive Definitions for the Dimensions of Bereavement

Dimension (Theme)	Constitutive Definition
Being stopped	The theme of bereavement that describes the interruption of life's usual flow following the death of a loved one. The theme is characterized by varying types and degrees of inability, frequently stated in terms of "I can't."
Hurting	A theme of bereavement characterized by a cluster of intensely painful emotions. Feelings of sorrow or sadness, usually accompanied by tearfulness and crying, are of such severity that they were referred to by most as "pain."
Missing	A theme of bereavement that describes the acute awareness of all that has been lost. Most frequently, "missing" includes the wishing or yearning for the loved one's presence in the face of the irreversible, permanent nature of the absence.
Holding	A theme of selective preservation encompassing the bereaved one's desire to maintain all, particularly that which was good, from the loved one's lost existence or, in some cases, to leave what one could behind.
Seeking	A theme of bereavement that describes a search for help. The search for help takes the form of seeking comfort and meaning.
Change	A theme about bereavement that describes the dynamic, change-inducing character of bereavement.
Expectations	The theme that describes a sense of "rightness" or "oughtness" that hovers over bereavement.
Inexpressibility	The theme that refers to the felt inadequacy of words to describe the experience of personal bereavement.
Personal history	The theme within which the five core themes (being stopped, hurting, missing, holding, seeking) are embedded and which is essential for understanding bereavement's quality. Understanding the bereaved's history, who the loved one was, what that person meant to the survivor, how they were together, what their hopes, dreams, shared experiences were, and the nature of the events surrounding the death are critical for understanding bereavement.

study participants to construct inductive hierarchies for all of the dimensions of bereavement except inexpressibility and personal history. The examples of verbatim responses for each dimension are the observations, and the nonrelational definitional proposition stating the constitutive definition for the dimension is the conclusion. An example is the inductive hierarchy that was constructed for the dimension of hurting.

Observation$_1$	Pain, I can't stand it.
Observation$_2$	There is no relief—hurt, hurt, hurt.
Observation$_3$	It really hit me.
Observation$_4$	I want to lick my wounds.
Observation$_5$	God is a gigantic practical joker who does things to people.
Observation$_6$	That great sadness did something to me. . . . Nothing could hurt more. I don't think *anything could hurt more.*
Conclusion	Hurting is a theme of bereavement characterized by a cluster of intensely painful emotions. Feelings of sorrow or sadness, usually accompanied by tearfulness and crying, are of such severity that they were referred to by most as "pain."

CONCEPTUAL-THEORETICAL-EMPIRICAL STRUCTURE

Examination of the titles of citations in Carter's discussion of the data analysis plan indicates that phenomenology served as the methodologic frame of reference for the research. Although Carter discussed the operations used for data analysis, she did not identify concepts or propositions that reflect the philosophic or substantive underpinnings of this method. A vertical proposition linking the methodologic frame of reference to the empirical indicators is, however, evident in Carter's statement that the framework for conducting the analysis was derived from recommendations by van Kaam, Taylor and Bogdan, and van Manen.

DIAGRAM

A diagram was constructed to illustrate the conceptual-theoretical-empirical structure for Carter's study (Fig. A–2). A second diagram was constructed to more fully illustrate the concept of bereavement by including its dimensions (Fig. A–3). This diagram depicts the embedding of the core themes in the contextual theme, personal history.

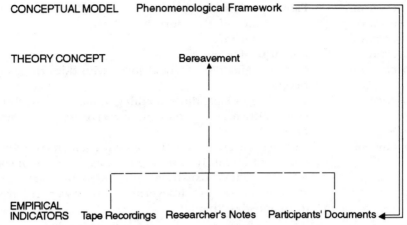

Figure A-2. Conceptual-theoretical-empirical structure for Carter's study (1989).

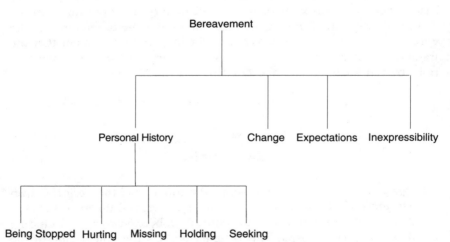

Figure A-3. The concept of bereavement and its dimensions.

EVALUATION OF THE RELATION BETWEEN THEORY AND RESEARCH

The stated intent of this study was to identify themes associated with bereavement obtained from individuals who had experienced the death of a loved one and to compare those themes with three existing theoretical perspectives of bereavement. The outcome of the research was generation of a theory of bereavement.

SIGNIFICANCE

The theory of bereavement meets the criterion of significance in part. The theoretical significance of the research is implied in the first sentence of the report, where Carter stated that "no single, general, universally accepted theoretical perspective on the phenomenon of bereavement exists." Carter went on to review the main ideas of three theoretical perspectives that she claimed are popular in the nursing literature. Furthermore, in the discussion section, Carter maintained that "none of the three theoretical perspectives examined in this study were found to provide a wholly adequate base for nursing care." It is unclear whether Carter's intent, then, was to develop a general theory that would be universally accepted and would be an adequate base for nursing care. The social significance of the research was not addressed.

Carter's theory of bereavement does deal with a phenomenon of interest to the discipline of nursing. In particular, the theory addresses a principle governing the life process, that of bereavement.

As is to be expected of the product of descriptive theory-generating research, the theory of bereavement does not predict with any precision. It does, however, enhance understanding of the multidimensional nature of bereavement.

INTERNAL CONSISTENCY

The theory of bereavement partially meets the criterion of internal consistency. Semantic clarity is evident in that bereavement is described in terms of nine dimensions and each dimension is defined clearly and concisely.

Semantic consistency for the dimensions of bereavement also is evident, inasmuch as each dimension is defined just once. Furthermore, there are no redundancies in the dimensions of the concept of bereavement.

A lack of semantic consistency is, however, evident in the review of the three theoretical perspectives. In this section of the report, three different terms are used: bereavement, mourning, and grief. Furthermore, the term grief is used in the title of the report. The use of the terms grief and mourning raises a question about exactly what phenomenon was addressed by the other theoretical perspectives and introduces confusion into an otherwise consistent research report.

The propositions of the theory reflect structural consistency. It is possible to construct inductive hierarchies for seven of the nine dimensions of the concept bereavement. The discussion of the two dimensions for which hierarchies cannot be constructed (inexpressibility and personal history) does, however, contain sufficient evidence to support the conclusions represented by their constitutive definitions.

PARSIMONY

Formalization of the theory of bereavement indicates that the theory meets the criterion of parsimony. The decision to identify bereavement as the single concept of the theory and the themes as dimensions of this concept, rather than identify the themes as separate concepts, yielded a description of the phenomenon of bereavement that is neither oversimplified nor excessively verbose.

TESTABILITY

The theory of bereavement meets the criterion of testability, inasmuch as it would be possible to test the theory by replicating the study by using the methodology employed by Carter. The actual questions asked during interviews would, however, have to be obtained from the investigator for a replication study. No hypotheses were generated by Carter, but a falsifiable hypothesis asserting that bereavement encompasses the nine dimensions identified in this study could be developed and tested. Testability could have been improved, however, if the investigator had indicated how many study participants experienced each dimension of bereavement.

OPERATIONAL ADEQUACY

The research design used to generate the theory of bereavement partially meets the criterion of operational adequacy. The sample was composed of adults who had experienced the death of a loved one, which provided the necessary prerequisite for bereavement. Understanding the representativeness of the sample would, however, have been improved if the causes of death had been listed. Furthermore, generalizability to the population of bereaved persons would have been enhanced if more males had been included in the sample.

The empirical indicators are appropriate qualitative measures for a phenomenological inquiry. Furthermore, the investigator's description of the data analysis plan and the method used to validate the findings indicates that the analysis was in keeping with the methodologic guidelines of phenomenological inquiry (Oiler, 1986). The report does not, however, include any discussion of how the investigator controlled for bias in data collection and analysis, which is an important feature of the phenomenological method.

EMPIRICAL ADEQUACY

The theory of bereavement meets the criterion of empirical adequacy for descriptive research using qualitative methods. The data presented in the form of verbatim comments from study participants support the conclusions regarding the dimensions of bereavement. Furthermore, by using a novel approach to establishment of empirical adequacy, Carter collected data that permitted a comparison of the study findings with the concepts of three alternative theories (the Freudian perspective, Kübler-Ross's stages of dying, and an existential-phenomenological perspective). In effect, she used the data from her study to extend consideration of empirical adequacy to the three alternative theories. Her discussion of the areas of agreement and disagreement between the dimensions of her theory and the major concepts of the three other theories suggests that her theory is more comprehensive. The inclusion of Kübler-Ross's stages of dying as an alternative description of bereavement must, however, be questioned, inasmuch as that theory deals with the person who is dying rather than the bereaved survivor.

PRAGMATIC ADEQUACY

The theory of bereavement meets the criterion of pragmatic adequacy. Carter identified guidelines for the nursing care of the bereaved. These guidelines are in the form of expectations regarding the various responses a bereaved person might display.

CONCEPTUAL-THEORETICAL-EMPIRICAL STRUCTURE

The methods used to collect and analyze the data from which the theory of bereavement was generated are in keeping with a phenomenological frame of reference. Inasmuch as concepts and propositions reflecting the philosophical or substantive elements of this frame of reference are not identified, evaluation of its credibility is not possible.

REFERENCES

Dubin, R. (1978). *Theory building* (rev. ed.). New York: The Free Press.

Carter, S. L. (1989). Themes of grief. *Nursing Research, 38*, 354–358.

Kaplan, A. (1964). *The conduct of inquiry.* San Francisco: Chandler.

Oiler, C. J. (1986). Phenomenology: The method. In P. L. Munhall & C. J. Oiler (Eds.), *Nursing research: A qualitative perspective* (pp. 69–84). Norwalk, CT: Appleton-Century-Crofts.

Willer, D., & Webster, M., Jr. (1970). Theoretical concepts and observables. *American Sociological Review, 35*, 748–757.

Analysis and Evaluation of Two Correlational Studies

THE RELATIONSHIP BETWEEN SOCIAL SUPPORT AND SELF-CARE PRACTICES

Patricia Hubbard
Ann F. Muhlenkamp
Nancy Brown

A two-study approach was used to investigate the relationship between individuals' perceived level of social support and their performance of specific, positive health practices. One sample consisted of 97 adults, age 55 and older, attending activities at a senior citizen's center. The second sample was comprised of adults attending a health fair. Subjects were surveyed using the Lifestyle Questionnaire and the Personal Resources Questionnaire. The primary study hypothesis — that a strong, positive association would be found between the social support and health practices variables — was upheld for both samples. A secondary hypothesis — that married participants would score significantly higher on both the social support and health practices instruments than would their nonmarried counterparts — was supported only among the senior center participants. An additional hypothesis generated for the senior center participants — that participants with a confidant would have significantly higher scores on both the social support and health practices instruments — was upheld.

Folk wisdom supports the belief that one's physical health and psychological well-being depend to a great extent on one's nurturing relation-

---

Patricia Hubbard, MS, is a research associate in the College of Nursing at Arizona State University, Tempe, AZ. Ann F. Muhlenkamp, PhD, is a professor of nursing in the College of Nursing at Arizona State University, Tempe, AZ. Nancy Brown, MS, is an instructor in the College of Nursing at Arizona State University, Tempe, AZ.

This work was supported in part by a grant NU00800-03 from the Division of Nursing, Department of Health and Human Services.

Reprinted from *Nursing Research*, *33*, 266–270, 1984.

ships. Not until recently, however, has research begun to document this important association between the supportiveness of the social environment and health. However, the actual mechanisms through which social support works to promote and maintain healthy functioning remain unclear. One possible explanation lies in the possibility that those people who are enmeshed in supportive social networks take better care of themselves by engaging in more positive health practices than do people with less supportive networks.

The link between health practices and health has been well-documented (USDHEW, 1979), and few would dispute the fact that a person's life-style has a significant impact on the individual's health. Syme (cited in Ferguson) pointed out that "many common ailments may not be so much medical problems as problems of living," and that "virtually every disease and ailment may be related to the way in which we conduct our lives" (1980, p. 7). In addition, there is increasing evidence that developing and maintaining supportive relationships may be as important to wellness as are other more commonly recognized health practices. Numerous studies have shown that good health and long life are positively related to a supportive social environment. In fact, people in supportive relationships have been found to have lower morbidity and mortality from all causes (Belloc & Breslow, 1972; Lynch, 1977).

REVIEW OF THE LITERATURE

Excellent reviews of the literature on social support are available (Cobb, 1976; Mitchell & Trickett, 1980; Norbeck, 1981). As Dimond and Jones (1983) noted in their conceptual analysis of social support, diverse definitions of the construct abound, yet these definitions converge on several points. Points in common include the idea of social support as a multifaceted construct comprised of the communication of positive affect, a sense of belonging or social integration, and elements of reciprocity. In addition, the construct may or may not encompass instrumental behavior. The approaches to defining social support usually proceed from a consideration of its source, such as who provides it; the functions it serves for people, such as affective need gratification or material aid; and the intimacy characteristics of the relationship, such as whether it is a confiding relationship (Mueller, 1980).

The literature concerning the relationship between social support and health generally has focused on two main ideas. Social support is viewed as either having some direct, protective influence on the person

(Cassel, 1974; Wolf, 1980) or as buffering the effects of stressful life events (Cobb, 1976; Dean & Lin, 1977; Lin, Ensel, Simeone, & Kuo, 1979; Tolsdorf, 1976). Thoits (1982), however, criticized the research that has tried to establish that social support acts as a buffer against stress. She pointed out that methodological deficits have plagued studies, including imprecise definitions, failure to treat social support as a multidimensional concept, and confounding of study results through the interactive effects of other variables with social support.

Other studies have linked social support and specific health practices. Berkman and Syme (1979) hypothesized several possible explanations for the positive relationship between social support and good health. According to one explanation, the socially isolated may be more likely to adopt self-destructive health practices. Another explanation is the possibility that social isolation may lead to depression, which, in turn, may predispose toward accidents or suicide. Finally, Berkman and Syme suggested that inadequate support may cause actual physiological changes that increase susceptibility to disease. Langlie (1977), in a survey of 383 Midwestern adults, found that appropriate indirect health risk behaviors such as use of a seat belt, exercise and nutrition behavior, medical and dental care, and various screening exams were associated with a social network characterized by high socioeconomic status and frequent interaction between nonkin. Pratt (1971) found that structural characteristics of the family influenced personal health maintenance practices. Coburn and Pope (1974) reported that SES positively affected health practices among their sample of Canadian male workers, and that group membership and participation were also significant indicators of health practices.

HYPOTHESES

The purpose of the current investigation was to explore the relationship between what people do to promote healthy life-styles and how they perceive their level of social support. The primary hypothesis was that a positive association would be found between the social support and health practice variables. Secondary hypotheses included that married participants would score significantly higher on both the social support and health practice instruments than would their nonmarried counterparts; and participants with a confidant would have higher scores on both the social support and the health practice instruments.

METHOD

To test these hypotheses, a descriptive survey approach was used. Two distinct samples are reported as Study 1 and Study 2.

The data from the two samples were not combined as the subjects' characteristics were so disparate — a relatively homogeneous group of senior citizens and a demographically heterogeneous group of health fair participants. Therefore, no statistical comparisons have been made between the groups. The second study is, in effect, a replication of the first for the purpose of demonstrating the robustness of the phenomenon under question.

Instruments

Social support is viewed as a multidimensional construct consisting of people as interpersonal resources who provide gratification of basic human needs in relationships. Adequacy of the individual's perceived level of social support was measured using Brandt and Weinert's (1981) Personal Resources Questionnaire (PRQ), Part II. This instrument was designed to tap five dimensions of social support proposed by Weiss (1974). These dimensional subscales are labeled intimacy, social integration, nurturance, worth, and assistance. The PRQ-II consists of 25 statements that are responded to on a 7-point Likert scale from *strongly agree* to *strongly disagree*. Brandt and Weinert (1981) reported a Cronbach's alpha of .89 on Part II of the PRQ and validity coefficients of between .30 and .44 ($p<.001$).

Positive health practices are specific activities performed that may affect one's health. The six kinds of practices considered in this study are nutrition, exercise, relaxation, safety, substance use, and prevention practices. The Lifestyle Questionnaire (Brown, Muhlenkamp, Fox, & Osborn, 1983; Muhlenkamp & Brown, 1983) was used to measure these activities. This instrument contains 24 items and includes 4 statements relating to each of the 6 health-practice categories. Items are scored on a 4-point Likert scale with responses ranging from *regularly* to *never*. Higher scores on the scale indicate more positive health practices.

Validity was established by Brown et al. (1983) through administering the Lifestyle Questionnaire to two samples who had also completed the first edition of the Stevens Point Health Assessment instrument (1980), which measures level of wellness. A correlation of .83 was found between the two instruments. Test-retest reliability was .88 at three weeks and .78 at four weeks. Cronbach's alpha was .76 on a sample of 383. The scale was found to be relatively free of social desirability response set.

In addition to data from these two instruments, routine sociodemographic data were collected to further describe the sample.

STUDY 1

Sample

The sample consisted of 97 volunteers who represented 88% of the individuals initially approached to participate at a senior citizen's center in a Southwest metropolitan area. Fifty-seven of the participants were female and 40 were male, ranging in age from 55 to 90, with a mean of 70. Ninety-seven percent of the participants were Caucasian and a majority (66%) were Protestant. The mean educational level was 13½ years, or just over 1 year of college. The mean annual income ranged from $10,000 to $14,000, identifying these people as more affluent than the majority of their agemates nationally. A social class variable was computed using Hollingshead's (1957) Two-Factor Index, which requires a listing for educational level and occupation. Although some of the subjects did not complete the income item, four of Hollingshead's five social classes were represented among the 59% of the subjects who were willing to provide the income data; none of the participants were members of the lowest class.

Results

Of the 175 possible points on the social support instrument (PRQ-II), the mean score among the senior adults was 135 (SD = 19). Because the literature links the presence of a confiding relationship to well-being, a yes/no response item was added at the end of the instrument: "Is there a person you confide in or talk to about yourself or your problems?" A similar item was included by Brandt and Weinert on Part I of the PRQ. A high percentage (91%) answered yes.

The mean Lifestyle score among this group was 80 (maximum score possible on this instrument was 96). Of the subscales, exercise had the lowest reported positive response, with a mean of 11 of the possible 16 points. The highest mean scores were on the relaxation and substance-use subscales. A significant, positive correlation of .37 ($p = .0002$) was found between the total scores of the PRQ and the Lifestyle Questionnaire.

Married participants reported significantly higher levels of perceived support than did nonmarried respondents and single individuals perceived themselves as the least supported. Those individuals who reported having a confidant scored significantly higher on both the PRQ ($t(8.5) = 3.06$; $p = .01$) and the Lifestyle Questionnaire ($t(95) = 2.05$; $p = .04$) than did participants lacking a confiding relationship. In addition, the presence of a confidant was significantly related to higher social class ($r = .32$; $p = .01$) and older age was positively related to the Lifestyle score ($r = .19$; $p = .06$). When the effects of social support, and other socioeconomic variables were assessed for their combined effect on positive health behavior, an R^2 of .20 resulted. Social support emerged as the most significant indicator, accounting for 14% of the variance in the Lifestyle Questionnaire. None of the additional variables included reached significance.

STUDY 2

Sample

This sample consisted of 133 individuals attending a health fair in a large metropolitan area. The health fair, sponsored by a local hospital, provided an opportunity to collect the desired data at two shopping malls over a four-day period. Approximately 65% of the participants approached volunteered to complete the questionnaires.

Of the 133 people participating in the study, 58 were female, 73 were male, and 2 did not specify their sex. Ages ranged from 15 to 77 years with a mean of 44 years. Participants were overwhelmingly Caucasian (95%); 3% were Asian and fewer than 1% were Black. Six marital status categories were represented: married (72%), single (14%), widowed (5%), divorced (5%), other unspecified (2%), and separated (1%).

Nine percent of the respondents did not graduate from high school and 24% reported having the equivalent of a high school education. Of the remainder, 36% had some college and 27% had a college or professional degree. Just over half (51%) of the participants were employed, whereas 23% were retired, 18% were either homemakers, volunteers, or students, and 6% were unemployed.

Of the 65% of the sample responding to the type of occupation item,

34% were employed in either professional, technical, or managerial positions. In addition, 18% were in clerical or sales positions, 8% were craftsmen, foremen, or operative personnel, and 5% were in service or labor-type occupations.

Results

The mean score on the PRQ-II among these health fair participants was 130 (SD = 20). The mean Lifestyle score was 68.1 (SD = 9), with mean subscale scores ranging from 8.5 for health promotion to 15.1 for substance use.

The overall correlation between social support and health practices was .57 ($p = .0001$). When the effects of social support and demographic variables were assessed for their combined impact upon positive health behavior using stepwise multiple linear regression techniques, the R^2 was .38. Social support was the most significant indicator and accounted for 34% of the variance in positive health practices.

Females had higher health practice scores ($\overline{x} = 70.8$; SD = 8.8) than did males ($\overline{x} = 66.0$; SD = 9.3). This difference was significant ($t(129) = 3.0$; $p = .003$). The mean social support score for females ($\overline{x} = 134.6$; SD = 20.96) was also higher than that of males ($\overline{x} = 126.0$; SD = 19.35); this difference was again significant ($t(129) = 2.43$; $p = .02$). No significant associations attributable to education, occupation, marital status, or age were discovered.

Table 1 shows the information obtained from the PRQ-II for both samples. Table 2 compares the two sample's responses on the Lifestyle Questionnaire.

TABLE 1. Comparison of Mean Social Support (PRQ) Scores

	SENIOR CENTER (n = 97)			HEALTH FAIR (n = 133)		
Subscale	$\overline{X}$	SD	Range	$\overline{X}$	SD	Range
Intimacy	27.66	5	11–35	27.06	6	9–35
Social integration	28.05	5	13–35	25.80	5	9–35
Nurturance	24.79	6	11–35	25.76	6	5–35
Worth	27.20	5	12–35	25.68	5	12–35
Assistance	26.99	5	5–35	25.82	5	5–35
PRQ total	134.69	19	66–175	130.11	20	76–175

TABLE 2. Comparison of Mean Health Practice (Lifestyle) Scores

Subscale	SENIOR CENTER ($n = 97$)			HEALTH FAIR ($n = 133$)		
	$\overline{X}$	SD	Range	$\overline{X}$	SD	Range
Exercise	11.44	3	4–16	9.53	3	4–16
Nutrition	13.29	2	7–16	12.11	3	4–16
Relaxation	14.75	1	12–16	11.57	3	4–16
Health promotion	12.16	4	4–16	8.53	4	4–16
Substance use	14.60	2	9–16	15.08	2	9–16
Safety	13.91	2	8–16	11.35	3	6–16
Lifestyle total	80.15	8	56–93	68.09	9	39–95

DISCUSSION

In view of the nonrandom nature of the two samples, the generalizations presented here are tentative. However, the primary hypothesis was supported by both studies. Considering the other numerous variables that undoubtedly affect this relationship, such as childrearing practices, cultural influences, personality characteristics, and health education programs, the strength of these correlations becomes even more meaningful. Although the literature implies that the effects of social support and health practices are interactive, as yet no causal relationship has been established between the variables. It is possible that people who take better care of themselves are more capable of attracting and maintaining supportive relationships. However, it seems just as likely that those people who have more adequate social support would tend to lead healthier lifestyles. Whether this link is or is not causal in nature, the relationship between the two is important, since intervention aimed at one may also affect the other.

The secondary hypothesis was only supported by the senior center study. Married individuals among this sample scored significantly higher on the PRQ-II than did their nonmarried counterparts. This finding suggests that the marriage relationship may be important to one's sense of having a socially supportive environment during later adulthood.

It is puzzling that marital status apparently did not make a difference in the health practices of these same subjects, since marital status may be viewed as one dimension of social support, and given the significant correlation between social support and health practices. It would appear that it is not only one's spouse that influences a person to perform positive health practices during later adulthood. Instead, it may be someone in an individual's larger social network that encourages good health practices. Included may be children, whom some of the nonmarried participants may not have available as support resources. However, both Langlie (1977) and Coburn and Pope (1974) argued that it is more likely the person's wider social network, exclusive of kin relationships, that is most likely to influence participation in positive health practices.

In the health fair sample, the mean age was 44, and marital status did not make a difference in either perceived level of social support or the number of health practices performed by the individuals. One possible interpretation of this finding is that marriage may not serve the same supportive function for younger people that it seems to for older adults. The wider social circle available to many young and midlife adults may provide adequate support regardless of marital status, particularly today when remaining single by choice is gaining more social approval.

Finally, the hypothesis that participants with a confidant would have higher scores on both the social support and the health practice instruments than would other subjects was upheld. However, data was only available for the senior center group. This finding supports the results of other researchers regarding the importance of a confidant to well-being (Dimond, 1979; Jordan & Meckler, 1982; Lowenthal & Haven, 1968). Although the identity of the confidant was not determined in the present study, such information would be valuable.

Several additional findings of interest emerged from the studies. Among the health fair participants, women had significantly higher scores on both the social support and the health practice instruments than did men. This is consistent with a cultural norm that encourages women to be more emotionally engaged in relationships than men. This difference also supports the research of Langlie (1977) and Mechanic and Cleary (1980), which found that women generally take better care of themselves than do men. In contrast, no significant differences based upon sex were found in the senior center sample. This finding is supported by Larson's (1978) review of research on the subjective well-being of older Americans in which no overall differences between women and men were revealed. It is possible that any differences existing between women and men at younger ages in regard to either social support or health practices disappear later in life.

Both samples could be considered limited at first glance — the senior center sample because of the social nature of the setting as well as the affluence of the participants and the health fair sample because of these individuals' motivation to attend such screening services. However, since the correlations between social support and health practices were strong for both samples, the problem of a social bias affecting the senior center study seems minimal. Furthermore, the mean Lifestyle scores for both groups were consistent with previous sample results, including Brown et al. (1983),* suggesting that affluence and motivation are also relatively unimportant.

In conclusion, these studies have affirmed the importance of social support as a variable in health-related behavior. Specifically, social support has been shown to be related to health practices among two samples of volunteer subjects. Although it is known that social support has a significant relationship to health, Cobb (1976) cautioned that it does not provide a panacea. Many other known and unknown variables are also vital to optimal health. Continuing exploration of the ways in which social support contributes to well-being appears to be a promising avenue of investigation with potential benefits for all ages.

IMPLICATIONS

Most nursing efforts to foster health have been directed toward the individual's assessed intrapersonal resources. This research provides evidence that it may be equally useful to focus on the interpersonal resources available to the person, since these may have an important influence on performance of positive health practices. In order to do this, nurses need the ability to assess the kind and amount of support needed by an individual, as well as to identify creative ways of encouraging the use of available supports.

Systematic assessment and intervention directed toward incorporating the social environment as a significant determinant of health status have been lacking (Norbeck, 1982). A greater awareness of the significance of social support to health and ways that it may be used in practice settings will be valuable contributions to nursing. Future research should focus on determining whether the relationship between social support and positive health practices is consistent across other samples.

---

*To convert the Lifestyle score in Brown et al. (1983) to the current scoring method, multiply the mean subscale score by the number of items in the subscale as necessary.

REFERENCES

Belloc, N. B., & Breslow, L. (1972). Relationship of physical health status and health practices. *Preventive Medicine, 1*, 409–421.

Berkman, L., & Syme, S. L. (1979). Social networks, host resistance, and mortality: A nine-year follow-up study of Alameda County residents. *American Journal of Epidemiology, 109*, 186–203.

Brandt, P., & Weinert, C. (1981). The PRQ—a social support measure. *Nursing Research, 30*, 277–280.

Brown, N., Muhlenkamp, A., Fox, L., & Osborn, M. (1983). The relationship between health beliefs, health values, and health-promotion activity. *Western Journal of Nursing Research, 5*, 155–163.

Cassel, J. (1974). Psychosocial processes and stress: Theoretical formulation. *International Journal of Health Services, 4*, 471–481.

Cobb, S. (1976). Social support as a moderator of life stress. *Psychosomatic Medicine, 38*, 300–314.

Coburn, D., & Pope, C. R. (1974). Socioeconomic status and preventive health behavior. *Journal of Health and Social Behavior, 15*, 67–77.

Dean, A., & Lin, N. (1977). The stress buffering role of social support. *The Journal of Nervous and Mental Disease, 165*, 403–417.

Dimond, M. (1979). Social support and adaptation to chronic illness: The case of maintenance hemodialysis. *Research in Nursing and Health, 2*, 101–108.

Dimond, M., & Jones, S. L. (1983). Social support: A review and theoretical integration. In P. L. Chinn (Ed.), *Advances in nursing theory development* (pp. 235–249). Rockville, MD: Aspen Systems Corp.

Ferguson, T. (1979–80, Winter). Friends and health. *Medical Self-Care*, pp. 3–7.

Hollingshead, A. B. (1957). *Two-factor index of social position*. Unpublished manuscript. (Available from author, P.O. Box 1965, Yale Station, New Haven, CT 06520).

Jordan, J., & Meckler, J. R. (1982). The relationship between life change events, social supports, and dysmenorrhea. *Research in Nursing and Health, 5*, 73–79.

Langlie, J. K. (1977). Social networks, health beliefs, and preventive health behavior. *Journal of Health and Social Behavior, 18*, 244–260.

Larson, R. (1978). Thirty years of research on the subjective well-being of older Americans. *Journal of Gerontology, 33*, 109–125.

Lifestyle Assessment Questionnaire. (2nd ed.). (1980). University of Wisconsin: Stevens Point Institute for Lifestyle Improvement.

Lin, N., Ensel, W., Simeone, R., & Kuo, W. (1979). Social support, stressful life events & illness: A model and an empirical test. *Journal of Health & Social Behavior, 20*, 108–119.

Lowenthal, M. F., & Haven, C. (1968). Interaction and adaptations: Intimacy as a critical variable. *American Sociological Review, 33*, 20–30.

Lynch, J. (1977). *The broken heart: The medical consequences of loneliness*. New York: Basic Books.

Mechanic, D., & Cleary, P. D. (1980). Factors associated with the maintenance of positive health behavior. *Preventive Medicine, 9*, 805–814.

Mitchell, R. E., & Trickett, E. S. (1980). Task force report: Social networks as mediators of social support. *Community Mental Health Journal, 16*, 27–44.

Mueller, D. (1980). Social networks: A promising direction for research on the relationship of the social environment to psychiatric disorder. *Social Science and Medicine, 14A*, 147–161.

Muhlenkamp, A., & Brown, N. (1983). *The Development of an Instrument to Measure Health Practices.* Paper presented at the American Nurses' Association Council of Nurse Researchers Conference, Minneapolis.

Norbeck, J. (1981, July). Social support: A model for clinical application and research. *Advances in Nursing Science*, pp. 43–59.

Norbeck, J. (1982, December). The use of social support in clinical practice. *Journal of Psychosocial Nursing and Mental Health Services*, pp. 22–29.

Pratt, L. (1971). The relationship of socioeconomic status to health. *American Journal of Public Health, 2*, 281–291.

Thoits, P. A. (1982). Conceptual, methodological, and theoretical problems in studying social support as a buffer. *Journal of Health and Social Behavior, 23*, 145–159.

Tolsdorf, C. (1976). Social networks, support, and coping: An exploratory study. *Family Process, 15*, 401–417.

U.S. Department of Health, Education, and Welfare. (1979). *Healthy people: The surgeon general's report on health promotion and disease prevention.* (DHEW Publ. (PHS) No. 79-55-71). Washington, DC: U.S. Government Printing Office.

Weiss, R. S. (1974). The provisions of social relationships. In Z. Rubin (Ed.), *Doing unto others* (pp. 17–26). Englewood Cliffs, NJ: Prentice-Hall.

Wolf, S. (1980). Social forces, neural mechanisms and health. *Psychosomatics, 1*, 843–850.

Analysis of Theory

The stated purpose of Hubbard, Muhlenkamp, and Brown's (1984) research was to explore the relationship between what people do to promote healthy life styles and how they perceive their level of social support. Although the investigators indicated that a descriptive survey approach was used, the relationship between social support and health practices was tested by means of correlational procedures. Therefore, the study may be classified as correlational research designed to test explanatory theory.

CONCEPT IDENTIFICATION AND CLASSIFICATION

Analysis of the research report revealed that an explanatory theory of social support and health practices was tested. The theory, as presented in the report, encompasses four concepts: social support, health practices, marital status, and confidant.

The concept social support is a variable because it has a continuous range of scores. It may be classified as a construct in Kaplan's (1964) schema and Willer and Webster's (1970) schema because it was invented for research purposes and can be inferred only through subjects' responses to a questionnaire. Social support may be classified as a relational unit in Dubin's (1978) schema because it involves an interaction between an individual and others who provide support.

Health practice is a variable because it takes scores ranging from regularly to never; it may be classified as construct in the Kaplan and Willer and Webster schemas because it is an abstract idea that can be observed only through subjects' responses to a questionnaire, and it may be classified as an associative unit in Dubin's schema because it can take the absent value of "never."

Marital status also is a variable. The dimensions considered in this study are married, single, widowed, divorced, separated, and unspecified other. This concept may be classified as directly observable in Kaplan's schema and as observable in Willer and Webster's schema because it is determined by subjects' statements about their marital status. In Dubin's schema, it is a relational unit because it involves a comparison of one person with another and its ascription involves an interaction between the properties wife and husband.

In this study, confidant is a variable with two dimensions — having a confidant and not having a confidant. The concept may be classified as directly observable in Kaplan's schema and as observable in Willer and Webster's schema because it is determined by subjects' statements that they have or do not have a person to confide in. Confidant is a relational unit in Dubin's schema because it involves an interaction between an individual and a person in whom the individual confides.

PROPOSITION IDENTIFICATION AND CLASSIFICATION

Nonrelational and relational propositions making up the theory of social support and health practices are evident in the research report. The constitutive definitions listed in Table A–5 may be classified as nonrelational definitional propositions. The operational definitions listed in Table A–5 also may be classified as nonrelational definitional propositions; they are not, strictly speaking, part of the theory. Rather, they link the concepts of the theory with their respective empirical indicators.

Constitutive definitions for social support and health practices are given in the research report. Constitutive definitions for marital status and confidant are not given, but they are self-evident. Operational defini-

TABLE A–5. Concepts, Definitions, and Empirical Indicators for the Theory of the Relationship between Social Support and Health Practices

Concept	Constitutive Definition	Operational Definition	Empirical Indicator
Social support	A multifaceted construct consisting of the communication of positive affect, a sense of belonging or social integration, and elements of reciprocity. In this study, "social support" is viewed as a multidimensional construct consisting of people as interpersonal resources who provide gratification of basic human needs in membership	Adequacy of the individual's perceived level of social support was measured by the Personal Resources Questionnaire, Part II	Personal Resources Questionnaire, Part II scores

Health practices	Positive health practices are specific activities performed that may affect one's health	The six kinds of practices considered in this study are nutrition, exercise, relaxation, safety, substance use, and prevention practices. The Lifestyle Questionnaire was used to measure these activities	Lifestyle Questionnaire scores
Marital status	No definition given	The six marital status categories included in the study are: married, single, widowed, divorced, separated, other unspecified	No specific empirical indicator given. Apparently an item included in the routine sociodemographic data that were collected
Confidant	No definition given	Presence of a confiding relationship was measured by the question: "Is there a person you confide in or talk to about yourself or your problems?"	Yes/no response to item about a confidant added at the end of the Personal Resources Questionnaire, Part II

tions for all four concepts can be extracted from the report. Explicit empirical indicators are identified for social support, health practices, and confidant. No specific empirical indicator is identified for marital status, although the report does state that routine sociodemographic data were collected. It seems likely that marital status was an item included in these data. The concepts, constitutive definitions, operational definitions, and empirical indicators are presented in Table A–5.

Relational propositions that appear to be central to the theory are listed below in the form in which they are stated in the report. Propositions 1 through 8 are located in the introductory and literature review sections of the report. Proposition 9 is located in the results section.

1. Those people who are enmeshed in supportive social networks take better care of themselves by engaging in more positive health practices than do people with less supportive networks.
2. A person's life-style has a significant impact on the individual's health.
3. Good health and long life are positively related to a supportive social environment.
4. Other studies have linked social support and specific health practices.
5a. Appropriate indirect health risk behaviors . . . were associated with a social network characterized by high socioeconomic status.
5b. Appropriate indirect health risk behaviors . . . were associated with frequent interaction between nonkin.
6. Structural characteristics of the family influenced personal health maintenance practices.
7. SES positively affected health practices.
8. Group membership and participation were also significant indicators of health practices.
9. The literature links the presence of a confiding relationship to well-being.

Propositions 1 to 4 concern the relationship between social support and health. They can be combined and stated formally as the following proposition, which asserts that a relationship exists and is positive in direction.

There is a positive relationship between social support and health practices.

Propositions 5a and 7 concern the relationship between socioeconomic status and health practices. The two statements can be combined and stated more formally as the following proposition, which asserts that a relationship exists and is positive in direction.

Socioeconomic status is positively related to health practices.

Propositions 5b and 8 concern the relationship between interaction with others and health practices. The two propositions can be combined and stated as follows. This formal proposition asserts that a relationship exists and is positive in direction.

There is a positive relationship between nonkin and group interaction and health practices.

Proposition 6 states that there is a relationship between family structure and health practices. This proposition indicates that a relationship exists. No other assertions about the relationship can be made on the basis of information given in the research report.

Proposition 9 states that there is a positive relationship between having a confidant and well-being. This proposition asserts that a relationship exists and is positive in direction.

Three hypotheses, stated in general empirical indicators terms, are given in the research report:

1. There is a positive association between the social support and health practice variables.
2. Married participants will score significantly higher on both the social support and health practice instruments than would their nonmarried counterparts.
3. Participants with a confidant will have higher scores on both the social support and the health practice instruments.

The three hypotheses can be stated more formally in terms of specific empirical indicators, and the multiple relationships inherent in hypotheses 2 and 3 can be separated. The formalized hypotheses are listed below.

1. There is a positive relationship between scores on the Personal Resources Questionnaire, Part II and the Lifestyle Questionnaire.

2a. There is a positive relationship between the sociodemographic datum of marital status and scores on the Personal Resources Questionnaire, Part II (PRQ-II) such that married subjects will have higher scores on the PRQ-II than nonmarried subjects.

2b. There is a positive relationship between the sociodemographic datum of marital status and scores on the Lifestyle Questionnaire such that married subjects will have higher scores on the Questionnaire than nonmarried subjects.

3a. There is a positive relationship between the response to the confidant question and scores on the Personal Resources Questionnaire, Part II (PRQ-II), such that subjects responding "Yes" to the confidant question will have higher scores on the PRQ-II than subjects responding "No."

3b. There is a positive relationship between the response to the confidant question and scores on the Lifestyle Questionnaire, such that subjects responding "Yes" to the confidant question will have higher scores on the Questionnaire than subjects responding "No."

HIERARCHY OF PROPOSITIONS

The hypothesis-testing nature of the study indicates that a hierarchy of propositions would be deductive. The propositions given in the research report do not lend themselves to hierarchical arrangement as axioms and theorems. However, the following hierarchy can be constructed for hypothesis 1.

Axiom$_1$ If social support is positively related to health practices, and

Axiom$_2$ if social support is measured by the Personal Resources Questionnaire, Part II, and

Axiom$_3$ if health practices are measured by the Lifestyle Questionnaire,

Hypothesis   then there is a positive relationship between scores on the Personal Resources Questionnaire, Part II and the Lifestyle Questionnaire.

Hierarchies cannot not be constructed for hypotheses 2a, 2b, 3a, and 3b because the research report does not contain explicit theoretical propositions that state relationships between marital status and social support and health practices or between having a confidant and social support and health practices.

CONCEPTUAL-THEORETICAL-EMPIRICAL STRUCTURE

The term self-care, which frequently is associated with Orem's (1991) Self-Care Framework, appears in the title of the research report. There is, however, no other mention of this term in the report. Furthermore, the assumptions underlying the research are not explicit.

DIAGRAMS

A diagram of the theoretical proposition dealing with the relationship between social support and health practices is presented in Figure A–4. This proposition was tested by hypothesis 1. Conceptual maps for the relationships tested by hypotheses 2a, 2b, 3a, and 3b are given in Figure A–5. Figure A–5 depicts the relationships as stated in the hypotheses.

Inasmuch as the frame of reference guiding the research was not identified, a diagram of the conceptual-theoretical-empirical structure could not be developed.

EVALUATION OF THE RELATION BETWEEN THEORY AND RESEARCH

The stated intent of this research was to explore the relationship between perceived social support and promotion of healthy life-styles. The re-

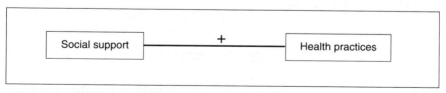

Figure A–4. Diagram of the relationship between social support and health practices.

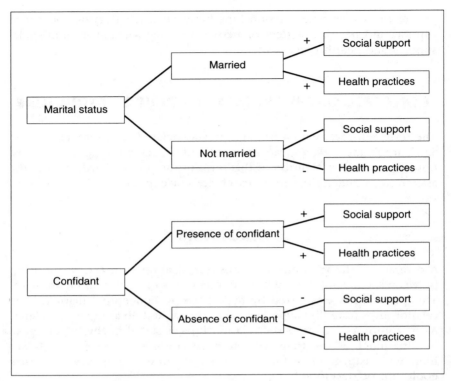

Figure A–5. Conceptual maps of the relationships of marital status and confidant to social support and health practices.

search went beyond the stated intent by testing relationships between marital status and social support and health practices, having a confidant and social support and health practices, and demographic variables and health practices. The report includes findings from two separate tests of the theory with two distinct samples.

SIGNIFICANCE

The theory of social support and health practices partially meets the criterion of significance. The theory deals with phenomena that are of interest to the discipline of nursing. More specifically, the theory deals with human behavior (individuals' health practices) in interaction with the environment (people making up social support networks). The research findings provide some precision in the estimate of the magnitude of the relationship between social support and health practices and contribute to our understanding of influences on health care practices. It is noteworthy that the investigators reported the results of multiple regression analyses of the relative influence of social support and demographic variables on health practices. The findings for both samples indicate that social support is the most significant indicator. These findings could be used to develop a theory that predicts with more precision in future research.

Additional evidence of theoretical significance is not evident. An attempt was made to establish the theoretical significance of the theory through a brief statement indicating that research has only recently focused on the important association between environmental stressors and health. There is, however, no indication in the report that this research extends or fills gaps in knowledge of the relationship between social support and health practices. The literature review and discussion sections imply that the findings duplicate previous research. The investigators might have commented on the value of replicating previous research. To their credit, they did note that their conduct of two studies represented replication that could demonstrate the robustness of the relationship between social support and health practices. The social significance of the theory is not addressed.

INTERNAL CONSISTENCY

The theory of social support and health practices meets some but not all the requirements of the internal consistency criterion. Semantic clarity is achieved through operational definitions for all four concepts. Semantic consistency is evident in that definitions of the concepts were consistent throughout the report. The investigators were careful to resolve differences in the various definitions of social support found in the literature by identifying the points on which the diverse definitions converge. There is a potential for confusion in the apparently interchangeable use of the terms social support, supportive social networks, interaction between nonkin, and group membership and participation, as well as of the terms health, well-being, health practices, indirect health risk behaviors, and health maintenance practices.

Moreover, there are some concept redundancies. The concepts marital status and confidant appear to be redundant with social support. In fact, the investigators noted that marital status is one dimension of social support. And having a person to confide in or talk to about problems (the operational definition for confidant) is part of a social support network. Furthermore, marital status and confidant may be redundant in that the confidant could be the spouse of a married subject. That could not be ascertained because the investigators did not determine the identity of the confidant.

Structural consistency in the report is problematic. Although there is no apparent mixing of inductive and deductive logic, there is evidence of discontinuity and redundancy in the propositions. The relationship between marital status and health practices must be inferred through proposition 6, which states the relationship between family structural characteristics and personal health maintenance practices. Here the inference would be that marital status is one family structural characteristic. Then the relationship tested by hypothesis 2b could be developed through the following deductive process. The deduction does not, however, yield the directional relationship stated in the hypothesis.

$Axiom_1$	If family structural characteristics are related to health practices, and
$Axiom_2$	if marital status is a family structural characteristic,
Theorem	then marital status is related to health practices.

The relationship between confidant and health practices must be inferred through proposition 9, which states the relationship between presence of a confiding relationship and well-being. In this case, the inference would have to be that well-being is positively related to health practices. The deduction leading to the relationship tested by hypothesis 3b would be as follows:

$Axiom_1$	If presence of a confiding relationship is related to well-being, and
$Axiom_2$	if well-being is positively related to health practices,
Theorem	then presence of a confiding relationship is positively related to health practices.

Furthermore, there are no propositions linking marital status or confidant with social support, although these relationships were tested by hypotheses 2a and 3a. As noted above, redundancies are evident in that, theoretically, both marital status and confidant can be considered dimensions of social support. The apparent multicollinearity makes interpretation of the correlations between marital status and social support and confidant and social support problematic (Pedhazur, 1982).

PARSIMONY

Formalization of the theory of social support and health practices indicates that, in general, the theory meets the criterion of parsimony. However, the narrative report could have been more concise, and the above-mentioned redundancies and interchangeable use of terms should have been avoided.

TESTABILITY

The theory of social support and health practices meets the criterion of testability. The concepts can be observed through the instruments used for data collection. Most of the propositions are measurable by means of their statements as hypotheses. The assertions of direction were tested by means of directional hypotheses. The hypotheses are falsifiable as stated in the report.

Explicit hypotheses are not given for some propositions that appear to be central to the theory. These include (1) the statements of relationships between socioeconomic status and health practices and (2) interaction with others (nonkin and group) and health practices. It is likely that the relationship between socioeconomic status and health practices was tested in the multiple regression analysis that included socioeconomic variables, as well as in the correlational analyses of occupation and education with health practices. Furthermore, it is likely that the relationship between nonkin and group interactions and health practices was tested through the hypothesis of a relationship between social support and health practices.

OPERATIONAL ADEQUACY

The research design used to test the theory of social support and health practices meets the criterion of operational adequacy. It is noteworthy that the research report included findings from two different samples.

Although these were nonrandom samples, the investigators claimed that the findings suggest that any bias introduced by the social class homogeneity of the senior center sample was minimal. They also noted that approximately 65 percent of the health fair participants volunteered for the study.

Congruence between constitutive and operational definitions of social support and health practices is evident. The research instruments used to measure social support and health practices have satisfactory reliability. The validity of the Lifestyle Questionnaire is satisfactory. The reported validity coefficients for the Personal Resources Questionnaire, Part II, are statistically significant but quite low. The psychometric properties of the empirical indicators for marital status and confidant are not included in the research report, but validity and reliability frequently are assumed for such variables. The study report indicates that research procedures and data analysis techniques typically employed in correlational studies were used.

EMPIRICAL ADEQUACY

Some parts of the theory of social support and health practices meet the criterion of empirical adequacy. The study findings suggest that there is indeed a positive relationship between social support and health practices. The investigators noted that in view of the many other variables that can affect the relationship between social support and health practices, the strength of the correlations found in the two study samples included in the report ($r = .37$, $r = .57$) is meaningful and strong. A meta-analysis of the findings yielded an average effect size for the two samples of $r = .47$. Given that Cohen (1977) considered a correlation of .30 to be a moderate effect size and a correlation of .50 to be a large effect size, the strength of the relationship may be classified as relatively strong.

The investigators considered alternative substantive explanations for the findings, in that they noted that it may be that people who maintain positive health practices attract and maintain supportive relationships or that those who have adequate social support tend to lead healthier lifestyles. On the basis of these comments, the relationship between social support and health practices may be classified as symmetrical. The empirical adequacy of this assertion must be tested in future research.

The empirical adequacy of the relationships between confidant and social support and health practices is limited because the relationships have been tested in just one sample. The empirical adequacy of the relationship between marital status and social support is highly questionable because the findings from the two samples differed. The investigators did not offer alternative methodologic explanations for their findings, although they might have cited the aforementioned problem of multicollinearity. They did offer alternative substantive explanations for the findings, although they did not indicate a willingness to reject the hypothesis of a relationship between marital status and social support despite the negative results in one study. Finally, the empirical adequacy of the relationship between marital status and health practices was not demonstrated in this study.

The conclusions of the study do not go beyond the data. The investigators commented that their findings affirm the association between social support and health-related behavior, although they were careful to point out that given the nonrandom samples, generalizations are tentative and additional research is needed to determine the scope of the theory.

PRAGMATIC ADEQUACY

The theory of social support and health practices meets the initial requirement of pragmatic adequacy in that its applicability in nursing practice is discussed. In particular, the investigators commented that intervention aimed at either social support or health practices could affect the other concept. They also commented that systematic assessment and intervention related to social support is needed. The theory requires further testing before findings can serve as a basis for practice.

CONCEPTUAL-THEORETICAL-EMPIRICAL STRUCTURE

No conceptual model or other frame of reference that might have guided the study was identified in the report. The use of the term self-care was limited to the report title and cannot be associated with any particular perspective.

REFERENCES

Cohen, J. (1977). *Statistical power analysis for the behavioral sciences*. New York: Academic Press.

Dubin, R. (1978). *Theory building* (rev. ed.). New York: The Free Press.

Hubbard, P., Muhlenkamp, A. F., & Brown, N. (1984). The relationship between social support and health care practices. *Nursing Research, 33,* 266–270.

Kaplan, A. (1964). *The conduct of inquiry*. San Francisco: Chandler.

Orem, D. E. (1991). *Nursing: Concepts of practice* (4th ed.). St. Louis: Mosby Year Book.

Pedhazur, E. J. (1982). *Multiple regression in behavioral research* (2nd ed.). New York: Holt, Rinehart & Winston.

Willer, D., & Webster, M., Jr. (1970). Theoretical concepts and observables. *American Sociological Review, 35,* 748–757.

UNCERTAINTY AND ADJUSTMENT DURING RADIOTHERAPY

Norma J. Christman

The relationships among uncertainty, hope, symptom severity, control preference, and psychosocial adjustment were examined in persons having radiotherapy for cancer. After 15 days of radiotherapy, both uncertainty (17%) and hope (16%) explained significant amounts of the variance in adjustment. At the end of treatment, uncertainty (18%), hope (11%), and symptom severity (7%) all significantly increased the explained variance in adjustment. Greater uncertainty and less hope were associated with more adjustment problems; symptom severity increased the explanation of adjustment difficulty at treatment completion. There was no evidence that uncertainty had positive effects in this sample. Findings also showed that control preference was unrelated to the concepts of interest in this sample.

Uncertainty results from cognitive appraisal (Lazarus & Folkman, 1984) of an event for which the outcome is unclear or the cues are inadequate,

Norma J. Christman, PhD, RN, is an associate professor at the College of Nursing, University of Kentucky, Lexington.

This study was conducted while Dr. Christman was an American Nurses' Foundation Scholar and a postdoctoral Fellow in the Department of Behavioral Science, University of Kentucky. The research was supported in part by an ANF Competitive Grant Award and in part by a National Institute of Mental Health Research Training Grant, T32 MH15730, to the Department of Behavioral Science. Revision of this manuscript was partially supported by a grant, R29 NR01830-01, from the National Center for Nursing Research and the National Cancer Institute, National Institutes of Health.

Reprinted from *Nursing Research, 39,* 17–20, 47, 1990.

unfamiliar, contradictory, or numerous (Budner, 1962; McIntosh, 1974). Appraisal determines whether the event is perceived as stressful or benign (Lazarus & Launier, 1978). Events characterized by the features of uncertainty frequently may be appraised as stressful (Mishel, 1981) with coping responses impeded because the outcome is unclear or because of difficulty in assigning meaning to the cues (Lazarus & Launier, 1978; Shalit, 1977). On the other hand, uncertainty may have positive effects when it permits reassuring interpretation of cues (Davis, 1960–61; Lazarus & Folkman, 1984). Thus, in some situations, certainty may be more aversive than uncertainty.

Dealing with uncertainty is described as a major task faced by persons in health care environments (Cohen & Lazarus, 1979). Uncertainty is characterized also as a feature of living with cancer (Cassileth, Zupkin, Sutton–Smith, & March, 1980; Comaroff & Maguire, 1981; Mages & Mendelsohn, 1979; Wortman & Dunkel–Schetter, 1979). Though not directly related to uncertainty, the experience of cancer and its treatment were found to generate high levels of distress and difficulty in coping (Freidenbergs et al., 1981–82; Greer & Silberfarb, 1982; Krouse & Krouse, 1982; Meyerowitz, Heinrich, & Schag, 1983). The diagnosis of cancer may be certain, but treatment efficacy, as well as the effect treatment may have on activities of daily life, are often less clear. Perhaps as a way of dealing with uncertainty, cancer patients frequently devise ways of monitoring their disease and its response to treatment (Leventhal & Nerenz, 1983; Lewis, Haberman, & Wallhagen, 1986). Even though cancer treatment is stressful, cessation of treatment was associated with increased emotional distress (Andersen, Karlsson, Anderson, & Tewfik, 1984; Andersen & Tewfik, 1985; Burish & Lyles, 1983; Peck & Boland, 1977); without continued treatment, uncertainty about tumor recurrence may increase. The side effects of treatment may also create uncertainty when such symptoms are misinterpreted as signs of treatment failure (Krant, 1981; Peck & Boland).

The potential positive effects of uncertainty, that is, hope, in cancer patients have been examined in two studies. Cassileth et al. (1980) reported that hope was positively related to medical status and preference for active involvement in treatment. Mishel, Hostetter, King, and Graham (1984) reported that hope was unrelated to seriousness of illness but that it was negatively associated with uncertainty.

Thus, current evidence indicates that uncertainty may be stressful and may influence coping and adjustment to illness and its treatment. The relationship between uncertainty and hope and the influence of both on adjustment require further study. In situations characterized as uncertain, personal factors may influence appraisal and coping more than the objective features of the event (Lazarus & Folkman, 1984). For example, individual differences in preference for control, stage of disease, or site of cancer may modify the impact of these variables on adjustment.

The notion of control has been viewed as a primary motivation for much of human behavior (White, 1959) and has received considerable attention in studies of responses to stressful events (Averill, 1973). There is some evidence that perceived control positively influenced psychosocial adjustment in cancer patients (Follick, Smith, & Turk, 1984; Lewis, 1982; Taylor, Lichtman, & Wood, 1984). However, perception of control was reported also as stress inducing (Averill; Folkman, 1984). Recently, efforts have been directed toward identifying individual differences that modify responses to the availability of control (Auerbach, Martelli, & Mercuri, 1983; Sime & Libera, 1985). The meaning of a control response to the individual and the context within which control is available may modify responses to the availability of control (Averill). A situation involving a high degree of uncertainty may be differentially stressful to persons who vary in their preference for control (Krantz, Baum, & Wideman, 1980). Persons who prefer control in a situation that offers little possibility for control may feel less hope, experience more stress, and have more adjustment problems than persons who do not desire control.

The purpose of this study was to examine the influence of uncertainty, hope, preference for control, and symptom severity on psychosocial adjustment while undergoing radiation therapy for cancer. Both uncertainty and symptom severity were expected to be positively related to adjustment problems across phases of the treatment experience. In addition, the data were examined to determine: (a) if there was evidence of a positive relationship between uncertainty and hope and (b) if preference for control was related to uncertainty, hope, or adjustment problems. Lastly, the usefulness of these variables in explaining the variation in adjustment beyond that explained by site and stage of disease was examined.

METHOD

Sample

Patients receiving external beam radiotherapy for cure or control of their cancer were sought for inclusion in the sample. Patients were excluded who had brain involvement, were receiving palliative treatment, were on concurrent chemotherapy, or had a psychiatric diagnosis. A total of 68 patients met the criteria for inclusion. Eight patients refused to take part. Most cited the distance they traveled each day for treatment, or the time required to complete the measures, as the reasons for their unwillingness to participate. Three patients were lost to the study due to complications necessitating changes in their treatment plan and two patients withdrew from the study. The final sample included 55 patients whose ages ranged from 27 to 79 years ($M = 55$, $SD = 14.26$). The majority were white (98%, $n = 53$), female (76%, $n = 42$), married (75%, $n = 41$), within 3 months of diagnosis (86%, $n = 47$), and all had been rated above the 80% level on the Karnofsky Performance Status Scale (Grieco & Long, 1984). None had received prior radiation treatment. Forty-five percent ($n = 25$) had less than a high school education; 29% ($n = 16$) had attained a high school diploma; 15% ($n = 8$) had some college or vocational training; and 11% ($n = 6$) had a college or graduate degree. Over half the sample (53%, $n = 29$) were homemakers or retired. Of those employed outside the home, the majority were in skilled or unskilled occupations ($n = 21$). Site and stage of cancer varied across the sample (Table 1).

TABLE 1. Number and Percent of Subjects by Site and Stage of Cancer

Variables	n	%
SITE		
Cervix	15	27.3
Uterus	12	21.8
Prostate	5	9.1
Lymphatics	5	9.1
Head-neck	3	5.5
Breast	10	18.2
Other	5	9.1
STAGE[a]		
I	20	36.4
II	21	38.2
III	8	14.5
IV	1	1.8

[a]Staging data were unavailable for 5 subjects.

Instruments

The Mishel (1981) Uncertainty in Illness Scale (MUIS) was used as the measure of uncertainty. The MUIS is a 34-item scale with a 5-point Likert format ranging from *strongly agree* to *strongly disagree*. It measures uncertainty about diagnosis, prognosis, treatment, symptoms, and relationships with caregivers. The scale is composed of four subscales: ambiguity, alpha .91; complexity, alpha .75; deficient information, alpha .71; and unpredictability, alpha .70. Construct, discriminant, and convergent validity have been reported (Mishel, 1981, 1984). The largest and most reliable subscale, the ambiguity subscale, was used in all analyses to increase measurement precision. More recent psychometric evaluation of the MUIS indicated that the deficient information and unpredictability subscales were unstable across multiple populations (M. H. Mishel, personal communication, October 1987, January 1989).

Hope was measured with the Beck Hopelessness Scale (BHS). The BHS (Beck, Weissman, Lester, & Trexler, 1974) is a 20-item scale with a true – false response format measuring negative expectations about one's self and future and has been widely used as an indicator of hope. In scoring the scale, lower scores indicate more hope. Internal consistency of the scale was reported as .93 and concurrent and construct validity were established (Beck et al.).

The Krantz Health Opinion Survey (KHOS) was the indicator of a general preference for control in health care. The scale contains 16 items with a binary agree – disagree response format. The Information subscale (I) measures the desire to ask questions and to obtain information about medical decisions. The Behavioral Involvement subscale (B) measures attitudes toward self-treatment and behavioral involvement in medical care. The KHOS demonstrated internal consistency of .77, with I and B scale alpha coefficients reported as .74 and .76, respectively; test – retest reliability was reported as .74 for the total scale, .71 for the B scale, and .59 for the I scale (Krantz et al., 1980). Predictive, construct, and discriminant validity have been reported for the KHOS (Krantz et al.; Smith, Wallston, Wallston, Forsberg, & King, 1984).

Symptom severity was measured using a modification of the Symptom Distress Scale (McCorkle & Young, 1978). Symptoms common during radiation therapy (King, Nail, Kreamer, Strohl, & Johnson, 1985) were listed. Subjects identified the symptoms they had experienced during the past week and rated the severity of each symptom on a 5-point scale ranging from *not at all bad* to *extremely bad*. Subjects also listed any other symptoms not included on the scale. Few patients reported such symptoms, and those reported (e.g., runny nose) were unrelated to the primary diagnosis or to the treatment.

Adjustment was measured with the Psychosocial Adjustment to Illness Scale (PAIS) self-report form. The PAIS (Derogatis & Lopez, 1983; Morrow, Chiarello, & Derogatis, 1978) is a 46-item multidimensional scale designed to assess psychological and social adjustment to illness in seven domains: health care orientation, vocational environment, domestic environment, sexual relationships, family relationships, social environment, and emotional distress. Each item has four response options scored from zero to 3; higher scores indicate more adjustment problems. The internal consistency estimates range from .85 for the emotional distress subscale to .47 for the health care orientation subscale; criterion and construct validity were reported (Derogatis & Lopez). The health care orientation domain was omitted from calculation of total adjustment scores because several of these items are conceptually similar to those contained in the KHOS, particularly the behavioral involvement subscale.

Procedure

Potential subjects were identified from patients scheduled for treatment in the radiation therapy department of a university medical center. Medical records were reviewed to identify patients who met the inclusion criteria. Patients were approached following their 1st, 15th, or last treatment and written informed consent was sought. For subjects entering the study at their 1st treatment (Time 1), responses to the measures were also obtained following their 15th treatment (Time 2) and their last treatment (Time 3). For those entering at their 15th treatment, responses to the measures were also obtained following their last treatment. This enabled assessment of responses over time, a large enough sample to assess relationships among several measures at Time 2 and Time 3, and assessment of the potential effects of repeated testing. Responses to the MUIS, BHS, symptom severity, and PAIS were obtained at each time of measurement. Presentation of the MUIS, BHS, and PAIS were randomly varied. Symptom severity was assessed last at each time of measurement. The KHOS was administered at the 1st time of measurement for each subject.

RESULTS

Initially, the data were examined for potential effects due to missing data. Three subjects at Time 1, 5 at Time 2, and 6 at Time 3 failed to provide complete data on the PAIS. Also, 2 subjects produced unusable data on the KHOS, another 2 on the BHS, and staging data were unavailable for 5 subjects. No subject had missing data on all these variables. Examination of the data indicated no systematic differences between subjects with complete data and those with incomplete data on any of the other variables.

The mean scores for uncertainty, hope, and adjustment problems remained relatively stable across the course of treatment (Table 2). Symptom severity increased at the time of the 15th treatment and remained at this level at the last treatment reflecting the impact of radiotherapy side effects. The mean score for preference for control was 4.93 ($SD = 2.71$, $n = 53$).

Uncertainty and symptom severity were not consistently related to adjustment problems across the treatment phases. Patients who perceived their illness experiences as more uncertain also reported more adjustment problems only after their 15th, $r = .39$, $p < .02$, and last treatments, $r = .42$, $p < .01$. Symptom severity was positively associated with

TABLE 2. Means and Standard Deviations for Uncertainty, Hope, Adjustment Problems, and Symptom Severity by Time of Measurement

Variables	Treatment		
	1	15	Last
Uncertainty			
M	41.39	42.26	39.46
(SD)	(12.29)	(9.51)	(10.69)
n	39	46	55
Hope			
M	3.21	2.52	2.47
(SD)	(3.53)	(2.97)	(2.93)
n	39	46	53
Problems			
M	26.36	27.34	27.41
(SD)	(15.95)	(17.87)	(17.66)
n	36	41	49
Symptom			
M	4.82	8.59	8.20
(SD)	(4.48)	(7.07)	(6.85)
n	39	46	55

Note. n varied due to missing data.

adjustment problems after the 1st, $r = .37$, $p < .03$, and last, $r = .31$, $p < .05$, treatments but not after the 15th treatment, $r = .18$. After their 1st and 15th treatments, patients reporting their illness experiences as more uncertain also reported less hope, $r = .49$, $p < .01$, and $r = .44$, $p < .01$, respectively. By the last treatment, this relationship was in the same direction but no longer significant, $r = .22$. Less hope was consistently associated with more adjustment problems ($r = .38$, $p < .03$ after the 1st treatment, $r = .50$, $p < .01$ after the 15th treatment, and $r = .41$, $p < .01$ after the last treatment).

Individual differences in preference for control in health care showed little relationship to uncertainty, hope, or adjustment problems. There was only one significant correlation. At the end of treatment, patients who reported desiring more behavioral involvement in their care also reported more uncertainty, $r = .34$, $p < .02$. Inspection of the scattergrams depicting the relationship between these variables suggested that the emergence of a relationship at treatment completion was most likely caused by the responses of two patients who scored at or near the upper end of the range on both variables. In this sample, little evidence supported the notion that control preference influenced perceived uncertainty, hope, or adjustment problems. Thus, control preference was eliminated from further analyses.

Hierarchical multiple regression was used to identify the predictors of problems in adjustment following 15 treatments and at treatment completion (Table 3). Stage of disease (i.e., I, II, or III) and site of cancer (i.e., genitourinary or other) were dummy coded (Cohen & Cohen, 1983) and entered into the regression equations first. After the 15th treatment both uncertainty (17%) and hope (16%) significantly increased the amount of explained variance. After the last treatment, uncertainty (18%), hope (11%), and symptom severity (7%) significantly increased the amount of explained variance. At both these times during the course of treatment, perceiving one's illness experiences as more uncertain and feeling less hopeful were predictive of more problems in adjustment. By the end of treatment, greater symptom severity was also predictive of adjustment difficulties. At both times, site and stage of cancer explained 5% or less of the variance and neither contributed significantly to the prediction of adjustment problems. The relative homogeneity of the sample with respect to prognosis may account for the lack of variation associated with site or stage of cancer.

Comparison of mean scores for patients who responded one, two, or three times to the measures indicated no differences associated with the number of times measured. Because mean scores do not explain whether

TABLE 3. Hierarchical Regression of Uncertainty, Hope, and Symptom Severity on Psychosocial Adjustment After 15 Treatments and the Last Treatment

Variables	R^2	R^2 Change	Beta	df	F
15 TREATMENTS ($n = 39$)					
Stage	.01	.01	−.10	1	<1
Site	.01	.00	.01	1	<1
Uncertainty	.18	.17	.42	1	7.39**
Hope	.34	.16	.46	1	8.28***
Symptoms	.34	.00	.05	1	<1
Entire model				33	3.47**
LAST TREATMENT ($n = 44$)					
Stage	.01	.01	−.08	1	<1
Site	.05	.04	−.20	1	1.64
Uncertainty	.23	.18	.43	1	9.36***
Hope	.34	.11	.34	1	6.64**
Symptoms	.41	.07	.27	1	4.24*
Entire model				38	5.17***

*$p < .05$, **$p < .02$, ***$p < .01$

the addition of subjects affected the obtained relationships, the regression analyses were repeated for subjects measured only two times and for those measured three times, and the results were compared. For data obtained at both the 15th and the last treatment, the variance accounted for by each variable and the overall explained variance varied by 3% or less, which did not alter the interpretation of the findings. Thus, repeated exposure to the same instruments did not affect the mean responses or the nature of the obtained relationships.

DISCUSSION

Both perceiving cues about illness experiences as vague or unclear and feeling less hopeful were predictive of more psychosocial adjustment problems in patients receiving radiotherapy for cancer. Consistent with the findings of Mishel et al. (1984) in women undergoing initial treatment for gynecologic cancer, patients who found the cues about their cancer and its treatment with radiation difficult to interpret experienced less hope and more disruption in their emotional state and daily life activities.

There was no evidence that uncertainty facilitated hope in this sample of patients undergoing active treatment. It may be that positive effects of uncertainty are more operative once treatment is completed. At this time patients must deal with the probabilities associated with treatment effectiveness. Because in many instances treatment effectiveness is uncertain, patients may be more inclined to interpret posttreatment uncertainty positively to bolster feelings of hopefulness. The decrease in the strength of the relationship at treatment completion found in this study may reflect the beginning of such a process. Confirmation of this interpretation requires more long-term study of patients' responses to radiotherapy.

Contrary to previous findings (Cassileth et al., 1980), there was little support for a relationship between hope and preference for control. In fact, there was little evidence indicating that preference for control, as measured in this study, influenced any of the measures obtained. One or more of several factors may explain the absence of effects for control preference.

The binary response format of the KHOS presents a forced choice that could affect measurement error. This response format also restricts the range of possible scores and could have attenuated the obtained relationships. Since the initial psychometric properties of the KHOS were reported (Krantz et al., 1980), other investigators have modified the binary response format to a Likert format (Rock, Meyerowitz, Maisto, & Wallston, 1987; Smith et al., 1984). While such modification increased the range of possible scores, it only slightly improved the internal consistency estimates (Smith et al.). It is unclear whether increasing the KHOS subscale score ranges would have significantly affected the relationships obtained in this study given their generally low magnitude. Perhaps the lack of effects for control preference are real rather than a result of measurement problems.

When in a situation that presents little possibility of control, persons who prefer control may modify their expectations for control in that situation. People may discriminate those events in which they can exert control from those they cannot and alter their expectations and behavior accordingly. In this case, general health-related control preferences should have little influence on responses to illness and its treatment. If perceptions of the specific event do modify expectations and behavior, situation-specific measures of control preference may be more useful in understanding control and how it influences responses (Smith et al., 1984).

That symptom severity was a significant predictor of adjustment at treatment completion is not surprising. Some symptoms such as fatigue are cumulative over the course of treatment (Haylock & Hart, 1979) and may have more impact at the end of treatment. The positive relationship between symptom severity and adjustment problems at the beginning of treatment most likely reflects the effects of symptoms due to prior surgery, diagnostic procedures, or chemotherapy. The lack of a relationship between these two variables after the 15th treatment is more difficult to explain, since this is the time when the major treatment side effects begin (King et al., 1985). Perhaps, it is not the initial impact of the side effects but their continuation over time that has more influence on adjustment.

There is growing evidence that symptoms and their interpretation may explain a variety of responses to illness and its treatment (Leventhal & Nerenz, 1983). More careful study of the impact of symptoms, especially those due to treatment, is necessary and holds promise for identifying approaches for intervention. For example, do patients interpret fatigue as a side effect of radiotherapy or as a sign of disease progression? Helping patients to correctly interpret symptoms (Leventhal & Johnson, 1983; King et al., 1985) may limit their impact on adjustment, reducing uncertainty and facilitating hope.

REFERENCES

Andersen, B. L., Karlsson, J. A., Anderson, B., & Tewfik, H. H. (1984). Anxiety and cancer treatment: Response to stressful radiotherapy. *Health Psychology*, *3*, 535–551.

Andersen, B. L., & Tewfik, H. H. (1985). Psychological reactions to radiation therapy: Reconsideration of the adaptive aspects of anxiety. *Journal of Personality and Social Psychology*, *48*, 1024–1032.

Auerbach, S. M., Martelli, M. F., & Mercuri, L. G. (1983). Anxiety information, interpersonal impacts, and adjustment to a stressful health care situation. *Journal of Personality and Social Psychology*, *44*, 1284–1296.

Averill, J. R. (1973). Personal control over aversive stimuli and its relationship to stress. *Psychological Bulletin*, *80*, 286–303.

Beck, A. T., Weissman, A., Lester, D., & Trexler L. (1974). The measurement of pessimism. *Journal of Consulting and Clinical Psychology*, *42*, 861–865.

Budner, S. (1962). Intolerance of ambiguity as a personality variable. *Journal of Personality*, *30*, 29–50.

Burish, T. G., & Lyles, J. N. (1983). Coping with the adverse effects of cancer treatments. In T. G. Burish & L. A. Bradley (Eds.), *Coping with chronic disease* (pp. 159–189). New York: Academic Press.

Cassileth, B. R., Zupkis, R. V., Sutton-Smith, K., & March, V. (1980). Information and participation preferences among cancer patients. *Annals of Internal Medicine, 92,* 832–836.

Cohen, J., & Cohen, P. (1983). *Applied multiple regression/correlation analysis for the behavioral sciences.* Hillsdale, NJ: Lawrence Erlbaum.

Cohen, F., & Lazarus, R. S. (1979). Coping with the stresses of illness. In G. C. Stone, F. Cohen, & N. E. Adler (Eds.), *Health psychology — a handbook* (pp. 217–254). San Francisco: Jossey-Bass.

Comaroff, J., & Maguire, P. (1981). Ambiguity and the search for meaning: Childhood leukemia in a modern clinical context. *Social Science and Medicine, 15B,* 115–123.

Davis, F. (1960–61). Uncertainty in medical prognosis: Clinical and functional. *American Journal of Sociology, 66,* 41–47.

Derogatis, L. R., & Lopez, M. C. (1983). *The Psychosocial Adjustment to Illness Scale: Administration, scoring and procedures manual.* Riderwood, MD: Clinical Psychometric Research.

Folkman, S. (1984). Personal control and stress and coping processes: A theoretical analysis. *Journal of Personality and Social Psychology, 46,* 839–852.

Follick, M. J., Smith, T. W., & Turk, D. C. (1984). Psychosocial adjustment following ostomy. *Health Psychology, 3,* 505–517.

Friedenbergs, I., Gordon, W., Hibbard, M., Levine, L., Wolf, C., & Diller, L. (1981–82). Psychosocial aspects of living with cancer. *International Journal of Psychiatry in Medicine, 11,* 303–329.

Greer, S., & Silberfarb, P. M. (1982). Psychological concomitants of cancer: Cancer state of research. *Psychological Medicine, 12,* 563–573.

Grieco, A., & Long, C. J. (1984). Investigation of the Karnofsky Performance Status as a measure of quality of life. *Health Psychology, 3,* 129–142.

Haylock, P. J., & Hart, L. K. (1979). Fatigue in patients receiving localized radiation. *Cancer Nursing, 2,* 461–467.

King, K. B., Nail, L. B. Kreamer, K., Strohl, R. A., & Johnson, J. E. (1985). Patients' descriptions of the experience of receiving radiation therapy. *Oncology Nursing Forum, 12*(4), 55–61.

Krant, M. J. (1981). Psychological impact of gynecological cancer. *Cancer, 48,* 608–612.

Krantz, D. S., Baum, A., & Wideman, M. (1980). Assessment of preferences for self-treatment and information in health care. *Journal of Personality and Social Psychology, 39,* 977–990.

Krouse, H. J., & Krouse, J. H. (1982). Cancer as crisis: The critical elements of adjustment. *Nursing Research, 31,* 96–101.

Lazarus, R. S., & Folkman, S. (1984). *Stress, appraisal, and coping.* New York: Springer.

Lazarus, R. S., & Launier, R. (1978). Stress-related transactions between person and environment. In L. A. Pervin & M. Lewis (Eds.), *Perspectives in interactional psychology* (pp. 287–327). New York: Plenum.

Leventhal, H., & Johnson, J. E. (1983). Laboratory and field experimentation: Development of a theory of self-regulation. In P. J. Wooldridge, M. H. Schmitt, J. K. Skipper & R. C. Leonard (Eds.), *Behavioral science and nursing theory* (pp. 189–262). St. Louis: Mosby.

Leventhal, H., & Nerenz, D. R. (1983). A model for stress research with some implications for the control of stress disorders. In D. Meichenbaum & M. E. Jaremko (Eds.), *Stress reduction and prevention* (pp. 5–38). New York: Plenum.

Lewis, F. M. (1982). Experienced personal control and quality of life in late-stage cancer patients. *Nursing Research, 31,* 113–119.

Lewis, F. M., Haberman, M. R., & Wallhagen, M. I. (1986). How adults with late-stage cancer experience personal control. *Journal of Psychosocial Oncology, 4*(4), 27–42.

Mages, N. L., & Mendelsohn, G. A. (1979). Effects of cancer on patients' lives: A personological approach. In G. C. Stone, F. Cohen, & N. E. Adler (Eds.), *Health psychology — a handbook* (pp. 255–284). San Francisco: Jossey-Bass.

McCorkle, R., & Young, K. (1978). Development of a symptom distress scale. *Cancer Nursing, 1*, 373–378.

Meyerowitz, B. E., Heinrich, R. L., & Schag, C. C. (1983). A competency-based approach to coping with cancer. In T. G. Burish & L. A. Bradley (Eds.), *Coping with chronic disease* (pp. 113–135). New York: Academic Press.

Mishel, M. H. (1981). The measurement of uncertainty in illness. *Nursing Research, 30*, 258–263.

Mishel, M. H. (1984). Perceived uncertainty and stress in illness. *Research in Nursing & Health, 7*, 163–171.

Mishel, M. H., Hostetter, R., King, B., & Graham, V. (1984). Predictors of psychosocial adjustment in patients newly diagnosed with gynecologic cancer. *Cancer Nursing, 7*, 291–299.

Morrow, G. R., Chiarello, R. J., & Derogatis, L. R. (1978). A new scale for assessing patients' psychosocial adjustment to medical illness. *Psychological Medicine, 8*, 605–610.

Peck, A., & Boland, J. (1977). Emotional reactions to radiation treatment. *Cancer, 40*, 180–184.

Rock, D. I., Meyerowitz, B. E., Maisto, S. A., & Wallston, K. A. (1987). The derivation and validation of six multidimensional health locus of control scale clusters. *Res. in Nurs. & Health, 10*, 185–195.

Shalit, B. (1977). Structural ambiguity and limits to coping. *Journal of Human Stress, 3*(4), 32–45.

Sime, A. M., & Libera, M. B. (1985). Sensation information, self-instruction and responses to dental surgery. *Research in Nursing & Health, 8*, 41–47.

Smith, R. A., Wallston, B. S., Wallston, K. A., Forsberg, P. R., & King, J. E. (1984). Measuring desire for control of health care processes. *Journal of Personality and Social Psychology, 47*, 415–426.

Taylor, S. E., Lichtman, R. R., & Wood, J. V. (1984). Attributions, beliefs about control, and adjustment to breast cancer. *Journal of Personality and Social Psychology, 46*, 489–502.

White, R. W. (1959). Motivation reconsidered: The concept of competence. *Psychological Review, 66*, 297–333.

Wortman, C. B., & Dunkel-Schetter, C. (1979). Interpersonal relationships and cancer: A theoretical analysis. *Journal of Social Issues, 35*, 120–155.

Analysis of Theory

The stated purpose of Christman's (1990) study was to examine the influence of the set of variables uncertainty, hope, preference for control, and symptom severity on psychosocial adjustment while undergoing radiotherapy for cancer. The usefulness of this set of variables in explaining the variation in adjustment beyond that explained by site of cancer and stage of disease also was examined. The study may be classified as correlational research designed to test an explanatory theory.

CONCEPT IDENTIFICATION AND CLASSIFICATION

Analysis of the research report revealed that an explanatory theory of influences on psychosocial adjustment was tested in the situation of radiotherapy for cancer. The theory encompasses seven concepts: uncertainty, hope, symptom severity, preference for control, site of cancer, stage of disease, and psychosocial adjustment.

All seven concepts are variables. Each concept has a range of either nominal (site of cancer, stage of disease) or interval (uncertainty, hope, symptom severity, preference for control, psychosocial adjustment) level scores.

Uncertainty may be classified as a construct in both Kaplan's (1964) and Willer and Webster's (1970) schemas because it is an abstract term that can be observed only through subjects' responses to a questionnaire. This concept may be classified as enumerative in Dubin's (1978) schema because all subjects demonstrated some degree of uncertainty.

Hope also may be classified as a construct in Kaplan's and Willer and Webster's schemas because it is such an abstract concept. It may be classified as an associative unit in Dubin's schema because hope could take an absent value (hopelessness) in this study.

Preference for control is another construct in Kaplan's and Willer and Webster's schemas; it was invented for research purposes and can be observed only through subjects' responses to a questionnaire. It may be classified as a relational unit in Dubin's schema because, as measured in this study, it represents a combination of the properties desire to ask questions to obtain information and attitudes toward self-involvement in medical care.

Symptom severity may be classified as an indirect observable term in Kaplan's schema because it cannot be directly observed, yet it is not as abstract as a construct. It may be classified as a construct in Willer and Webster's schema because it cannot be observed directly without reference to the subjects' reports of the presence and severity of their symptoms. This concept may be classified as an associative unit in Dubin's schema because, as measured in this study, it was possible to have no symptoms.

Both site of cancer and stage of disease may be classified as directly observable in Kaplan's schema and as observable in Willer and Webster's schema. Each of these concepts is determined by subjects' statements regarding the site and stage of their cancer or by a report in the hospital record. Both concepts may be classified as enumerative in Dubin's schema because all subjects had cancer.

Psychosocial adjustment may be classified as a theoretical term in Kaplan's schema because it is a complex, global property; it may be classified as a construct in Willer and Webster's schema because it is so abstract. Psychosocial adjustment may be classified as a summative unit in Dubin's schema because of its complexity.

PROPOSITION IDENTIFICATION AND CLASSIFICATION

Nonrelational and relational propositions making up the theory of influences on psychosocial adjustment during radiotherapy for cancer are evident in the research report. One statement about uncertainty may be classified as a nonrelational existence proposition:

Uncertainty is characterized also as a feature of living with cancer.

This statement can be formalized as follows:

The phenomenon of uncertainty occurs when a person has cancer.

Another statement about uncertainty may be classified as a nonrelational proposition that asserts level of existence. The statement is:

Without continued treatment, uncertainty about tumor recurrence may increase.

Formalized, this proposition asserts:

A high level of uncertainty about recurrence may be present when cancer treatment is not continued.

Additional nonrelational propositions can be extracted from the research report to provide the constitutive and operational definitions for all of the concepts except site of cancer and stage of disease. These nonrelational definitional propositions are listed in Table A-6. The

TABLE A–6. Concepts, Definitions, and Empirical Indicators for the Theory of Influences on Psychosocial Adjustment during Radiotherapy for Cancer

Concept	Constitutive Definition	Operational Definition	Empirical Indicator
Uncertainty	Uncertainty results from cognitive appraisal of an event the outcome of which is unclear or for which the cues are inadequate, unfamiliar, contradictory, or numerous. Events characterized by features of uncertainty frequently can be appraised as stressful with coping responses impeded because the outcome is unclear or because of difficulty in assigning meaning to the cues. Uncertainty encompasses ambiguity, complexity, deficient information, and unpredictability.	The Mishel Uncertainty in Illness Scale was used as the measure of uncertainty. It measures uncertainty about diagnosis, prognosis, treatment, symptoms, and relationships with caregivers.	Mishel Uncertainty in Illness Scale
Hope	Hope is the potential positive effect of uncertainty. Hope is defined as expectations about one's self and future.	Hope was measured with the Beck Hopelessness Scale.	Beck Hopelessness Scale

(Continued)

TABLE A–6. Concepts, Definitions, and Empirical Indicators for the Theory of Influences on Psychosocial Adjustment during Radiotherapy for Cancer (Continued)

Concept	Constitutive Definition	Operational Definition	Empirical Indicator
Symptom severity	Symptom severity is defined as the severity of symptoms common during radiation therapy.	Symptom severity was measured by using a modification of the Symptom Distress Scale.	Modified Symptom Distress Scale
Preference for control	Control has been viewed as a primary motivation for much of human behavior. Preference for control encompasses desire to ask questions and to obtain information about medical decisions as well as attitudes toward self-treatment and behavioral involvement in medical care. Preference for control encompasses desire to ask questions and to obtain information about medical decisions as well as attitudes toward self-treatment and behavioral involvement in medical care.	Preference for control was measured by the Krantz Health Opinion Survey.	Krantz Health Opinion Survey

Site of cancer	No definition given.	The sites of cancer represented in the study sample included cervix, uterus, prostate, lymphatics, head-neck, breast, and other.	No specific empirical indicator given. Apparently a question asked of subjects or obtained from the hospital record.
Stage of disease	No definition given.	The stages of cancer represented in the study sample included I, II, III, and IV.	No specific empirical indicator given. Apparently a question asked of subjects or obtained from the hospital record.
Psychosocial adjustment	Psychosocial adjustment encompasses psychological and social adjustment to illness in terms of health care orientation, vocational environment, domestic environment, sexual relationships, family relationships, social environment, and emotional distress.	Psychosocial adjustment was measured with the Psychosocial Adjustment to Illness Scale.	Psychosocial Adjustment to Illness Scale

operational definitions are not part of the theory; they are the vertical propositions that link the theory concepts to the empirical indicators.

Constitutive definitions for uncertainty, hope, symptom severity, preference for control, and psychosocial adjustment are given in the research report. Furthermore, operational definitions and empirical indicators are explicitly identified for all of these concepts. The constitutive definitions were formalized by combining statements about single concepts in the introductory section of the report with statements about the concepts that appear in the instruments section. The operational definitions for site of cancer and stage of disease can be extracted from a table [Table 1] included in the research report. It seems likely that the empirical indicator for both of these concepts was the subject's response to a question or a report contained in the hospital record.

Relational propositions that appear to be central to the theory of influences on psychosocial adjustment during radiotherapy for cancer are listed below in the words used in the report. All of these propositions are found in the introductory section of the report.

1. The side effects of treatment may also create uncertainty when such symptoms are misinterpreted as signs of treatment failure.
2. The potential positive effects of uncertainty, that is, hope. . . .
3. Hope was positively related to medical status and preference for active involvement in treatment.
4. Hope . . . was negatively associated with uncertainty.
5. Uncertainty . . . may influence . . . adjustment to illness and its treatment.
6. Individual differences in preference for control, stage of disease, or site of cancer may modify the impact of [uncertainty and hope] on adjustment.
7. Perceived control positively influenced psychosocial adjustment.
8a. Persons who prefer control in a situation that offers little possibility for control may feel less hope than persons who do not desire control.
8b. Persons who prefer control in a situation that offers little possibility for control may have more adjustment problems than persons who do not desire control.
9. Both uncertainty and symptom severity were expected to be

positively related to adjustment problems across the phases of the treatment experience.

10. In addition, the data were examined to determine: (a) if there was evidence of a positive relationship between uncertainty and hope and (b) if preference for control was related to uncertainty, hope, or adjustment problems.

11. Lastly, the usefulness of these variables in explaining the variation in adjustment beyond that explained by site and state of disease was examined.

Proposition 1 deals with the relationship between symptoms and uncertainty. It indicates that the asymmetrical, sequential, and probabilistic relationship between symptoms and uncertainty is contingent on interpretation of the symptoms.

Propositions 2 and 4 concern the relationship between uncertainty and hope. These two statements can be combined into the following proposition asserting that a relationship exists and is negative in direction, asymmetrical, and sequential.

There is a negative, asymmetrical, and sequential relationship between uncertainty and hope.

Propositions 3 and 8a concern the relationship between preference for control and hope. Taken together, these statements indicate that the probabilistic, positive relationship between preference for control and hope is contingent on the possibility of control in a situation.

Proposition 5 deals with the relationship between uncertainty and adjustment; it asserts that a relationship exists, is asymmetrical, and probabilistic.

Proposition 6 addresses the relationship of uncertainty and hope with adjustment; it asserts that the asymmetrical relationship of uncertainty and hope with adjustment is contingent on preference for control, site of cancer, and stage of disease.

Propositions 7 and 8b concern the relationship between preference for control and adjustment; taken together, they indicate that the probabilistic, positive relationship between preference for control and adjustment is contingent on the possibility of control in a situation.

Propositions 9 to 11 can be restated as hypotheses using concept names.

Hypothesis$_1$	There is a positive relationship between uncertainty and psychosocial adjustment across the phases of the treatment experience.
Hypothesis$_2$	There is a positive relationship between symptom severity and psychosocial adjustment across the phases of the treatment experience.
Hypothesis$_3$	There is a positive relationship between uncertainty and hope.
Hypothesis$_4$	Preference for control is related to uncertainty.
Hypothesis$_5$	Preference for control is related to hope.
Hypothesis$_6$	Preference for control is related to psychosocial adjustment.
Hypothesis$_7$	Uncertainty, hope, symptom severity, and preference for control explain the variation in psychosocial adjustment beyond that explained by site of cancer and stage of disease.

HIERARCHY OF PROPOSITIONS

The hypothesis-testing nature of the study indicates that hierarchies of propositions would be deductive. The propositions given in the research report do not, however, lend themselves to hierarchical arrangement as axioms and theorems.

In contrast, sufficient information is given in the report to develop hierarchies of axioms and hypotheses for hypotheses$_{1-6}$. The hierarchy for hypothesis$_1$ serves as an example.

Axiom$_1$	If there is a positive relationship between uncertainty and psychosocial adjustment, and
Axiom$_2$	if uncertainty is measured by the Mishel Uncertainty in Illness Scale, and
Axiom$_3$	if adjustment is measured by the Psychosocial Adjustment to Illness Scale,
Hypothesis$_1$	then there is a positive relationship between scores on the Mishel Uncertainty in Illness Scale and the Psychosocial Adjustment to Illness Scale.

A complete hierarchy cannot be developed for Hypothesis₇ because empirical indicators are not explicitly identified for site of cancer and stage of disease.

CONCEPTUAL-THEORETICAL-EMPIRICAL STRUCTURE

The research report contains no statements regarding a substantive or methodologic frame of reference for the study.

DIAGRAM

A diagram was constructed to illustrate the influences on psychosocial adjustment during radiotherapy for cancer (Fig. A-6). This inventory of determinants, or causes, depicts the six concepts that are regarded as antecedents of psychosocial adjustment. The absence of any explicit frame of reference for the study did not permit the construction of a diagram of the conceptual-theoretical-empirical structure.

EVALUATION OF THE RELATION BETWEEN THEORY AND RESEARCH

The stated intent of this study was to determine the relationship of the set of variables (uncertainty, hope, preference for control, symptom sever-

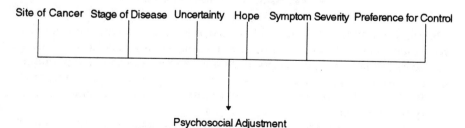

Figure A–6.   Inventory of determinants of psychosocial adjustment.

ity, site of cancer, and stage of disease) to psychosocial adjustment in the situation of radiotherapy for cancer.

SIGNIFICANCE

The theory of influences on psychosocial adjustment during radiotherapy for cancer meets the criterion of significance only in part. The theoretical significance of the research is not addressed directly. Although the investigator states that "the relationship between uncertainty and hope and the influence of both on adjustment require further study," it is unclear exactly how the study extends or fills in gaps in knowledge. The social significance of the research is addressed through the investigator's comment that "dealing with uncertainty is . . . a major task faced by persons in health care environments." The extent of psychosocial adjustment problems in the situation of radiotherapy for cancer is not, however, discussed.

The theory deals with a phenomenon of interest to the discipline of nursing. In particular, the theory addresses the patterning of human behavior (psychosocial adjustment) in interaction with the environment (radiotherapy) during a critical life situation (cancer). Furthermore, the research findings provide some precision regarding the magnitude of the hypothesized relationships and enhance our understanding of variables that are related to psychosocial adjustment.

INTERNAL CONSISTENCY

The theory of influences on psychosocial adjustment during radiotherapy for cancer meets the criterion of internal consistency only in part. There are no redundancies in concepts; each one represents a separate phenomenon. Furthermore, semantic clarity is evident in that the meaning ascribed to each concept is either explicitly stated in the report or can easily be extracted.

Semantic consistency for most of the concepts is evident. A lack of semantic consistency is, however, evident in the use of the terms stage of disease and stage of cancer. The substitution of disease for cancer certainly is minor and creates no serious confusion, but it is pointed out to emphasize the need to use a concept name consistently throughout the report. Another inconsistency is the interchangeable use of the terms adjustment, adjustment problems, adjustment difficulties, and psychosocial adjustment.

The propositions of the theory do not reflect structural consistency. Proposition 5 provides a partial rationale for hypothesis$_1$. The hypothesized positive direction of the relationship between uncertainty and adjustment is not, however, accounted for in the narrative dealing with proposition 5.

No propositions given in the research report directly support hypothesis$_2$. A partial rationale for this hypothesis is provided only when a deductive hierarchy is created from proposition 1 (axiom$_1$) and proposition 5 (axiom$_2$). The hierarchy is as follows:

Axiom$_1$	If symptoms are related to uncertainty, and
Axiom$_2$	if uncertainty is related to adjustment,
Hypothesis$_2$	then symptoms are related to adjustment.

The hierarchy does not, however, account for the hypothesized positive direction of the relationship. Moreover, the intervening variable of interpretation of symptoms from proposition 1 is not accounted for in hypothesis$_2$.

Propositions 2 and 4 provide the basis for hypothesis$_3$. There is, however, some confusion regarding the sign of the relationship. Proposition 2 states that hope is a positive effect of uncertainty, whereas proposition 4 presents empirical evidence of a negative relationship. The rationale for the hypothesized positive direction is, therefore, not clear.

The basis for hypothesis$_4$ is not evident. The research report contains no statements that could provide a rationale for the relationship between preference for control and uncertainty.

Propositions 3 and 8a support the development of hypothesis$_5$. The hypothesis does not, however, reflect the positive direction of the relationship between preference for control and hope noted in the propositions. Furthermore, it does not account for the intervening variable of possibility of control.

Propositions 7 and 8b undergird hypothesis$_6$, which, however, fails to account for the intervening variable of possibility of control or the positive direction of the relationship between preference for control and adjustment noted in the propositions.

The basis for hypothesis$_7$ is not clear. Proposition 6 asserts that preference for control, site of cancer, and stage of disease are intervening variables in the contingent relationship of uncertainty and hope with adjustment. Hypothesis$_7$, however, asserts that preference for control, site of cancer, and stage of disease are directly related to adjustment. Thus, the intervening variables identified in proposition 6 are not accounted for in hypothesis$_7$.

PARSIMONY

Formalization of the theory of influences on psychosocial adjustment during radiotherapy for cancer indicates that the theory meets the criterion of parsimony. A parsimonious set of concepts and propositions emerged from the study results. The concept preference for control was eliminated, and propositions including this concept were modified or eliminated. Furthermore, the study results suggested that site of cancer and stage of disease could be eliminated as theory concepts.

TESTABILITY

The theory of influences on psychosocial adjustment during radiotherapy for cancer meets the criterion of testability. With the exception of site of cancer and stage of disease, the concepts of the theory were connected to empirical indicators by means of operational definitions, and the propositions were measurable. Dummy coding permitted inclusion of site of cancer and stage of disease in the statistical analyses.

However, as noted in the discussion of internal consistency, the hypotheses did not fully reflect the contingent relationships asserted by some of the propositions. The hypotheses were falsifiable as stated.

OPERATIONAL ADEQUACY

The research design used to generate the theory of influences on psychosocial adjustment during radiotherapy for cancer partially meets the criterion of operational adequacy. The sample was of adults who were receiving external beam radiotherapy for cure or control of cancer. The number of subjects available at each treatment time is, however, small for a study that tested the influence of six independent variables (uncertainty, hope, preference for control, symptom severity, site of cancer, stage of disease) on psychosocial adjustment.

The identified empirical indicators are valid and reliable measures of the concepts. A potential source of confusion arises between the wording of hypotheses including the concept psychosocial adjustment and the scoring of its empirical indicator. Thus, it is important to note that higher scores on the Psychosocial Adjustment to Illness Scale indicate more adjustment problems.

The statistical analyses are appropriate techniques to test the hypotheses. The investigator did not, however, employ repeated measures statistical procedures that could have yielded informative data regarding changes in concept scores across the phases of the treatment experience.

EMPIRICAL ADEQUACY

The theory of influences on psychosocial adjustment during radiotherapy for cancer does not meet the criterion of empirical adequacy. None of the hypothesized relationships were supported by the results of the data analysis. A comparison of the hypothesized relationships and the actual findings is given in Table A–7.

Alternative substantive explanations are offered for the findings addressing the relationship between uncertainty and hope and for the findings involving preference for control. An alternative methodological explanation for the preference for control results also is offered. This explanation focuses on potential measurement error associated with the scoring format for the Krantz Health Opinion Survey.

PRAGMATIC ADEQUACY

The theory of influences on psychosocial adjustment during radiotherapy for cancer meets an initial requirement of the criterion of pragmatic adequacy. The investigator recommends additional study of the impact of symptoms that are due to treatment for illness. She also notes that the findings of future research hold promise for development of interven-

TABLE A–7. Comparison of Hypothesized Relationships and Study Findings

Hypothesis	Study Findings	Conclusion
1. Uncertainty is positively related to adjustment problems across phases of the treatment experience.	Uncertainty was not consistently related to adjustment problems across the treatment phases. Patients who perceived their illness experiences as more uncertain also reported more adjustment problems only after their 15th and last treatments.	$Hypothesis_1$ not supported
2. Symptom severity is positively related to adjustment problems across phases of the treatment experience.	Symptom severity was not consistently related to adjustment problems across the treatment phases. Symptom severity was positively associated with adjustment problems after the 1st and last treatments, but not after the 15th treatment.	$Hypothesis_2$ not supported
3. There is a positive relationship between uncertainty and hope.	After their 1st and 15th treatments, patients reporting their illness experiences as more uncertain also reported less hope. By the last treatment, this relationship was in the same direction but no longer significant.	$Hypothesis_3$ not supported
4–6. Preference for control is related to uncertainty, hope, or adjustment problems.	Individual differences in preference for control in health care showed little relationship to	$Hypotheses_{4-6}$ not supported

7. Uncertainty, hope, symptom severity, and preference for control explain the variation in adjustment beyond that explained by site and stage of disease.

uncertainty, hope, or adjustment problems. There was only one significant correlation. At the end of treatment, patients who reported desiring more behavioral involvement in their care also reported more uncertainty.

After the 15th treatment, both uncertainty and hope significantly increased the amount of explained variance. After the last treatment, uncertainty, hope, and symptom severity significantly increased the amount of explained variance. At both these times during the course of treatment, perceiving one's illness experiences as more uncertain and feeling less hopeful were predictive of more problems in adjustment. By the end of treatment, greater symptom severity also was predictive of adjustment difficulties. At both times, site and stage of cancer explained 5% or less of the variance and neither contributed significantly to the prediction of adjustment problems.

Hypothesis$_7$ not supported

tions that might help patients to correctly interpret treatment-related symptoms, which in turn might reduce uncertainty and facilitate hope.

CONCEPTUAL-THEORETICAL-EMPIRICAL STRUCTURE

Although the connections between the theoretical and empirical components of the study are evident in the form of the operational definitions, no conceptual model or other frame of reference for the study is evident. Thus, further evaluation of the conceptual-theoretical-empirical structure is not possible.

REFERENCES

Dubin, R. (1978). *Theory building* (rev. ed.). New York: The Free Press.

Christman, N. J. (1990). Uncertainty and adjustment during radiotherapy. *Nursing Research, 39,* 17–20, 47.

Kaplan, A. (1964). *The conduct of inquiry.* San Francisco: Chandler.

Willer, D., & Webster, M., Jr. (1970). Theoretical concepts and observables. *American Sociological Review, 35,* 748–757.

Analysis and Evaluation of Two Experimental Studies

PROMOTING AWARENESS: THE MOTHER AND HER BABY

Susan K. Riesch
Sharlyn K. Munns

This study considered the problem of how to increase a mother's awareness of her infant's behavior and her own behavior as a beginning step toward the promotion of quality interaction between mother and infant. The impact of informing 108 mothers of term infants and 32 mothers of preterm infants about: (a) neonatal interactive, motoric, state control, and response to stress behavior patterns; and (b) maternal behavior to enhance and support infant behavior was tested with four groups. In describing the behavior that occurred during a feeding session, mothers in two treatment groups reported significantly more of their own behavior than that of their neonate. They more closely resembled the trained observers' report of the behavior than did mothers in two control groups. Recommendations include incorporating an educative treatment in plans of nursing care for mothers and infants and further research to determine the optimal timing and long-term effects of such an intervention.

Bowlby's (1969) ethological-evolutionary theory of attachment specifies that the infant-mother bond emerges and is consolidated during the first year of life. The early maternal-neonatal interaction, its importance to the child's future development, and the capabilities of the

Susan K. Riesch, DNSc, is an associate professor at the School of Nursing, University of Wisconsin-Milwaukee. Sharlyn K. Munns, MS, Peoria, Illinois. The authors acknowledge the contributions of Nancy Wright, Denise Linde, and Nancy Maynard in the initial design and data collection phases of this study, and Dr. Jacqueline Clinton for assistance with data analysis and preparation of this manuscript.

This study was supported by the Faculty Research Development, DHHS, Division of Nursing 5R01-NU00648-03.

Reprinted from *Nursing Research*, 33, 271–276, 1984.

neonate as a contributor to that interaction have been investigated and reported extensively in the literature (Ainsworth & Bell, 1974; Ainsworth, Blehar, Waters, & Wall, 1978; Schaffer, 1977). However, incorporation of this knowledge as a nursing intervention has been investigated less thoroughly, especially with respect to the premature infant (Brown, LaRossa, Aylward, Davis, Rutherford, & Bakeman, 1980).

Several studies demonstrated that structuring the maternal-infant interaction or providing structured interventions to promote interaction affected the interaction. Field (1977, 1980) and Field, Dempsey, Hallock, and Shuman (1978) devised a number of manipulations designed to inform mothers about social interaction with infants and to facilitate the interactions between mothers and their premature infants. In one of Field's (1977) early studies, she asked mothers to imitate their infants rather than attempt to keep their infants' attention. As a result of this direction, the study mothers decreased their activity and became increasingly responsive to their infants' behaviors. Likewise, by asking the mothers to repeat their phrases and to be silent during their infants' gaze aversion, Field noted that the mothers were increasingly sensitive to the behavioral cues of their infants and increasingly responsive to their signals.

The effect of demonstrating infant social capabilities as an intervention to promote maternal-infant interaction was studied by Anderson (1981) with full-term infants and by Widmayer (1979) with preterm infants. Anderson compared the effects of three specific strategies upon the quality of the interaction between newly delivered mothers and their full-term infants. These strategies included providing information to mothers about (1) neonatal behavior, (2) neonatal behavior coupled with a demonstration of the behavior, and (3) neonatal care and equipment. Anderson found that informing mothers of the behavioral characteristics of neonates enhanced the quality of the interaction (as measured by the Price [1975] Maternal Infant Adaptation Scale), but that coupling the information with a demonstration of the neonatal behavior through the performance of the Brazelton (1973) Neonatal Behavioral Assessment Scale (BNBAS) significantly enhanced the interaction between mother and infant. The third strategy, providing information on neonatal care and equipment, did not influence the interaction.

Similar findings were reported by Widmayer (1979), although the sample consisted of mothers and their preterm infants. Widmayer reported that mothers of preterm infants who observed the administration of the BNBAS shortly after birth and who were asked to complete the Field et al. (1978) Mother's Assessment of the Behavior of Her Infant scale (MABI) at birth and weekly for four weeks performed significantly better than a preterm control group. The mothers and infants in the treatment group were judged to have more optimal ratings for feeding and face-to-face interactions than those in the control group. Widmayer's findings suggested that the mothers' observations of the BNBAS administered with the healthy preterm infant and the weekly completion of the MABI during the first month may act together to elicit optimal interaction behaviors.

Using Broussard and Hartner's (1970) Neonatal Perception Inventory (NPI) as the basis for intervention, Hall (1980) demonstrated a relationship between a structured, informative in-home nursing intervention concerning infant behavior and primiparas' perceptions of their normal full-term infants. An individualized instruction plan was developed for each subject based upon the subject's specific perception of her infant within the six categories of the NPI: crying, feeding, vomiting, sleeping, eliminating, and patterns of eating and sleeping. Postintervention, the NPI scores increased significantly for the experimental group, suggesting that teaching about normal infant behavior during the early phase of the puerperium had a positive influence on mothers' perceptions of the neonate.

Brown et al. (1980) studied the effects of a nursery-based educative intervention with healthy premature infants and their black, socially disadvantaged mothers. These authors failed to find either short-term or long-term effects of the interventions with the infants and their mothers.

The question studied was: What is the effect of providing mothers with information about the social capabilities of newborn infants and about the methods mothers can use to elicit those capabilities upon their observations of, and responses to, neonatal social behaviors?

The findings reported here are the compilation of two studies. The initial study consisted of examining the impact of an educative nursing intervention upon the observations and responses of mothers of full-term infants. The second study was a replication with a sample of preterm infants. The initial study is referred to as the term study and the second study is referred to as the preterm study.

METHOD

Sample

All women who delivered their neonates without complication at two university-affiliated urban medical centers in a midwestern city during the study period were eligible for the term study. Sample criteria excluded high-risk or ill mothers and infants. Thus mothers with chronic diseases, teen mothers (aged 17 years and under), or mothers who required a cesarean birth were excluded. Although 169 mother-infant dyads met the criteria during the study period and agreed to participate, only 108 formed the study sample. Most potential subjects were lost due to early discharge, unforeseen complications such as phototherapy or feeding problems, and scheduling mishaps between the investigators and subjects. For the total sample of mothers in the term study, the mean age was 22.8 years with a minimum age of 18 and maximum age of 41. Half the mothers had delivered their first baby, about one third their second, and the remaining mothers their third baby or more. The largest number of children previously delivered by any participant was five. About equal numbers of mothers were married as not married, and chose rooming-in as not rooming-in. Approximately one third of the mothers breastfed their infants. Approximately three quarters of the mothers did not attend childbirth preparation classes. Fifty-four of the subjects and their infants served as the treatment group, and the remaining 54 subjects as the control group.

For the preterm study, all women whose infants were born during the study period at the same institutions and whose infants met the following criteria were invited to participate in the preterm study. The criteria for the preterm study were: (a) gestational age 34 to 37 weeks, (b) singleton birth, (c) absence of physical malformation, and (d) absence of serious medical complications at 72 hours of age such as respiratory distress requiring respirator assistance, sepsis, convulsions, or severe acid-base imbalance. Thus the sample constituted a group of preterm infants who had relatively good medical prognosis. Mothers of the infants who qualified as participants were free of chronic illness or mental retardation. Forty-eight subjects and their infants agreed to participate. A total of 32 mother-infant dyads participated in the study. The treatment and control groups each included 16 mother-infant dyads. The chief reason for subject attrition in the preterm study was inability to contact the dyad after hospital discharge.

The mean age of the mothers was 25.2 years with a minimum age of 18 and maximum age of 37. More than half the mothers were primiparous; about one fifth delivered their second baby, another fifth their third baby, and the remaining their fourth baby. Most were married and most chose rooming-in during the hospitalization. About half chose to breastfeed their infants and about half attended prenatal classes.

Subjects for both studies signed an informed consent after full explanation of the study's purpose and procedures. Both the term and preterm studies were reviewed and approved by the committees for the protection of human subjects at the medical institutions and the university.

Instrument

The Behavioral Checklist, developed by Riesch, Wright, Linde, and Maynard (1978), consisted of two parts: (a) a checklist of 22 neonatal social behaviors and 16 maternal social behaviors, and (b) two interview questions to elicit maternal report of her own behavior and that of her neonate. Items were selected for the neonatal behavioral checklist from the four behavioral dimensions of the BNBAS: interactive, motoric, state control, and response to stress. Behaviors that could be observed readily during interaction between mother and infant, occurred without examiner stimulation, and were representative of the four BNBAS dimensions were chosen for inclusion on the checklist. The behaviors are summarized in Table 1.

TABLE 1. Neonatal Behavioral Categories

Category	ITEM	
	Brazelton	Checklist
Interactive behavior	Orientation Alertness Cuddliness Consolability	Focusing Smiling Cooing Eye-to-eye contact Alerting/brightening Head toward stimuli
Motor behavior	Reflexes Pull-to-sit Motor maturity Defensive reaction Hand-to-mouth Activity	Stretching Nestling Hand-to-mouth
State control	Habituation Predominant state Peak of excitement Lability of states Rapidity of buildup Irritability Self-quieting	Head away from stimuli Closing eyes Diminution of activity (i.e., wiggling, crying, etc.) Quiet, lack of body movement Nonnutritive sucking
Response to stress	Tremulousness Skin color Startles	Tremors Change in skin color Startles

The two interview questions asked were: (a) What, in the last 10 minutes, did you notice your baby do? and, (b) What, in these last 10 minutes, did you do that you think the baby noticed? Probes, such as "Tell me more," "What do you mean by . . . ," or repeating the mothers' responses were used to gather additional comments relative to the mother's report of the infant's and her own behavior.

Interrater reliability was established in pilot situations through simultaneous data collector observation of 40 different inpatient maternal-infant interaction episodes. Random combinations of the data collectors observed whether or not each maternal and each neonatal behavior on the checklist occurred. An interrater reliability coefficient of .80 or better was maintained for each item throughout the pilot and study phases of the research.

Intrarater reliability was established using videotapes of maternal-infant interactions. The videotaped interaction constituted documented evidence of whether or not a behavior occurred. The same data collector rated the same interaction on two different occasions. The intrarater agreement ranged from .96 to 1.00. Content validity of the instrument was attained using a panel of experts prepared at the doctoral level in parent-child nursing and developmental psychology.

Demographic data included variables that were most likely to influence the early maternal-infant interaction: age of the mother; marital status; infant feeding method; childbirth preparation; parity; and rooming-in.

The nursing intervention or treatment was an audiotape with accompanying text to which the subject listened in the privacy of her room, during a time mutually agreed upon by the mother and investigator. Visitors, care providers, phone calls, and other distractions were postponed during the listening period. Specifically, the tape described a neonate's ability to demonstrate protective reflexes (cough, blink, sneeze); to habituate to sound, light, or motion; to self-quiet through touch, nestling, fist sucking; and to attend to animate and inanimate objects. Appropriate actions the mother could use to elicit or support the neonatal behavior were described, such as, positioning, stroking, rocking, and gazing. The text of the tape was conversational and versions that referred to either the male or female infant were used according to the infant's gender. The printed text of the taped message was left with the mother upon conclusion of the listening period. In the term study, the intervention occurred within 48 hours of the infant's birth. In the preterm study, the intervention occurred within five days of the infant's birth.

An observation of maternal-infant interaction during a feeding episode, which occurred 24 to 72 hours after the intervention, was the posttest measure. The interaction between the dyads was observed continuously for 10 minutes. Mothers were instructed to feed the infants as they normally did and were reminded that they would be asked about the baby's and their own behavior at the conclusion of the 10 minutes. For those observed in the hospital, a Do Not Disturb — Research in Progress sign was posted on the room's door to keep distractions at a minimum. If fathers of the infants were present either at the home or hospital observation, they were invited to remain. TV sets, in either setting, usually remained on with the volume lowered.

Each mother indicated to the researcher when the feeding began. The researcher then observed and recorded on the checklist whether or not the neonatal and maternal behaviors occurred. The interaction was observed for 10 minutes. In most instances the investigator was positioned obliquely to the dyad, seated, and out of the direct line of vision of the mother. If the mother made inquiries during the observation, the inquiries were deferred to the period following the observation. After the 10 minutes, the mother was asked to report the infant's behavior and her own behavior. The information provided by the mother's report was recorded verbatim, then coded on the checklist by two investigators to insure agreement since the mother's exact words often needed interpretation before recording.

Procedure

All eligible subjects were approached to be study participants during their hospital stay. A member of the research team visited the units daily to seek subjects. Upon agreement to participate, subjects were assigned randomly to either the treatment or control groups. Mothers in the treatment groups received the nursing intervention designed to inform them of the social capabilities of newborn infants and appropriate actions to stimulate, quiet, or support the neonate's ability to self-stimulate or self-quiet. Those in the control groups received usual and customary nursing care (e.g., physical care, demonstration of infant feeding, bathing, and care procedures).

The postintervention observations of the term infants and mothers occurred during the evening feeding on the second or third day of life while the observations of the preterm infants and mothers occurred in the home two to four days after discharge. The average age of the term infant at posttest was 70 hours, the average age of the preterm infant at posttest was 192 hours.

RESULTS

The treatment and control groups in both studies were found to be similar statistically in terms of age of mother, marital status, infant feeding method, childbirth preparation, parity, and rooming-in. There were no significant differences in the variances of the independent variables among the treatment and control groups. Thus the assumption of homogeneity of variance was met and comparisons of the independent variables between groups were analyzed using the student t test.

The treatment group differed significantly from the control group on the posttest measure. The mean number of neonatal behavioral cues reported by mothers in the treatment group was significantly greater than those reported by mothers in the non-treatment group in both the term ($t(106) = 6.10$, $p = .0001$) and preterm ($t(30) = 3.26$, $p = .003$) studies. Similarly, the mean number of maternal self-reported responses in the treatment group was significantly greater than the maternal self-reported responses in the nontreatment group in both the term ($t(106) = 6.29$, $p = .0001$) and preterm ($t(30) = 2.68$, $p = .01$) studies.

To test for congruence between nurse observation and mother report of both maternal and infant behaviors, the sum of all the neonatal and maternal behaviors that occurred as reported by the mother and observed by the nurse after the 10-minute feeding session was tabulated for each mother-infant dyad. The nurse was considered the standard for the behavior that occurred during the feeding session. A ratio of nurse to mother reports was calculated for each participant — one ratio for the report of infant behavior and one ratio for the report of mother behavior. The ratios of nurse-observed behaviors to mother-reported behaviors in the control group was compared to the ratios in the treatment group.

The mean ratio of nurse-observed infant behaviors to mother-reported infant behaviors in the treatment group was significantly less than in the control groups of the term ($t(106) = 4.25$, $p = .001$) and the preterm ($t(30) = 4.18$, $p = .0001$) studies. The mean ratio of nurse-observed mother behavior to mother-reported mother behavior was significantly less in the treatment groups than in the control groups of both the term ($t(106) = 5.94$, $p = .005$) and the preterm studies

$(t(30) = 3.74, p = .001)$. The reports of infant and mother behavior by mothers in the treatment groups were more congruent with the nurses' observations than were those reported by mothers in the control group.

Influence of Demographic Characteristics

To assess the degree to which the treatment and the demographic characteristics influenced the mother report of infant behavior and mother behavior in both the term and preterm studies, a forward, stepwise multiple regression analysis was performed. The independent variables included the treatment and the social characteristics of the dyad: maternal age, type of rooming, method of feeding, prenatal preparation, and parity.

For the term study, only two variables were correlated significantly with mother report of infant behavior: treatment and marital status (Table 2). Together, treatment and marriage accounted for 32.9% of the variance in mother report. Inspection of the betas revealed that both variables had a positive effect on the mother report of infant behavior and that both explained a significant amount of the variance.

Only the variables of treatment and prenatal preparation were correlated significantly with the mother report of mother behavior in the term study (Table 2). Together, the treatment and prenatal preparation factors accounted for a significant amount of variance in mother report of mother behavior, 33.3%. The betas demonstrated the positive effect of the variables on mother report of mother behavior.

TABLE 2. Explanation for Variance in Mother Report of Behavior in the *Term* Study (N = 108)

Independent Variable	Multiple r	r^2	r^2 Change	Beta	F Change
Infant behavior					
Treatment	.55	.30	.30	.55	42.57*
Marital status	.57	.33	.03	.17	24.24*
Mother behavior					
Treatment	.55	.30	.30	.55	43.22†
Prenatal preparation	.58	.33	.03	.18	24.76†

*p = .0001; †p = .0000

**TABLE 3. Explanation for Variance in Mother Report of
Behavior in the *Preterm* Study (N = 32)**

Independent Variable	Multiple r	r^2	r^2 Change	Beta	F Change
Infant behavior					
Treatment	.49	.24	.24	.43	9.71†
Maternal age	.55	.30	.06	.03	8.60†
Mother behavior					
Marital status	.59	.34	.34	.40	10.70‡
Prenatal preparation	.63	.40	.06	.28	7.57†
Treatment	.68	.46	.06	.42	3.85*

*p = .0342; †p = .0006; ‡p = .0001

For the preterm group, the variables of treatment and maternal age were correlated significantly with mother report of infant behavior. Together these factors accounted for 30.1% of the variance in mother report. Inspection of the betas indicated a positive effect (Table 3). Variance in the mother report of mother behavior is best explained by the variables of marital status, prenatal preparation, and treatment. Together, these factors accounted for 46.0% of the variance in mother report, treatment being the least significant of the three. The betas indicated that being married, attending childbirth classes, and receiving the nursing treatment had a positive effect (Table 3).

Mothers most frequently reported their infants' interactive behavior, that is attending behavior. Infant response to stress behaviors was reported second most frequently, and motor behaviors were reported third most frequently in both the term and preterm studies. State control behavior, particularly habituating behavior, was reported the least frequently of the four dimensions of infant behavior. In addition, the nurses observed habituation behaviors less frequently in the preterm infant than in the term infant.

Mothers of the term infants reported most frequently that their infants noticed the mother's touching, vocalizing, and eye-to-eye contact during the feeding interaction. Mothers of the preterm infants reported most frequently that their infants noticed changes in maternal stimuli, maternal patting and stroking, and other forms of maternal touching.

DISCUSSION

Mother Report of Infant Behavior

Mothers who were assigned to the treatment groups of the term and preterm studies reported significantly more of their infants' behavior during a 10-minute feeding session than mothers assigned to either of the control groups. The results of these studies suggest that mothers are especially receptive to information regarding their infants' interactive capabilities during the early puerperium and that mothers develop an awareness of their own behavioral responses toward their infants. The findings of the term study support Rubin's concept of a taking-in phase during the early postpartal period (Rubin, 1961). For the two or three days after the birth of her child, Rubin contended that a mother is passive and most receptive to learning about her new role. Rather than focusing on the intricacies of the interaction between the mother and her newborn and judging it appropriate or not, the findings of the term study suggest that care should be taken to provide structure and intervention that positively influence the interaction. Information on the social capabilities of newborn infants is suggested as a positive influence.

Application of Rubin's paradigm to the preterm infant is less clear. In the preterm study, the intervention was applied at the infant's fifth day of life as opposed to the term infant's third day of life. Whether or not the mother of the preterm infant experiences the passivity described by Rubin for a time beyond that thought typical for the mother of a term baby is an area for further research. Certainly the mothers of the preterm infants displayed a receptivity to the information similar to that of the term infant mothers. Yet whether this is a finding in support of Rubin's concepts is still in question.

Caplan (1957) noted that intervention during the early puerperium had a much greater effect upon influencing the attitudes of family members than it did at periods of stability of emotional functioning. More recent studies tend to support Caplan's contention. Other investigators found that providing information to mothers about the behavioral characteristics of their infants during the early postpartal period was a positive influence on mothers' perceptions of their newborn infants (Broussard & Hartner, 1970; Hall, 1980), and can actually enhance interaction behaviors during feeding and face-to-face interactions (Anderson, 1981; Widmayer, 1979). The term and preterm studies support Caplan's contention, though further study is recommended to determine the best timing for the intervention, whether that be in the early puerperium as Caplan and others suggested or if a later intervention is equally effective. Further study is also recommended to determine the duration of the effects of treatment provided in this research and of the treatments provided in studies by Anderson (1981), Hall (1980), and Widmayer (1979).

Mother Report of Mother Behavior

Mothers who received the intervention to inform them of the neonate's social capabilities and of the maternal behaviors to enhance and support their infants reported significantly more of their own behavior than did mothers who did not receive the treatment. Awareness of one's own behavior undoubtedly was a significant factor in the mother's reporting of her own behavior that her infant noticed. The new mother is concerned about how she will perform her new role; she needs to meet her own expectations and those of others in the performance of her maternal role (Rubin, 1967). The mother's expectations may or may not be realistic. Unrealistic expectations may serve as a detriment to a mother's accomplishments. Informing the mother of the responses she can initiate in order to enhance or support her particular infant may relieve some of her role uncertainty, thus allowing her to interact freely with her infant.

Mother-Nurse Agreement

As a trained observer, the nurse was used as a standard for the purpose of examining what particular behaviors occurred during the interaction. Mothers in the treatment groups attained the same degree of observational skill toward themselves and their infants as did the trained observer. Thus, interventions which require the mother to analyze her behavior and that of the infant as a prerequisite for learning a particular procedure or parenting skill are within the scope of the early postpartum.

Infant habituating behaviors were the major source of discrepancy between the mother and the nurse. This finding suggests habituating behavior in infants is not as readily observable or impressive as is the interactive, response to stress, and motoric behaviors, or it may suggest that the study mothers were not well-informed on this aspect of the behavioral repertoire as a result of the intervention. Since habituation behaviors were noted less frequently in the preterm infant, it is suggested that the preterm infant has less ability to modify the effects of external stimuli. Because habituation behavior has important implications for the synchrony and reciprocity of behavior between two individuals, this finding should be investigated further.

Sociodemographic Influences

The experimental nursing treatment used in these studies accounted for significant portions of the variance of mother report of infant and mother behavior in the term and preterm groups. Thus, the simple procedure of informing mothers of infant's social capabilities and of maternal behaviors that stimulate and support the infant's sociality is a strong recommendation of this study. Particular maternal social characteristics, such as marital status, prenatal preparation, and maternal age along with the intervention, explained significant amounts of variance in mother report of infant and mother behavior. These findings are congruent with the literature.

Marriage is one form of social support to the new mother. Though not all unmarried women are without significant support, Hansen and Bjerre (1977) and Minde, Trehub, Corter, Boukydis, Celhoffer, and Marton (1978) noted that women with poor support systems were judged to have greater difficulties with the mother-child relationship than married women. It is suggested that the nurse determine the degree of social support the mother has available to her, the marital partner being one form of that support, and plan interventions to capitalize upon the dyad's interactional potential.

Prenatal preparation accounted for more variance than did the treatment in the preterm mother's report of her own behavior. There is little published research to support this finding other than the positions of Littlefield and Siebert (1978) and Bonovich (1981) that mothers who attend such classes have an opportunity to clarify any misconceptions they may have related to infant care, characteristics, and behavioral potential. Those mothers who do not participate in prenatal preparation may benefit from an individualized nursing demonstration of effective neonatal and maternal behavior in the postpartum period.

In the preterm study only, a significant amount of variance in the mother's report of her infant's behavior was accounted for by the treatment and by maternal age. The older the mother, the more infant behaviors she was able to report. This finding is congruent with that of Jones, Green, and Krauss (1980) and Mercer (1981), who observed that younger mothers held their preterm infants fewer minutes, were less sensitive, and less consistent in responding to their infants than were more mature mothers. It is suggested that the less mature mother may need an intervention of greater intensity than was provided in this study.

In both the preterm and term studies, considerable variance in mother report of mother and infant behavior is left unaccounted for. Since it is well documented that the infant is a social being and contributes markedly to the interaction with mother (Als, 1977; Brazelton, 1973; Wolff, 1966), it is suggested that a direct measure of the infant's contribution, such as the BNBAS, be included in future studies.

A limitation of the research is the difference between the preterm and term studies in timing and setting of the treatment and the posttest. The term group received the treatment sooner after birth than did the preterm group. In addition, posttest measures occurred in the hospital for the term group, whereas those measures occurred in the infant's home for the preterm group.

CONCLUSION

As a result of a nursing intervention to inform mothers of the behavioral potential of newborn infants and maternal behaviors to enhance this potential, mothers of term and preterm infants were able to report significantly more observations of their own behavior and that of the infant than mothers who did not receive the intervention. Because interaction is based upon the continuous interpretation of cues and responses between two persons, it must be determined that the cues and responses can at least be observed and labelled. After treatment the mothers in this study could identify and articulate the social behaviors of their infants and the behaviors the mothers themselves exhibited which they thought were observed by their infants.

It is suggested that information relative to the infants' interactional potential and the maternal behaviors that support and enhance that potential be included in all standard plans of maternal-neonatal nursing care. Further research is needed to determine whether such actions indeed promote the maternal-infant bond or have lasting effects relative to the development of the maternal-child relationship.

REFERENCES

Ainsworth, M. D. S., & Bell, S. M. (1974). Mother-infant interaction and the development of competence. In K. Connolly & J. Brunder (Eds.), *The growth of competence* (pp. 49–67). New York: Academic Press.

Ainsworth, M. D. S., Blehar, M., Waters, E., & Walls, S. (1978). *Patterns of attachment.* Hillsdale, NJ: Lawrence Erlbaum Associates.

Als, H. (1977). The newborn communicates. *Journal of Communication, 27,* 67–73.

Anderson, C. J. (1981). Enhancing reciprocity between mother and neonate. *Nursing Research, 30,* 89–93.

Bell, R. Q. (1974). Contributions of human infants to caregiving and social interaction. In M. Lewis & L. A. Rosenblum (Eds.), *The effect of the infant on its caregiver* (pp. 1–19). New York: John Wiley & Sons.

Bonovich, L. (1981). Participation: the key to learning for patients in antepartal clinics. *Journal of Obstetrical, Gynecological, and Neonatal Nursing, 10,* 75–79.

Bowlby, J. (1969). *Attachment and loss: Vol. 1. Attachment.* New York: Basic Books.

Brazelton, T. B. (1973). *Neonatal behavioral assessment scale.* Philadelphia: J. B. Lippincott Co.

Broussard, E. R., & Hartner, M. S. (1970). Maternal perception of the neonate as related to development. *Child Psychiatry and Human Development, 1,* 16–25.

Brown, J. V., LaRossa, M. M., Aylward, G. P., Davis, D. J., Rutherford, P. K., & Bakeman, R. (1980). Nursery-based intervention with prematurely born babies and their mothers: Are there effects? *The Journal of Pediatrics, 97,* 487–491.

Caplan, G. (1957). Psychological aspects of maternity care. *American Journal of Public Health, 47,* 25–31.

Field, T. M. (1977). Effects of early separation, interactive deficits, and experimental manipulation on infant-mother face-to-face interaction. *Child Development, 48,* 763–771.

Field, T. M., Dempsy, J., Hallock, N., & Shuman, H. (1978). The mother's assessment of the behavior of her infant. *Infant Behavior and Development, 1,* 156–167.

Field, T. M. (1980). Interactions of preterm and term infants with their lower and middle class teenage and adult mothers. In T. M. Field, S. Goldberg, D. Stern, & A. M. Sostek (Eds.), *High-risk infants and children* (pp. 33–51). New York: Academic Press.

Greenberg, M., Rosenburg, I., & Lind, J. (1973). Mothers rooming-in with their newborns: Its impact upon the mother. *American Journal of Orthopsychiatry, 43,* 783–788.

Hall, L. A. (1980). Effect of teaching primiparas' perceptions of their newborn. *Nursing Research, 29,* 317–322.

Hansen, E., & Bjerre, I. (1977). Mother-child relationship in low birthweight groups. *Child: Care, Health and Development, 3,* 93–103.

Jones, F. A., Green, A. H., & Krauss, D. R. (1980). Maternal responsiveness of primiparous mothers during the post-partum period: Age differences. *Pediatrics, 65,* 579–584.

Littlefield, V., & Siebert, G. (1978). The group approach to problem-solving for pregnant diabetic women. *The American Journal of Maternal Child Nursing, 3,* 274–280.

Mercer, R. T. (1981). A theoretical framework for studying factors that impact on the maternal role. *Nursing Research, 30,* 73–77.

Minde, K. K., Trehub, S., Corter, C., Boukydis, C., Celhoffer, L., & Marton, P. (1978). Mother-child relationship in the premature nursery: An observational study. *Pediatrics, 61,* 373–379.

Price, G. (1975). *Influencing maternal care through discussion of videotapes of maternal-infant feeding interaction.* Unpublished doctoral dissertation, Boston University.

Riesch, S., Wright, N., Linde, D., & Maynard, N. (September 22, 1978). *A model to study the effectiveness of a specific nursing intervention on mother-infant interaction.* Paper presented at the First Annual Research Day, University of Wisconsin-Milwaukee School of Nursing.

Rubin, R. (1961). Puerperal change. *Nursing Outlook, 9,* 753–755.

Rubin, R. (1967). Attainment of maternal role. Part 1. Process. *Nursing Research, 16,* 237–245.

Schaffer, H. R. (Ed.). (1977). *Studies in mother-infant interaction.* New York: Academic Press.

Widmayer, S. M. (1979). *An intervention for mothers and their preterm infants.* Unpublished doctoral dissertation, University of Miami.

Wolff, P. (1966). The courses, controls, and organization of behavior in the neonate. *Psychological Issues, 5,* 1–99.

Analysis of Theory

The stated purpose of Riesch and Munns's (1984) research was to determine the effect of providing mothers with information about the social capabilities of their newborn infants and the methods mothers can use to elicit those capabilities on their observations of and responses to neonatal social behaviors. The study may be classified as experimental research designed to test predictive theory.

CONCEPT IDENTIFICATION AND CLASSIFICATION

The research tested a predictive theory of infant and maternal social behaviors. The theory encompasses several concepts: information about infant and maternal social behaviors; six sociodemographic influences, including age of mother, marital status, infant-feeding method, childbirth preparation, parity, and rooming-in; infant behavior; and mother behavior.

The concept information about infant and maternal social behaviors is a variable because it has two dimensions: provision of information and no information. It may be classified as directly observable in Kaplan's (1964) schema and as observable in Willer and Webster's (1970) schema because the experimental nursing intervention can be heard via audiotape and the printed text of the tape can be read. The concept may be classified as an associative unit in Dubin's (1978) schema because the experimental treatment group received the information and the control group did not.

Age of mother is a variable because it has a range of scores. It may be classified as directly observable in Kaplan's schema and as observable in Willer and Webster's schema because it can be observed through the subject's report of her age. This concept may be classified as an enumerative unit in Dubin's schema because it is always present.

Marital status also is a variable. The dimensions considered in this research are married and not married. The concept may be classified as directly observable in Kaplan's schema and as observable in Willer and Webster's schema because it is determined by subjects' statements about their marital status. It may be classified as a relational unit in Dubin's schema because it involves a comparison of one person with another and its ascription involves an interaction between the properties wife and husband.

Infant-feeding method also is a variable with two dimensions—breastfed and bottle fed. This concept also may be classified as directly observable in Kaplan's schema and as observable in Willer and Webster's schema because the method of feeding can be seen by an observer. It may be classified as an enumerative unit in Dubin's schema because all infants in the study were, of course, fed and were observed during a feeding episode.

Childbirth preparation is another variable with two dimensions: attended prenatal preparation for childbirth classes or did not attend such classes. It may be classified as directly observable in Kaplan's schema and as observable in Willer and Webster's schema because it is determined by the subject's statement about class attendance. The concept may be classified as an associative unit in Dubin's schema because some subjects attended classes and some did not.

Parity is a variable with a range of scores. It may be classified as directly observable in Kaplan's schema and as observable in Willer and Webster's schema because it is determined by each subject's statement about how many children she has delivered. It may be classified as an enumerative unit in Dubin's schema because all mothers in this research had delivered at least one child.

Rooming-in is a variable with two dimensions: rooming-in or not rooming-in. It also may be classified as directly observable in Kaplan's schema and as observable in Willer and Webster's schema because it is determined by the subject's statement about the rooming arrangement or by patient chart notation. It may be classified as an associative unit in Dubin's schema because some subjects had rooming-in and others did not. It may also be classified as a relational unit because rooming-in involves an interaction between mother and infant.

Infant behavior is a variable with a range of scores; it may be classified as directly observable in Kaplan's schema and as observable in Willer and Webster's schema because the behaviors of interest can be seen by the mother and the investigator. It may be classified as a relational unit in Dubin's schema because it is conceptualized in this research as a response to or interaction with the mother's behavior or other external cues.

Mother behavior also is a variable with a range of scores. Like infant behavior, it may be classified as directly observable in Kaplan's schema and as observable in Willer and Webster's schema because the behaviors of interest are directly experienced by the mother and can be seen by the investigator. It too may be classified as a relational unit in Dubin's schema because it is conceptualized in this research as a response to or interaction with the infant's behavior.

PROPOSITION IDENTIFICATION AND CLASSIFICATION

The theory of infant and maternal social behaviors contains several nonrelational propositions and one relational proposition. The definitions given in Table A–8 may be classified as nonrelational propositions, although the operational definitions are technically not part of the theory but do serve as links between the concepts and their empirical indicators.

Constitutive definitions for information about infant and maternal social behaviors, infant behavior, and mother behavior can be extracted from the research report. A constitutive definition for sociodemographic influences is given. Although constitutive definitions for the six sociodemographic variables are not explicit, they are self-evident. Operational definitions for all concepts are given or can be extracted from the narrative report. Empirical indicators are identified for information about infant and maternal social behaviors, infant behavior, and mother behavior, but not for the sociodemographic variables. It seems likely that a personal data form was used to record the sociodemographic variables. The concepts, their definitions, and the empirical indicators are listed in Table A–8.

The one relational proposition given in the report alludes to the existence of relationships between information about infant and maternal social behaviors and infant behavior and mother behavior. As stated in the report, it is as follows:

> Providing structured interventions to promote interaction affected the interaction.

TABLE A–8. Concepts, Definitions, and Empirical Indicators for the Theory of Infant and Maternal Social Behaviors

Concept	Constitutive Definition	Operational Definition	Empirical Indicator
Information about infant and maternal social behaviors	An educative nursing intervention focusing on social capabilities of newborn infants and methods mothers can use to elicit those capabilities	The experimental treatment consisted of subjects listening to an audiotape that described a neonate's ability to demonstrate protective reflexes, to habituate to sound, light, or motion, to self-quiet through touch, nestling, fist sucking, and to attend to animate and inanimate objects. The audiotape also described appropriate actions the mother could use to elicit or support the neonatal behavior, such as positioning, stroking, rocking and gazing. Subjects also received a printed text of the taped message. The control group subjects received usual and customary nursing care (e.g., physical care, demonstration of infant feeding, bathing, and care procedures)	*Experimental treatment:* Audiotape and printed text *Control treatment:* Usual and customary nursing care

(Continued)

TABLE A–8. Concepts, Definitions, and Empirical Indicators for the Theory of Infant and Maternal Social Behaviors (Continued)

Concept	Constitutive Definition	Operational Definition	Empirical Indicator
Sociodemographic influences	Demographic data included variables that were most likely to influence the early maternal-infant interaction: age of the mother, marital status, infant feeding method, childbirth preparation, parity, and rooming-in	Operational definitions are given or can be extracted from the report for each sociodemographic variable	No specific empirical indicators are given for the variables
Age of mother	No definition given	Apparently, age of mother in years	
Marital status	No definition given	Categorized as married or not married	
Infant-feeding method	No definition given	Apparently categorized as breastfed or bottle fed	
Childbirth preparation	No definition given	Apparently categorized as attended or did not attend prenatal preparation for childbirth classes	

Parity	No definition given	Number of children delivered	
Rooming-in	No definition given	Categorized as rooming-in or not rooming-in	
Infant behavior	Social behavior exhibited by a neonate while being fed by the mother	In this study, infant behavior was measured by the 22 neonatal social behaviors and the interview question "What, in the last 10 minutes, did you notice your baby do?" on the Behavioral Checklist	Behavioral Checklist scores for neonatal social behaviors. Mother's response to interview question about her neonate's behavior
Mother behavior	Social behavior exhibited by a mother while feeding her neonate	In this study, mother behavior was measured by the 16 maternal behaviors and the interview question "What, in these last 10 minutes, did you do that you think the baby noticed?" on the Behavioral Checklist	Behavioral Checklist scores for maternal social behaviors. Mother's response to interview question about her behavior

The narrative discussion of this proposition suggests that the relationship is asymmetrical and positive in direction. However, no explicit assertions are made about the relationship prior to presentation of the research results.

Although no hypotheses are stated explicitly, they can be extracted from the report of statistical tests given in the results section. They are stated below in null form using concept names.

- There is no difference in the number of neonatal behavioral cues reported by the mothers in the experimental treatment group and those in the control group.
- There is no difference in the number of maternal self-reported responses given by subjects in the experimental treatment group and those in the control group.
- There is no difference in the ratio of nurse-observed infant behaviors to mother-reported infant behaviors for the experimental and control groups.
- There is no difference in the ratio of nurse-observed mother behavior to mother-reported mother behavior for the experimental and control groups.
- There is no relationship between the set of independent variables, information about infant and maternal social behaviors, age of mother, marital status, infant-feeding method, childbirth preparation, parity, and rooming-in and the dependent variable, mother report of infant behavior.
- There is no relationship between the set of independent variables, information about infant and maternal social behaviors, age of mother, marital status, infant-feeding method, childbirth preparation, parity, and rooming-in and the dependent variable, mother report of mother behavior.

HIERARCHY OF PROPOSITIONS

The hypothesis-testing nature of the research indicates that a hierarchy of propositions should be deductive. The propositions given in the research report do not, however, lend themselves to hierarchical arrangement as axioms and theorems. Furthermore, because hypotheses are not stated explicitly, hierarchies of axioms and hypotheses cannot be constructed.

CONCEPTUAL-THEORETICAL-EMPIRICAL STRUCTURE

The research seems to be based on the assumption that the infant-mother bond emerges and is consolidated during the first year of life. This assumption, which is part of Bowlby's (1969) ethologic-evolutionary theory of attachment, apparently provided the conceptual frame of reference for the research. No propositions were given, however, to explicate the link between this perspective and the concepts of the theory.

DIAGRAM

An inventory of determinants can be constructed for the theory of infant and maternal social behaviors. The inventory presented in Figure A–7 depicts the seven independent variables as antecedents of the two dependent variables, infant behavior and mother behavior. Given the lack of an explicit linkage between Bowlby's concept of the infant-maternal bond and the theory concepts, a diagram of the conceptual-theoretical-empirical structure could not be developed.

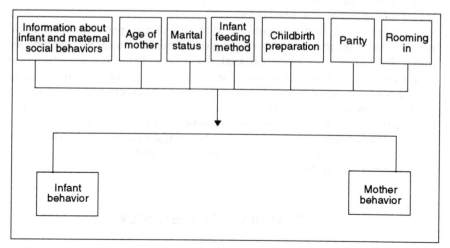

Figure A–7.   Inventory of determinants of infant and mother behaviors.

EVALUATION OF THE RELATION BETWEEN THEORY AND RESEARCH

The stated intent of this research was to determine the effect of a nursing intervention about infant and maternal social behaviors on infant and mother behaviors. The research also tested the influence of sociodemographic influences on infant and mother behaviors. The report includes the findings from two tests of the theory. One test used a sample of full-term infants and their mothers; the other was a replication with a sample of preterm infants and their mothers.

SIGNIFICANCE

The theory of infant and maternal social behaviors meets the criterion of significance. The investigators established the theoretical significance of their research by noting the paucity of studies designed to test interventions based on knowledge of early maternal-infant interactions.

The theory deals with phenomena of considerable interest to the discipline of nursing as well as to other disciplines concerned with human development. Of particular significance is the fact that the theory deals with the effect of a nursing process (the experimental treatment) on client behavior (infant and mother behaviors) that may have some bearing on health status (the developing mother-child relationship). Social significance was not addressed.

The research findings indicate that the theory predicts with some precision and increases understanding of influences on infant and mother social behaviors. The statistical analyses revealed that the experimental treatment consistently accounted for a significant amount of variance in the dependent variables and had a positive effect on mother-reported infant and mother behaviors. These analyses also revealed that sociodemographic variables do not have consistent effects across dependent variables or samples. The findings could be used to develop a theory or theories that predict with greater precision and expand explanatory power in future studies.

INTERNAL CONSISTENCY

The theory of infant and maternal social behaviors meets most of the requirements for the criterion of internal consistency. Semantic clarity and consistency are evident. The operational definitions of the six socio-demographic variables provide the needed specificity for the research. No concept redundancies are evident.

The structural consistency of propositions appears to be satisfactory; but there are discontinuities in the proposition sets. No specific propositions directly supporting the implicit hypotheses are included in the report. The only proposition given concerns the relationship between structured interventions and interaction. It must be inferred that the experimental treatment represents a structured intervention and that infant and mother behaviors represent interaction. Furthermore, although no propositions that could provide a rationale for inclusion of the sociodemographic variables are included in the report, the variables are frequently regarded as influences of maternal and infant behavior. There are no redundant propositions.

PARSIMONY

Formalization of the theory of infant and maternal social behavior indicates that the theory meets the criterion of parsimony. The narrative research report could have been expanded to include explicit presentation of propositions undergirding the statistical tests that were performed.

TESTABILITY

The theory of infant and maternal social behaviors meets the criterion of testability in a general way. The concepts can be observed empirically. Although specific empirical indicators for the sociodemographic variables are not given, it can be assumed that a personal data form was used to record the required information. Unstated propositions making up the theory were tested by means of hypotheses implicit in the statistical procedures. Although specific hypotheses are not stated, and although it is not known whether the statistical tests are one- or two-tailed, it seems likely that the implicit hypotheses could be falsified.

OPERATIONAL ADEQUACY

The research design used to test the theory of infant and maternal social behaviors meets the criterion of operational adequacy. The description of the research procedures indicates that the posttest-only control group design (Campbell & Stanley, 1963) was used. Random assignment of subjects was appropriately done, and evidence of the equivalence of the experimental and control groups for the two samples included in the report is presented.

The research instrument used to measure infant and mother behaviors appears to be valid. Reliability coefficients are satisfactory. The description of the experimental treatment indicates that it provides appropriate information about infant and maternal social behaviors. The comparison of nurse-observed and mother-reported infant and mother behaviors indicates that the two methods of measuring the dependent variables are essentially equivalent. The experimental and control group treatments seem sufficiently different so that any differences in the dependent variable could be attributed to experimental effect. The research procedures appear to be appropriate for experimental research. The data analysis techniques also are appropriate. In fact, Campbell and Stanley pointed out that the t test is the optimal statistic for the posttest-only control group design. The use of multiple regression analysis is appropriate to determine various influences on the dependent variables.

EMPIRICAL ADEQUACY

Some parts of the theory of infant and maternal social behaviors meet the criterion of empirical adequacy. The findings of the two studies indicate that the experimental effect was consistent across samples (full-term and preterm) and across dependent measures (infant behavior and mother behavior). The effects of the sociodemographic variables, however, were not consistent. Alternative methodologic explanations are not offered, but substantive explanations for the findings are given. The investigators compare their findings to Rubin's (1961) theory of postpartum taking-in and question the generalizability of Rubin's theory to maternal – preterm infant interaction. They also introduce other concepts that could have accounted for or enhanced understanding of their findings, including habituation, social support, and the infant's contribution to maternal-infant interaction. The limitations of the research are considered and the conclusions do not go beyond the data.

A meta-analysis of the findings of the two reported studies reveals a mean effect size of $r = .51$ for the effect of the experimental treatment on mother-reported infant behavior and a mean effect size of $r = .46$ for the effect of the experimental treatment on mother-reported mother behavior. The formula used for the calculations is: $r = t^2/(t^2 + df)$, where t is the obtained t test value and df is the associated degrees of freedom (i.e., $n_1 + n_2 - 2$) (Rosenthal, 1984). These calculations indicate that the experimental effect is relatively strong (Cohen, 1977) and that the proposition stating a relationship between information about infant and maternal social behaviors and mother-reported infant behavior and mother behavior is adequate.

PRAGMATIC ADEQUACY

The theory of infant and maternal social behaviors meets the initial requirements for the criterion of pragmatic adequacy. An educative nursing intervention was based on the findings of previous research, tested in two clinical situations, and found to have statistically and socially significant effects.

The innovative nursing intervention was developed for and tested with mothers of infants. The research findings suggest that the intervention is appropriate for mothers of full-term and preterm neonates. Although other requirements of pragmatic adequacy are not discussed in the report, it seems reasonable to conclude that further testing is needed to determine the feasibility of widespread adoption of the intervention and its congruence with clients' expectations. Furthermore, though nurses certainly have the legal ability to use the intervention and measure the outcomes, potential sources of resistance to this innovative nursing practice would have to be identified prior to its adoption in a health care setting.

The social significance of the intervention can be estimated quantitatively by use of the binomial effect size display developed by Rosenthal and Rubin (1982) and discussed in Chapter 4. Using the mean effect sizes given above, it can be shown that the number of mother-reported infant behaviors increased from a rate of 24 percent for the control group to 75 percent for the experimental treatment group. Similarly, the rate increased from 27 to 73 percent for mother-reported mother behaviors. It can be concluded, then, that the intervention leads to impressive and favorable outcomes.

CONCEPTUAL-THEORETICAL-EMPIRICAL STRUCTURE

The influence of Bowlby's (1969) assumption regarding the infant-maternal bond on this theory-testing research is not explicit. Furthermore, Bowlby's perspective is not mentioned in the discussion of the research results. Thus, the credibility of this frame of reference cannot be evaluated.

REFERENCES

Bowlby, J. (1969) *Attachment and loss. Vol. 1. Attachment.* New York: Basic Books.

Campbell, D. T., & Stanley, J. C. (1963). *Experimental and quasi-experimental designs for research.* Chicago: Rand McNally.

Cohen, J. (1977). *Statistical power analysis for the behavioral sciences.* New York: Academic Press.

Dubin, R. (1978). *Theory building* (rev. ed.). New York: The Free Press.

Kaplan, A. (1964). *The conduct of inquiry.* San Francisco: Chandler.

Pedhazur, E. J. (1982). *Multiple regression in behavioral research* (2nd ed.). New York: Holt, Rinehart & Winston.

Riesch, S. K., & Munns, S. K. (1984). Promoting awareness. *Nursing Research, 33,* 271–276.

Rosenthal, R. (1984). *Meta-analytic procedures for social research.* Beverly Hills, CA: Sage.

Rosenthal, R., & Rubin, D. B. (1982). A simple, general purpose display of magnitude of experimental effect. *Journal of Educational Psychology, 74,* 166–169.

Rubin, R. (1961). Puerperal change. *Nursing Outlook, 9,* 753–755.

Willer, D., & Webster, M., Jr. (1970). Theoretical concepts and observables. *American Sociological Review, 35,* 748–757.

EFFECTS OF AEROBIC INTERVAL TRAINING ON CANCER PATIENTS' FUNCTIONAL CAPACITY

Mary G. MacVicar
Maryl L. Winningham
Jennie L. Nickel

The effect of a 10-week aerobic interval-training cycle ergometer protocol on the functional capacity (VO_2L_{max}) of 45 women receiving chemotherapy for treatment of Stage II breast cancer was studied. Subjects were stratified by baseline functional capacity (± 1 MET) and randomized to experimental (EX), placebo (PL), and control (CO) groups. EX subjects completed a 10-week, 3 times/week exercise training program; PL subjects participated in 10 weeks of nonaerobic stretching and flexibility exercises; the CO group maintained normal activities. The EX group showed significant, $p < .05$, improvement on pre- to posttest VO_2L_{max} as well as workload and test time compared to the PL and CO groups. The interval-training exercise intervention was effective in improving the functional capacity of Stage II breast cancer patients on adjuvant chemotherapy.

It has been estimated that one-third or more of the decline in functional capacity experienced by cancer patients, regardless of stage of disease, can be attributed to hypokinetic conditions that develop as a consequence of prolonged physical inactivity (Dietz, 1981; Hinterbuchner, 1978; Rosenbaum, 1982). The progressive loss of functional

Mary G. MacVicar, PhD, RN, is an associate professor in the College of Nursing and Comprehensive Cancer Center, The Ohio State University, Columbus. Maryl L. Winningham, PhD, is a research associate, College of Nursing, The Ohio State University, Columbus. Jennie L. Nickel, PhD, RN, is an assistant professor in the College of Nursing, the Ohio State University, Columbus.

This study was supported by National Institutes of Health grants RO1 NR 01078, National Center for Nursing Research, and P 3OCA 16058 14, National Cancer Institute.

The authors acknowledge the assistance of Carole Anderson, PhD, FAAN, and Bonnie Garvin, PhD, RN, in critically reviewing this manuscript.

Reprinted from *Nursing Research*, 38, 348–351, 1989.

capacity associated with physical inactivity is attributed to the rapid decline in efficiency of multiple physiological systems, most apparent initially, in the cardiorespiratory and muscular systems. With continued inactivity, other physiological systems lose effectiveness and additional impairments evolve, such as limited joint mobility caused by increased density of supportive collagen tissues around the joint, osteoporosis, impaired balance, paresthesia, and lower pain threshold (Vallbona, 1982; Wenger & Hellerstein, 1984).

Exercise during treatment has been recommended for those with cancer to prevent the physiological sequelae of disuse and to maintain functional capacity (Cobb, 1975; Rosenbaum, 1982; Villaneuva, 1975); however, empirical data on exercise response are not available. Exercise that stimulates the aerobic energy system has been effective in promoting functional capacity in select clinical populations. If it can be demonstrated that aerobic exercise improves the functional capacity of those with cancer, it could be a cost-effective intervention that could be used to maintain the capacity for self-care and physical independence. The purpose of this study was to determine the effect of an aerobic exercise training protocol on the functional capacity of women receiving chemotherapy for treatment of breast cancer.

LITERATURE REVIEW

The concept of functional capacity, defined as the highest metabolic rate the individual can achieve on exertion (Vallbona, 1982), has been used extensively in disability and rehabilitation research as an indicator of an individual's ability to engage in physical activity. It is a particularly useful concept for nursing and self-care because the emphasis is on residual abilities and restorative potential, rather than what has been lost or presumed to be lost (Kirby, 1984). The physical ability to engage in activity is a universal self-care requisite (Orem, 1980), and is a component of health promotion behaviors, particularly when undertaken with the aim of proving or maintaining one's health or well-being (Frank-Stromborg, 1986; Walker, Sechrist, & Pender, 1987). The ability to maintain physical independence and to perform self-care activities can be compromised or lost if the integrity of physiological systems is not maintained.

There is a direct relationship between oxygen uptake (VO_2L_{max}) and performance of physical activity. Maximal oxygen uptake is also an indicator of the highest metabolic rate an individual can achieve with exertion. For this reason, it is considered to be the most objective physiological indicator of functional capacity (Kirby, 1984). Maintenance of functional capacity requires physical activity using large muscle groups to promote adaptation of the aerobic biochemical energy system. Inactive deconditioned skeletal muscle loses oxidative (oxygen utilizing) capacity and requires more oxygen for performance of comparable work than does the conditioned muscle, a factor contributing to rapid fatigue and decline in endurance (Astrand & Rodahl, 1986; Wenger & Hellerstein, 1984). Physical activity is dependent on the conversion of food substrates, primarily carbohydrates and fats, to adenosine triphosphate (ATP), the major energy source for the muscles (Baldwin, 1983). The synthesis of ATP for sustained activity requires oxygen. Oxygen uptake and delivery must match the demand of working muscles, and are contingent on an effective integrated response of the cardiovascular and pulmonary systems as well as on the oxygen-extraction ability of muscle cells (Frontera & Adams, 1986; Nadel, 1985).

Aerobic activity, such as walking, cycling, or swimming, that uses large muscle groups improves the oxidative capacity of skeletal muscles, stimulates the general adaptation of the aerobic biochemical system, and results in measurable increments of oxygen uptake. Disease and/or treatment(s) can inhibit the exercise response at any one of several points in the oxygen transport system, which limits the degree to which functional capacity can be improved. Nevertheless, within these limitations, aerobic exercise training can still induce physiological adaptations in the aerobic energy system sufficient to improve functional capacity. Even in advanced disease states where patients generally experience an accelerated decline in functional capacity, an exercise intervention may minimize loss of functioning.

A number of studies on other chronically ill populations have used aerobic exercise as an intervention technique. The earliest and most extensive research was conducted on medically and surgically treated cardiac patients. Data from these studies showed improved functional capacity evidenced by increased cardiac output with associated increased oxygen uptake (Fletcher, 1984; Soloff, 1978). Aerobic exercise is now an accepted component of rehabilitation for individuals with heart disease and is being tested as an intervention for other clinical populations regardless of prognosis.

Aerobic exercise principles have been adapted to fit the disease- and treatment-specific needs for restorative training of end-stage renal patients. Whether exercised during or between hemodialysis treatments, there was improved functional capacity and reduced number of complaints of muscle cramping (Goldberg et al., 1983; Painter, 1988; Painter et al., 1986). Patients with pulmonary pathology also responded favorably to exercise interventions. Despite limited ventilatory capacity and efficiency, exercise intervention using large muscle groups induced an improved functional capacity (Freedman, 1979). Physical activity resulted in more efficient oxygen utilization by muscles and increased respiratory muscle endurance, thereby contributing to the ability for sustained activity (Canny & Levison, 1987; Fletcher, 1984). Rest and reduction of activity is often recommended for cancer patients who have complained of lack of energy, fatigue, or weakness. Although there are some clear contraindications to activity such as anemia and low platelet count (Winningham, MacVicar, & Burke, 1986), research data indicate that the absence of activity may generate its own constellation of impairments. Studies of exercise intervention tested on other samples of chronically ill populations have shown that decline in functional capacity is not necessarily inevitable. The critical issue is identification of the optimal level of activity that can be performed at lowest risk. The aim is to mitigate impairments associated with physical inactivity and to improve functional capacity during therapy rather than delaying intervention until therapy is completed.

METHOD

Sample

Sixty-two women with Stage II breast cancer on postsurgical standard chemotherapy protocols entered the study. Posttest data were lost on 3 subjects as a result of equipment breakdown; transportation problems caused 1 woman to leave the program, 2 were dropped from the study when they were placed on a cardiotoxic drug (doxorubicin), and 2 were released from the project when they developed extreme reactions to their chemotherapy. Nine subjects were reclassified to more advanced stages of disease during their participation and their data were excluded from this report. Data analysis is presented on the remaining 45 subjects. Table 1 presents selected demographic variables for the sample. Analyses of variance showed no statistically significant differences between the groups on preintervention age or weight, two variables that could affect exercise response.

Forty-one subjects were on protocols consisting of methotrexate, cyclophosphamide, and 5-fluorouracil. Of these 41 subjects, 18 also

TABLE 1. Marital, Educational and Occupational Status, Age, Height, and Weight of Exercising, Placebo, and Control Subjects

Variables	Exercisers ($n = 18$)	Placebos ($n = 11$)	Controls ($n = 16$)
Marital status			
Single	2	0	0
Married	10	10	11
Divorced/widowed	6	1	5
Educational status			
< High school	7	7	6
College/technical	9	4	8
Graduate/professional	2	0	2
Occupational status			
Housewife/retired	4	4	4
Clerical	8	4	9
Administrative/ managerial/ professional	6	3	3
Age	45.4 ± 10.2	46.1 ± 10.3	43.8 ± 9.3
Height	161.2 ± 7.0	155.4 ± 13.0	163.2 ± 6.0
Weight (kg)	69.9 ± 14.2	64.0 ± 8.8	65.7 ± 13.1

received vincristine; 26 received intermittent prednisone, and 2 also received tamoxifen. Four subjects were treated only with tamoxifen. Medical approval was required according to standard procedure for special populations (American College of Sports Medicine [ACSM], 1986). Subjects received a detailed review of the project including time required for participation, testing procedures, associated risks, and assurances of confidentiality prior to signing the consent form. All subjects were paid for their participation.

To evaluate the effect of the intervention, it was necessary to make groups as metabolically equivalent as possible because subjects with higher baseline VO_2L_{max} values may not show the same degree of improvement as those with low VO_2L_{max}. Therefore, subjects were stratified according to the highest metabolic value (± 1 MET — multiples of the resting metabolic rate of 3.5 milliliters of oxygen per kilogram of body weight) achieved at pretest and randomized to experimental (EX, $n = 18$), placebo (PL, $n = 11$), and control (CO, $n = 16$) groups. No subject participated in any other exercise or rehabilitation program during the 10-week data-collection period.

Measures

Functional capacity was measured by the highest oxygen uptake achieved at symptom-limited graded exercise pre- and posttest. Oxygen uptake is expressed as volume of inspired oxygen in liters per minute (VO_2L_{max}). Heart rate, workload, and maximum time to achieve VO_2L_{max} were also used to evaluate exercise response. Systolic and diastolic blood pressures were monitored for safety reasons, but are not considered to be reliable enough to evaluate functional capacity (Sinacore & Ehsani, 1985).

Pre- and posttest procedures were conducted with subjects pedaling at a rate of 50 rotations/minute on calibrated cycle ergometers with an increase in workload resistance of 25 watts every 2 minutes until the subject could not maintain the pedaling rate and/or indicated exhaustion. Expired air was collected through a nonrebreathing face mask and analyzed for fractions of oxygen, carbon dioxide, as well as respiratory volume. These data provided the basis for calculation of oxygen uptake (VO_2L_{max}) by the Beckman Metabolic Cart (Sensor Medics Corp., Anaheim, CA). Heart rate was monitored with a 12-lead electrocardiograph (EKG), and a mercury sphygmomanometer was used for blood pressure measurement. The 12-lead EKG tracing was monitored continuously; heart rate and blood pressure data were recorded at rest, during the last 25 seconds of each 2-minute interval, at maximal exertion, and during recovery.

Experimental Group (Intervention Protocol)

The aerobic exercise protocol intervention tested in this study was an interval training cycle ergometer protocol developed by Winningham (1983). Aerobic interval exercise training consists of alternating higher and lower exercise intensity which involves use of large muscle groups. Exercise intensity is expressed as a percentage of the highest metabolic rate or functional capacity (ACSM, 1986) achieved by an individual on an exercise test. Exercise intensity is best monitored by heart rate. In this study the subject was entered in the protocol at a workload that would induce a heart rate of 60–85% of the heart-rate reserve calculated from the highest heart rate achieved at pretest. A lower workload permits removal of some lactic acid that accumulates in the working muscles during the higher intensity segments, thereby avoiding premature fatigue (Astrand & Rodahl, 1986). Each exercise level was comprised of a specific ratio of high-to-low workload or resistance for a set number of minutes. With improved conditioning, time spent at lower intensity was reduced with increased time at higher intensity. Progression was possible without discomforting fatigue, muscle soreness, or postexercise stiffness, an important consideration for individuals with chronic disease.

Aerobic exercise sessions using the aerobic interval training protocol were conducted 3/week for 10 weeks. Missed sessions were either made up on weekends or an extra session was scheduled the following week. Each session began with a prescribed set of flexibility and stretching exercises. The sessions were carefully supervised and monitored by trained staff who recorded heart rate and blood pressures at 5- to 7-minute intervals to ensure that subjects remained within the prescribed exercise intensity and to evaluate training response to the protocol.

Placebo Group

Because some benefits could accrue simply from interaction with project staff, the PL group was included in the study to isolate this effect as much as possible. PL subjects met with staff for flexibility and stretching exercises. During the sessions, heart rate and blood pressure were taken at 5- to 7-minute intervals so that subjects would experience similar conditions, but without the aerobic interval training protocol.

Control Group

CO subjects were instructed to carry on with their normal activities. There was no interaction with project staff other than that which occurred at pre- and posttest data collection periods.

RESULTS

For each variable, an analysis of covariance, with the baseline measurement as the covariate, was used to compare changes in the response from the pre- to posttest values for the three groups. Results are presented in Table 2. There were significant differences between groups on pre- to

TABLE 2. Analysis of Covariance, Adjusted for Baseline Values on VO_2L_{max} Heart Rate, Maximum Test Time, and Maximum Workload

Variables	F	p
VO_2L_{max}	50.40	<.01
Heart rate	3.42	<.04
Maximum test time	24.19	<.01
Maximum workload	28.67	<.01

posttest functional capacity, heart rate, maximum test time, and maximum workload. A mean 40% improvement on functional capacity was achieved by the EX group from pre- to posttest (pretest = 1.02 VO_2L_{max}, posttest = 1.45 VO_2L_{max}), but no significant pre- to posttest changes were observed on any measure for the PL or CO groups. Posthoc pairwise comparisons among groups were also done using Tukey's multiple comparison method (Winer, 1971) with results presented in Table 3. The EX group was significantly, $p < .05$, different from PL and CO on functional capacity (VO_2L_{max}), maximum workload, and test time.

These data show that the intervention protocol was effective in promoting adaptation of the aerobic physiological energy systems of the EX subjects. Compared to the PL and CO groups, EX subjects could work longer and achieved higher intensity workloads at posttest. For heart rate there was a significant difference between the EX and CO groups, but not between the EX and PL groups. However, this may be a function of exposure to the project staff and greater familiarity with the concept of exercise during their participation in the stretching and flexibility workouts. In other words, they were more willing or perhaps more comfort-

TABLE 3. Tukey's Multiple Comparison for Differences Among Groups on VO_2L_{max}, Heart Rate, Maximum Test Time, and Workload

Variables And Group	Means	Group	Critical Values	Difference
VO_2L_{max}				
Experimental	0.425	EX vs. PL	0.152	0.477*
Placebo	−0.052	EX vs. CO	0.137	0.513*
Control	−0.088	PL vs. CO	0.156	0.036
Heart rate				
Experimental	8.23	EX vs. PL	9.95	7.57
Placebo	0.66	EX vs. CO	8.98	9.07*
Control	−0.84	PL vs. CO	10.24	1.50
Maximum test time				
Experimental	2.44	EX vs. PL	1.11	2.84*
Placebo	−0.40	EX vs. CO	1.00	2.23*
Control	0.21	PL vs. CO	1.16	−0.61
Maximum workload				
Experimental	34.64	EX vs. PL	15.62	40.73*
Placebo	−6.09	EX vs. CO	14.03	36.61*
Control	−1.97	PL vs. CO	15.99	−4.12

*Significant at $\alpha = .05$ level.

able in attempting greater exertion at posttest, compared to the CO group. It is important to emphasize that the deconditioned individual can have a heart rate that is as much as 40 beats per minute higher than the conditioned individual at the same higher workload (Ellestad, 1986). The fact that there was no statistical difference between EX and PL groups on heart rate must be assessed against the analysis showing statistically significant differences between the EX and PL groups on VO_2L_{max}, maximum workload, and test time.

DISCUSSION

The pre- to posttest increase in VO_2L_{max} achieved by the EX group, compared to the PL and CO groups, demonstrates improved functional capacity as well as increased workload and an increased test time. Despite differences in exercise modes, protocols, and measurement techniques, comparison of data from this study with data generated by research on other chronically ill populations is useful. The mean 40% improvement in functional capacity of exercising subjects in this study is comparable to documented gains made by samples of other chronically ill groups, for example, 15 to 21% improvement in functional capacity for end-stage renal patients (Painter, 1988), up to 16% improvement for those with pulmonary impairments (Freedman, 1979), and over 50% improvement for cardiac patients (Peterson, 1983).

The data support recommendations that interventions to improve functional capacity be implemented during therapy (Dietz, 1981). Although self-care activities or activities of daily living were not measured in this study, increases in functional capacity could improve the individual's potential ability for self-care and/or daily living activities; however, further research is needed to determine the relationship between functional capacity and self-care activities. Specifically, it would be important to determine which activities are relinquished with decline of functional capacity and which are resumed as functional capacity improves.

The aerobic interval training protocol should be tested with a larger sample of breast cancer patients as well as with patients diagnosed with different cancers, at more advanced stages of disease, and with other treatment modalities such as radiation therapy, and combination radiation/chemotherapy protocols. In particular, it is extremely important to identify not only exercise benefits but to delineate specific psychological and physiological variables that influence or compromise adaptation to the exercise stimulus. Recent therapeutic technology is enhancing the longevity of those with cancer; however, empirically based restorative training techniques have not been developed for this diverse clinical population. It is particularly important to develop intervention protocols that permit quantification of functional capacity so that nursing outcomes directed toward improvement of functioning can be measured more effectively.

REFERENCES

American College of Sports Medicine. (1986). *Guidelines for exercise testing and prescription* (3rd ed.). Philadelphia: Lea & Febiger.

Astrand, P., & Rodahl, K. (1986). *Textbook of work physiology* (3rd ed). New York: McGraw-Hill.

Baldwin, K. M. (1983). Structural and functional organization of skeletal muscle. In A. A. Bove & D. T. Lowenthal (Eds.), *Exercise medicine: Physiological principles and clinical applications* (pp. 3–18). San Diego: Academic Press.

Canny, G. J., & Levison, H. (1987). Exercise response and rehabilitation in cystic fibrosis. *Sports Medicine, 4,* 143–152.

Cobb, B. (1975). Medical and psychological problems in the rehabilitation of the cancer patient. In R. E. Hardy & J. G. Cull (Eds.), *Counseling and rehabilitation of the cancer patient* (pp. 24–62). Springfield, IL: Charles C. Thomas.

Dietz, J. H. (1981). *Rehabilitation oncology.* New York: John Wiley & Sons.

Ellestad, M. H. (1986). *Stress testing: Principles and practice* (3rd ed.). Philadelphia: F. A. Davis.

Fletcher, G. F. (1984). Long-term exercise in coronary artery disease and other chronic disease states. *Heart & Lung, 13,* 28–46.

Frank-Stromborg, M. (1986). Health promotion behaviors in ambulatory cancer patients: Facts or fiction. *Oncology Nursing Forum, 13*(4), 37–43.

Freedman, A. P. (1979). Pulmonary aspects of exercise. In D. T. Lowenthal, K. Bharadwaja, & W. W. Oaks (Eds.), *Therapeutics through exercise.* New York: Grune & Stratton.

Frontera, W. A., & Adams, R. P. (1986). Endurance exercise: Normal physiology and limitations imposed by pathological processes (part I). *The Physician and Sportsmedicine, 14*(8), 95–106.

Goldberg, A. P., Geltman, E. M., Gavin, J. R., Carney, R. M., Hagberg, J. M., Delmex, J. A., Naumovich, A., Oldfield, M. H., & Harter, H. R. (1986). Exercise training reduces coronary risk and effectively rehabilitates hemodialysis patients. *Nephron, 42*(4), 311–316.

Hinterbuchner, C. (1978). Rehabilitation of physical disability in cancer. *New York State Journal of Medicine, 78,* 1066–1069.

Kirby, R. L. (1984). The nature of disability and handicap. In J. V. Basmajian & R. L. Kirby (Eds.), *Medical rehabilitation* (pp. 14–18). Baltimore: Williams & Wilkins.

Nadel, E. R. (1985). Physiological adaptations to aerobic training. *American Scientist, 73,* 334–343.

Orem, D. E. (1980). *Nursing: Concepts of practice* (2nd ed.). New York: McGraw-Hill.

Painter, P. L. (1988). Exercise in end-stage renal disease. In K. B. Pandolf (Ed.), *Exercise and sport sciences reviews* (pp. 305–339). New York: MacMillan.

Painter, P. L., Nelson-Worel, J. N., Hill, M. M., Thornberg, D. R., Shelp, W. R., Harrington, A. R., & Weinstein, A. B. (1986). Effects of exercise training during hemodialysis. *Nephron, 43*(2), 87–92.

Peterson, L. H. (1983). *Cardiovascular rehabilitation.* New York: MacMillan.

Rosenbaum, E. H. (1982). Returning to activities of daily living. In *Western States Conference on Cancer Rehabilitation: Proceedings* (pp. 160–165). San Francisco: Bull Publishing Company.

Sinacore, D. R., & Ehsani, A. A. (1985). Measurements of cardiovascular function. In J. M. Rothstein (Ed.), *Measurement in physical therapy* (pp. 255–280). New York: Churchill Livingstone.

Soloff, P. H. (1978). Medically and surgically treated coronary patients in cardiovascular rehabilitation: A comparative study. *International Journal of Psychiatry in Medicine, 9*(1), 93–105.

Vallbona, C. (1982). Bodily responses to immobilization. In F. J. Kottke, G. K. Stillwell, & J. F. Lehman (Eds.), *Krusen's handbook of physical medicine and rehabilitation* (3rd ed.) (pp. 963–975). New York: Saunders.

Villaneuva, R. (1975). Rehabilitation needs of cancer patients. *Southern Medical Journal, 68*(2), 169–172.

Walker, S. N., Sechrist, K. R., & Pender, N. J. (1987). The Health-Promoting Lifestyle Profile: Development and psychometric characteristics. *Nursing Research, 36,* 76–81.

Wenger, N. K. L., & Hellerstein, H. K. (1984). *Rehabilitation of the coronary patient.* New York: John Wiley & Sons.

Winer, B. J. (1971). *Statistical principles in experimental design* (2nd ed.). New York: McGraw-Hill.

Winningham, M. L., MacVicar, M. G., & Burke, C. A. (1986). Exercise for cancer patients: Guidelines and precautions. *The Physician and Sportsmedicine, 14,* 125–134.

Winningham, M. L. (1983). *Effects of bicycle ergometry on functional status of women with breast cancer.* Unpublished doctoral dissertation, The Ohio State University, Columbus.

Analysis of Theory

The stated purpose of the study conducted by MacVicar, Winningham, and Nickel (1989) was to determine the effect of an aerobic exercise training protocol on the functional capacity of women receiving chemotherapy for treatment of breast cancer. The study may be classified as experimental research designed to test a predictive theory.

CONCEPT IDENTIFICATION AND CLASSIFICATION

Analysis of the research report revealed that a predictive theory of the effect of aerobic exercise on functional capacity was tested in the situation of Stage II breast cancer adjuvant chemotherapy treatment. The theory includes two concepts: aerobic interval exercise training and functional capacity.

Both concepts can be classified as variables. Aerobic interval exercise training, which is the independent variable, has three dimensions represented by the experimental, placebo, and control groups. Functional capacity, which is the dependent variable, has four dimensions, each of which has a range of scores. The dimensions of functional capacity are oxygen uptake (VO_2L_{max}), heart rate, workload, and maximum time to achieve VO_2L_{max}.

Aerobic interval exercise training may be classified as an observational term in Kaplan's (1964) schema because the treatment groups (experimental, placebo, control) can be directly observed. For the same reason, this concept may be classified as an observable in Willer and Webster's (1970) schema. It may be classified as an associative unit in Dubin's (1978) schema because the experimental group received the training, whereas the placebo and control groups did not.

Functional capacity is a theoretical term in Kaplan's schema because it is a complex, global concept encompassing several dimensions. It is a construct in Willer and Webster's schema because it is not directly observable; indeed, it is quite abstract. It is a summative unit in Dubin's schema because it encompasses several properties represented by the dimensions of oxygen uptake (VO_2L_{max}), heart rate, workload, and maximum time to achieve VO_2L_{max}.

PROPOSITION IDENTIFICATION AND CLASSIFICATION

The research report contains statements that may be classified as nonrelational and relational propositions. Constitutive and operational definitions for aerobic exercise and functional capacity are given in the research report, along with their empirical indicators. These statements, which may be classified as nonrelational definitional propositions, are listed in Table A–9. The operational definitions are, of course, not a part of the theory but serve as vertical propositions linking the concepts of the theory to the empirical indicators.

The constitutive definition, an experimental operational definition, and the empirical indicators for aerobic interval exercise training are evident in the research report. A constitutive definition is given for the abstract concept functional capacity. A measured operational definition identifies the dimensions of this concept as oxygen uptake, heart rate, workload, and maximum time to achieve VO_2L_{max}. A constitutive definition and a measured operational definition are given for oxygen uptake, and its empirical indicator is identified. Constitutive definitions are not evident for any of the other dimensions of functional capacity, although the definition of heart rate is self-evident. A measured operational definition and an empirical indicator are given for heart rate. A partial operational definition is given for workload. No operational definition is given for maximum time to achieve VO_2L_{max}. Moreover, empirical indicators are not identified for either workload or maximum time to achieve VO_2L_{max}.

The relational propositions that are central to the theory of the effect of aerobic exercise on functional capacity are listed below as they are stated in the research report.

1. It has been estimated that one-third or more of the decline in functional capacity experienced by cancer patients, regardless of stage of disease, can be attributed to hypokinetic conditions that develop as a consequence of prolonged physical inactivity.
2. The progressive loss of functional capacity associated with physical inactivity is attributed to the rapid decline in efficiency of multiple physiological systems, most apparent, initially, in the cardiorespiratory and muscular systems.
3. Exercise during treatment has been recommended for those with cancer to prevent the physiological sequelae of disuse and to maintain functional capacity.
4. Exercise that stimulates the aerobic energy system has been effective in promoting functional capacity in select clinical populations.
5. There is a direct relationship between oxygen uptake (VO_2L_{max}) and performance of physical activity.
6. Maintenance of functional capacity requires physical activity using large muscle groups to promote adaptation of the aerobic biochemical energy system.
7. Aerobic activity, such as walking, cycling, or swimming, that uses large muscle groups improves the oxidative capacity of skeletal muscles, stimulates the general adaptation of the aero-

TABLE A–9. Concepts, Definitions, and Empirical Indicators for the Theory of the Effect of Aerobic Exercise on Functional Capacity

Concept	Constitutive Definition	Operational Definition	Empirical Indicator
Aerobic interval exercise training	Aerobic interval exercise training consists of alternating higher and lower exercise intensity which involves use of large muscle groups.	Experimental group: The aerobic exercise protocol intervention was an interval training cycle ergometer protocol developed by Winningham (1983). Each exercise level was comprised of a specific ratio of high to low workload or resistance for a set number of minutes. With improved conditioning, time spent at lower intensity was reduced with increased time at higher intensity. Aerobic exercise sessions using the aerobic interval training protocol were conducted 3/wk for 10 wk. Missed sessions were either made up on weekends or scheduled as an extra session the following week. Each session began with a prescribed set of flexibility and stretching exercises. The sessions were carefully supervised and monitored	Experimental group: aerobic exercise protocol

by trained staff who recorded heart rate and blood pressures at 5- to 7-min intervals to ensure that subjects remained within the prescribed exercise intensity and to evaluate training response to the protocol.

Placebo group: Subjects met with staff for flexibility and stretching exercises. During the sessions, heart rate and blood pressure were taken at 5- to 7-min intervals so that subjects would experience similar conditions, but without the aerobic interval training protocol.

Control group: Subjects were instructed to carry on with their normal activities. There was no interaction with project staff other than that which occurred at pre- and posttest data collection periods.

Placebo group: flexibility and stretching exercises

Control group: normal activities

(Continued)

TABLE A–9. Concepts, Definitions, and Empirical Indicators for the Theory of the Effect of Aerobic Exercise on Functional Capacity (Continued)

Concept	Constitutive Definition	Operational Definition	Empirical Indicator
Functional capacity	The concept functional capacity is defined as the highest metabolic rate the individual can achieve on exertion. Exercise intensity is expressed as a percent of the highest metabolic rate or functional capacity achieved by an individual on an exercise test.	Functional capacity was measured by the highest oxygen uptake achieved at symptom-limited graded exercise pre- and posttests. Heart rate, workload, and maximum time to achieve VO_2L_{max} were also used to evaluate exercise response.	See empirical indicators for oxygen uptake and heart rate
Oxygen uptake	Maximal oxygen uptake also is an indicator of the highest metabolic rate an individual can achieve with exertion. For that reason, it is considered to be the most objective physiological indicator of functional capacity.	Oxygen uptake is expressed as volume of inspired oxygen in liters per minute (VO_2L_{max}). Pre- and posttest procedures were conducted with subjects pedaling at a rate of 50 rotations/min on calibrated cycle ergometers with an increase in workload resistance of 25 W every 2 min until the subject could not maintain the pedaling rate and/or indicated exhaustion. Expired air was collected	VO_2L_{max} scores as calculated by the Beckman Metabolic Cart

Heart rate	No definition given	through a nonrebreathing face mask and analyzed for fractions of oxygen, carbon dioxide, as well as respiratory volume. These data provided the basis for calculation of oxygen uptake (VO_2L_{max}) by the Beckman Metabolic Cart. Exercise intensity is best monitored by heart rate. Heart rate was monitored with a 12-lead electrocardiograph (EKG). The 12-lead EKG tracing was monitored continuously; heart rate data were recorded at rest, during the last 25 s of each 2-min interval, at maximal exertion, and during recovery	12-lead EKG tracing
Workload	No definition given	In this study, the subject was entered in the protocol at a workload that would induce a heart rate of 60–85% of the heart rate reserve calculated from the highest heart rate achieved at pretest	No empirical indicator given
Maximum time to achieve VO_2L_{max}	No definition given	No definition given	No empirical indicator given

bic biochemical system and results in measurable increments of oxygen uptake.

8. Disease and/or treatment(s) can inhibit the exercise response at any one of several points in the oxygen transport system, which limits the degree to which functional capacity can be improved.

9. Nevertheless, within these limitations, aerobic exercise training can still induce physiological adaptations in the aerobic energy system sufficient to improve functional capacity.

10. Even in advanced disease states in which patients generally experience an accelerated decline in functional capacity, an exercise intervention may minimize loss of functioning.

Propositions 1 to 4, 6, 9, and 10 concern the relationship between aerobic exercise and functional capacity. These statements can be combined and stated formally as the proposition given below. The narrative report suggests that the relationship not only exists but also is positive in direction, asymmetrical, and sequential.

> There is a positive, asymmetrical, and sequential relationship between aerobic exercise and functional capacity.

Propositions 5 and 7 concern the relationship between aerobic exercise and the functional capacity dimension of oxygen uptake. These statements can be combined and stated formally as the following proposition. As with the previous proposition, the narrative report indicates that the relationship exists, is positive in direction, is asymmetrical, and is sequential.

> There is a positive, asymmetrical, and sequential relationship between aerobic exercise and oxygen uptake.

Proposition 8 is a contingent relationship. The narrative report suggests that the positive, asymmetrical, and sequential relationship between exercise and functional capacity is contingent on disease and treatment.

No hypotheses are stated explicitly, although one can be extracted from the results section of the research report. This hypothesis, stated in a combination of concept names (functional capacity, heart rate, maximum test time, maximum workload) and an empirical indicator term (groups), is:

There are significant differences between groups on pre- to posttest functional capacity, heart rate, maximum test time, and maximum workload.

HIERARCHY OF PROPOSITIONS

The hypothesis-testing nature of the study indicates that any hierarchy of propositions would be deductive. The propositions given in the research report do not, however, lend themselves to arrangement as sets of axioms and theorems. Furthermore, a deductive hierarchy of axioms and the hypothesis cannot be developed because empirical indicators are not given for two of the dimensions of functional capacity.

It is possible to construct the following hierarchy based on level of abstraction; it illustrates the progression of the investigators' apparent line of reasoning from the more general terms physical inactivity and physical activity to the more specific term aerobic exercise and, finally, to the statement of the study purpose. The propositions are stated as given in the research report. The numbers are those used above for the initial list of relational propositions.

1. It has been estimated that one-third or more of the decline in functional capacity experienced by cancer patients, regardless of stage of disease, can be attributed to hypokinetic conditions that develop as a consequence of prolonged physical inactivity.
2. The progressive loss of functional capacity associated with physical inactivity is attributed to the rapid decline in efficiency of multiple physiological systems, most apparent, initially, in the cardiorespiratory and muscular systems.
3. Exercise during treatment has been recommended for those with cancer to prevent the physiological sequelae of disuse and to maintain functional capacity.
10. Even in advanced disease states in which patients generally experience an accelerated decline in functional capacity, an exercise intervention can minimize loss of functioning.
6. Maintenance of functional capacity requires physical activity using large muscle groups to promote adaptation of the aerobic biochemical energy system.
4. Exercise that stimulates the aerobic energy system has been effective in promoting functional capacity in select clinical populations.

8. Disease and/or treatment(s) can inhibit the exercise response at any one of several points in the oxygen transport system, which limits the degree to which functional capacity can be improved.

9. Nevertheless, within these limitations, aerobic exercise training can still induce physiological adaptations in the aerobic energy system sufficient to improve functional capacity.

5. There is a direct relationship between oxygen uptake (VO_2L_{max}) and performance of physical activity.

7. Aerobic activity, such as walking, cycling, or swimming, that uses large muscle groups improves the oxidative capacity of skeletal muscles, stimulates the general adaptation of the aerobic biochemical system, and results in measurable increments of oxygen uptake.

The purpose of this study was to determine the effect of an aerobic exercise training protocol on the functional capacity of women receiving chemotherapy for treatment of breast cancer.

CONCEPTUAL-THEORETICAL-EMPIRICAL STRUCTURE

The research apparently was guided by Orem's (1980) Self-Care Framework. The conceptual model concept of universal self-care requisites is linked to the theory concept of functional capacity through the following vertical proposition:

> The physical ability to engage in activity is a universal self-care requisite.

The concept aerobic interval exercise training is repeatedly referred to as an intervention in the research report. The following statement may be considered a vertical proposition linking the two terms:

> If it can be demonstrated that aerobic exercise improves the functional capacity of those with cancer, it could be a cost-effective intervention that could be used to maintain the capacity for self-care and physical independence.

Another statement may be considered a horizontal proposition at the conceptual model level. This proposition, which apparently provides the conceptual basis for the study hypothesis, is:

The ability to maintain physical independence and to perform self-care activities can be compromised or lost if the integrity of physiological systems is not maintained.

DIAGRAM

A diagram of the conceptual-theoretical-empirical structure for the theory of the effect of aerobic exercise on functional capacity was constructed (Fig. A–8). The question marks indicate that empirical indicators are not identified for two dimensions of functional capacity. In addition, an inventory of effects was constructed to illustrate the specific effects of aerobic interval exercise training on the dimensions of functional capacity (Fig. A–9).

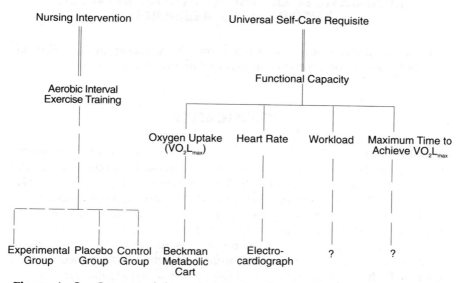

Figure A–8. Conceptual-theoretical-empirical structure for the theory of the effect of aerobic interval exercise training on functional capacity.

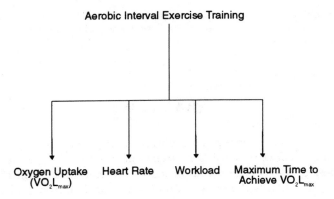

Figure A–9.   Inventory of effects of aerobic interval exercise training.

EVALUATION OF THE RELATION BETWEEN THEORY AND RESEARCH

The intent of the study was to test a predictive theory of the effect of aerobic exercise on four dimensions of functional capacity.

SIGNIFICANCE

The theory of the effect of aerobic exercise on functional capacity meets the significance criterion in part. The theoretical significance of the research is not addressed explicitly. The investigators do, however, imply that the study was designed to extend what is already known about the effect of aerobic exercise on functional capacity in various chronic illnesses to the situation of breast cancer chemotherapy treatment.

The social significance of the research is addressed in the first paragraph of the report, where the magnitude of decline in functional capacity that is due to inactivity is identified. The social significance of the research is further addressed by the investigators' comment that functional capacity "is a particularly useful concept for nursing and self-care because the emphasis is on residual abilities and restorative potential, rather than what has been lost or presumed to be lost."

The theory of the effect of aerobic exercise on functional capacity deals with a phenomenon of interest to the discipline of nursing by addressing a process (aerobic exercise) by which positive changes in health status (functional capacity) can be affected.

The theory predicts with some precision. More specifically, the study findings revealed a mean 40 percent improvement in functional capacity for experimental group subjects. Furthermore, the study findings enhance understanding of the effect of aerobic exercise on dimensions of functional capacity.

INTERNAL CONSISTENCY

The theory of the effect of aerobic exercise on functional capacity does not fully meet the internal consistency criterion. There are no redundancies in the concepts of the theory. Semantic clarity is, however, obscured because constitutive definitions are given only for aerobic interval exercise training, functional capacity, and the functional capacity dimension of oxygen uptake; the other dimensions are not defined.

Semantic consistency is not evident. First, aerobic interval exercise training is also referred to as aerobic exercise, aerobic activity, aerobic training, and aerobic interval training. Second, functional capacity is also referred to as exercise response, exercise intensity, and training response. Third, VO_2L_{max} is associated with functional capacity both directly [functional capacity (VO_2L_{max})] and indirectly [oxygen uptake (VO_2L_{max})]. Finally, the terms maximum test time and test time are introduced in the results section of the report. Apparently, these terms are used in place of maximum time to achieve VO_2L_{max}.

Furthermore, the propositions do not fully reflect structural consistency. The progression of statements dealing with the relationship between physical activity/inactivity and functional capacity to statements dealing with the relationship between aerobic exercise and functional capacity is a logical line of reasoning. However, the inclusion of several statements dealing with the relationship between aerobic exercise and functional capacity creates a redundancy. Paradoxically, no statement directly addresses the relationship between aerobic interval exercise training and the four dimensions of functional capacity (oxygen uptake, heart rate, workload, maximum time to achieve VO_2L_{max}). Moreover, the implied hypothesis does not account for the contingent relationship noted in proposition 8. Apparently, the intervening variables of disease and treatment were controlled by limitations on the sample with regard to type and stage of cancer and type of treatment.

PARSIMONY

The narrative presentation of the theory of the effect of aerobic exercise on functional capacity does not meet the criterion of parsimony. The lack of semantic consistency necessitated many readings of the research report prior to formalization. The decision to classify heart rate, workload, and maximum time to achieve VO_2L_{max} as dimensions of functional capacity, rather than as separate concepts, was difficult. The decision was based on the apparent equivalence of the terms exercise response and functional capacity in the narrative report. Furthermore, the redundant propositions precluded a parsimonious presentation of the theory. The formalized theory represents a more parsimonious set of concepts and propositions.

TESTABILITY

The theory of the effect of aerobic exercise on functional capacity partially meets the testability criterion. Operational definitions link aerobic interval exercise training, oxygen uptake, and heart rate with their respective empirical indicators, and the hypothesis extracted from the results section is falsifiable. In contrast, neither operational definitions nor empirical indicators are given for workload and maximum time to achieve VO_2L_{max}.

OPERATIONAL ADEQUACY

The research design used to generate the theory of the effect of aerobic exercise on functional capacity meets most of the requirements of the operational adequacy criterion. The sample was of adult women who were receiving chemotherapy for Stage II breast cancer. The statistical analyses were appropriate techniques for testing the hypothesis. Operational adequacy is, however, compromised by the lack of explicitly identified empirical indicators for workload and maximum time to achieve VO_2L_{max}.

EMPIRICAL ADEQUACY

The narrative report of results suggests that the investigators expected the mean scores of the experimental group to be different from those of the placebo and control groups for all four dimensions of functional capacity. Inasmuch as this expectation was not met for heart rate, the theory does not fully meet the criterion of empirical adequacy.

An alternative methodological explanation is given for the heart rate result. The investigators claimed that the exposure to project staff and familiarity with exercise may have resulted in greater willingness of the placebo group subjects to attempt greater exertion during testing. An alternative substantive explanation for the study findings is not offered.

PRAGMATIC ADEQUACY

The theory of the effect of aerobic exercise on functional capacity meets the pragmatic adequacy criterion. The study findings support the use of aerobic interval exercise training for women receiving adjuvant chemotherapy for Stage II breast cancer. The 40 percent improvement rate in functional capacity indicates that the exercise intervention is clinically meaningful.

CONCEPTUAL-THEORETICAL-EMPIRICAL STRUCTURE

The influence of Orem's Self-Care Framework on the research appears to be minimal. Universal self-care requisite is the only term taken directly from the vocabulary of this conceptual model of nursing. The exercise intervention is not conceptualized as a specific type of nursing care system or as a specific method of assisting within the context of Orem's model.

REFERENCES

Dubin, R. (1978). *Theory building* (rev. ed.). New York: The Free Press.

Kaplan, A. (1964). *The conduct of inquiry*. San Francisco: Chandler.

MacVicar, M. G., Winningham, M. L., & Nickel, J. L. (1989). Effects of aerobic interval training on cancer patients' functional status. *Nursing Research, 38,* 348–351.

Orem, D. E. (1980). *Nursing: Concepts of practice* (2nd ed.). New York: McGraw-Hill.

Willer, D., & Webster, M., Jr. (1970). Theoretical concepts and observables. *American Sociological Review, 35,* 748–757.

INDEX

Note: Page numbers followed by f indicate figures; page numbers followed by t indicate tables.